TINCTURE OF TIME

A CONCISE HISTORY OF MEDICINE

Ángel Rafael Colón, MD, MA
Professor Emeritus
Adjunct Professor to the Dean
Georgetown University
Washington, D.C.
and
Patricia Ann Colón, MA

Copyright © A.R. Colón, 2011
Second edition, 2013
Third edition, 2015
All rights reserved.
ISBN: 13-978-1466449282

Other books

Nurturing Children: A History of Pediatrics.
A History of Children: A Socio-Cultural Survey
  Across Millennia
The Boke of Children
The Child in the Iconography of Death

Pediatric Pathophysiology
Textbook of Pediatric Hepatology
An Outline of Pediatric Hepatology
El Niño Icterico

Cover: *Dr. Schnabel von Rom – the Plague Doctor*, engraving by Paul Fürst (1656). The plague doctor employed by the municipality treated both rich and poor. He walked among the sick in a long leather coat and a bird-like mask with crystal lenses. The beak of the mask held a sponge soaked in vinegar with dissolved cloves, amber, camphor, myrrh, storax and cinnamon, believed to obfuscate and disable the miasma they opined was responsible for the disease. The stick permitted examination for buboes without touching the patient. Note the death iconography at the tip of the stick – the winged hourglass. The precautions were futile, for most doctors attending plague victims themselves died suffocated with the same putrid signs and symptoms.

    Image courtesy of Wikimedia Commons and cover design by St.John William Colón.

Dedication: For the students of medicine at Georgetown University, with hopes that knowledge of the ancient and international foundations of their chosen vocation enriches their practice of medical science and art and contributes to the passion and compassion they dedicate to this profound and august profession.

o-o-o

The ageless admonition of Hippocrates, "*Ars longa, vita brevis, occasio praeceps, experimentum periculosum, iudicium difficile* – art is long, life short, the occasion fleeting, experience fallacious and judgment difficult" – remains as true today as when Hippocrates first made the observation, just as the classic dictum, "***Tincture of Time***" continues to prudently advise both physician and patient to defer on occasion to the healing processes of time and nature.

All the quotations in this manuscript have been acknowledged and used for scholarly and academic purposes only under the "Fair-use" guidelines of the United States copyright office.

Figures (Appendix I)

		page reference
1.	Acupuncture meridian lines	p. 11
2.	Chinese medical doll	p. 12
3.	Asklepios	p. 22
4.	Seven Ages of Man	p. 25
5.	Four Humors	p. 29
6.	*Hotel Dieu*	p. 58
7.	Urine color wheel	p. 58
8.	Phlebotomy man	pp. 59 and 67
9.	Astrologic man	p. 67
10.	Wound man	p. 67
11.	Fetus and Hemisection of coition	pp. 73 and 95
12.	*De Fabrica*	p. 73
13.	*Rewards of Cruelty*	p. 74
14.	Scultetus, *Armamentarium*	p. 77
15.	Tagliacozzi's rhinoplasty	p. 80
16.	Birthing chair	p. 82
17.	*De arte medica infantium*	p. 82
18.	Iatromechanics.	p. 90
19.	Phrenology	p. 103
20.	Hunter's obstetrical plate	p. 106
21.	Jenner's vaccination	p. 112
22.	Erhlich's WBC stains	p. 130
23.	Model of Laennec's stethoscope	p. 122
24.	Lister's spray	p. 139
25.	Incubator	p. 157
26.	MRI	p. 183
27.	*The Doctor*	p. 220

Table of Contents

INTRODUCTION   viii

1. ANCIENT MEDICINE   1
   Sumer, Egypt, Hebrew, India, Orient, New World

2. MEDICINE IN THE CLASSICAL PERIOD   19
   Greece and Rome

3. MEDIEVAL MEDICINE   37
   Arabic, Monastic, Pre-Renaissance

4. RENAISSANCE MEDICINE   65
   Incunabula, Art and anatomy

5. SEVENTEENTH CENTURY MEDICINE   84
   De Motu Cordis, Iatros schools

6. EIGHTEENTH CENTURY MEDICINE   99
   Enlightenment, Anatomists, *Accoucher*

7. NINETEENTH CENTURY MEDICINE   118
   Hospitals, Germ Theory, Anesthesia

8. WOMEN IN THE HISTORY OF MEDICINE   163

9. TWENTIETH CENTURY MEDICINE   179
   Laboratory centered medicine

APPENDICIES 207
    A: Oath of Hippocrates
    B: Code of Comportment
    C: Medical Poems
    D: Vitamins
    E: Nobel Prizes in Physiology and Medicine
    F: Origins of National Health Insurance
    G: Ophthalmology
    H: Spices
    I: Figures in text

BIBLIOGRAPHY 240

PROPER NAME INDEX 245

SUBJECT INDEX 261

Introduction

This concise introductory history of medicine is iatrocentric and Eurocentric, given that the underpinnings of modern medicine evolved in Europe. Nevertheless, it does incorporate a review of Persian and Oriental medicine and their important influences on Western thought. The primary goal is to introduce the reader to the many philosophical contortions through which the evolution of medicine passed and to inform the connections the giants of medicine had with each other over the centuries that lead to the extraordinary twenty-first century of compassionate healing.

For the medical student, the manuscript aims to balance the first two years immersion in scientific studies with an examination of medicine of the past that is both medically and culturally noteworthy and is imbued with a humanist's perspective that informs the practice of medicine with a passionate regard for the universality of the human condition:

> The humanist is not interested in the past merely because it is past. As the statistician likes a long series, not a short one, the humanist similarly likes the long accumulations from the past to illustrate the nature of man...*Plus ca change; plus ca reste.*
>
> Alan Gregg. *Bull NY Acad Med* 1941: 17, 83-99.

As the University of London's David Cannadine observed, a humanistic perspective

> makes plain the complexity and contingency of human affairs, and the range and variety of human experience, which teaches proportion, perspective, reflectiveness, breadth of view, tolerance of differing opinions and thus a greater sense of self- knowledge....[it] provides...the best antidote to the temporal parochialism which assumes that the only time is now, and the geographical parochialism which assumes that the only place is here.
> *Making History Now* (1999)

A consideration of humanist values complements William Osler's famous dictums of what he called the Four Apostolic Successions of Medicine, and we call the *ethos* of medicine:

> 1) No other profession can boast the same unbroken continuity of methods and ideals.
> 2) It has remarkable solidarity of ambitions, methods and work to observe phenomena, prevent disease, relieve suffering and heal.
> 3) It is a progressive science, changing and evolving.
> 4) It is singularly beneficent.
> *Counsels and Ideals*

With respect to medical progress one more observation as succinctly phrased by the editors of the *New England Journal of Medicine* in January of 2000 deserves mention:

> None of the developments [of medicine] was an isolated discovery or event; instead, each was a series of notable steps – some huge, some smaller – along a path that led to a crucial body of knowledge in a particular area. That is the usual way medical science progresses.

One can approach the history of medicine by examining seismic movements, famous personages, revolutionary concepts, social historiography and philosophical influences. We have chosen to organize the data by time periods, establishing the historical context at the beginning of each chapter that describes and explains the connections that informed advances in medicine as well as those that hindered progress. Medical history has numerable instances from antiquity onwards of medical truths that commonly continue to be recognized as valid and applicable to clinical practice and modern "discoveries" that in fact were known a millennium ago that until now had been lost to civilization.

The study of medicine allows little time in the day for other pursuits. This is the case for both students and for the most experienced and accomplished physicians. Practicing and teaching the art of medicine demands constant reading and learning of voluminous amounts of new information. There is much, however, to be learned from the past, and, with hope that students will be tempted to do just that, the book ends with a list that pertains to the history of medicine of sources that are eminently pleasurable to read.

x

I: Ancient Period

Timeline:

BCE
- 3500 Sumerian script
- 2600 Khufu rules Egypt
       Huang-Ti rules China
- 2500 Knossos founded
- 1925 Hittites conquer Babylonia
- 1860 Stonehenge
- 1728 Code of Hammurabi
- 1620 Explosion of Thera

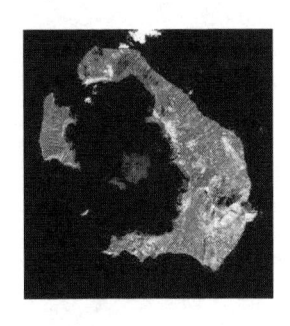

- 1304 Ramses II
- 1250 The Exodus
- 1000 Rig Veda
       David of Israel
- 814 Carthage founded
- 800 *Iliad* and *Odyssey*
- 563 Birth of Siddhartha – Buddha
- 551 Birth of K'ung Fu-tzu – Confucius
- 536 Babylonian captivity – *Talmud* begins
- 486 Xerxes the Great

Sumer: If a baby, while nursing, his flesh becomes flabby, even though his wet-nurse has milk; if he rejects the breast change to another [wet-nurse] for healing.
Traité akkadien de diagnostics et pronostic médicaux 36. (c. 1600 BCE)

Egypt: One having a dislocation in a vertebra of his neck, while he is unconscious of his two legs and his two arms, and his urine dribbles. An ailment not to be cured.
Edwin Smith Papyrus. Case 31. (c. 1600 BCE)

India: The child afflicted with *Skandapasmara* alternately loses and regains consciousness, looks violent with the hands and legs moving as if dancing, passes urine, stool and flatus, yawns and foams.
Susruta Samhita. Graha 2 (2nd century BCE)

Hebrews: *Askara* [diphtheria] is a much dreaded epidemic disease which usually attacks children, is located in the throat, and kills the patient by a painful death from suffocation.
Rabbi Ishmael ben R. Jose (fl. 2nd century), *Talmud*

Orient: Treating Red and Painful Eyes: Chan Jing suggest to use 7 pieces of *huang lian* [coptis root] in one cup of human milk to wash the eye. Another protocol uses cotton soaked with a solution containing 3 cups of *zhu li* [bamboo sap] and 1 cup of human milk to wipe the eye.
Ishimpo Scroll 25, no. 37 (c. 982 CE)

Ancient Medicine

The history of medicine is as old as the human cultures that began in the regions of the four great river civilizations – Euphrates, Nile, Indus and Yellow. Earliest records from millennia ago indicate there were elements of the art of healing. The quotations cited above, obviously based on clinical experience, appear arcane – unfathomable. On closer look, however, and cited in modern terminology, it becomes clear that man thousands of years ago was engaged in the medical arts and made observations that have stood the test of time. Except for the Sumerians who recognized cause and effect when a wet-nurse had insufficient breast milk, there is no indication there was an understanding of pathophysiological mechanisms, but the wisdom of the annotations cannot be disputed. The Egyptian *swnw* knew there was nothing he could do for a quadriplegic; the Indian *vaidya* gave a clear description of a grandmal seizure; the man from China recognized the healing properties of human breast milk for conjunctivitis; and the Hebrew knew membranous diphtheria suffocated.

The raison d'être to examine the ancients as far back as Mesopotamia, however outlandish medical methodology appears to the modern reader, is to understand the universal impulse since time immemorial to care for the sick, and the innate curiosity of the human mind to discover, innovate and control procedures that sustain and enhance life and to appreciate the thread of continuity in the present day that still motivates young and caring people to study medicine.

Ancient medicine is characterized by deistic beliefs that varied in every culture, but infused medical thinking everywhere with the apotropaic, designed to avert evil forces, the hermetic characterized by occult abstruseness, chthonic relating to the underworld of gods and spirits that caused disease and the theurgic pantheon of deities that protected all from illness. Early cultures undoubtedly were primitive and riddled with superstitions. It is striking, nonetheless, to realize that thousands of years ago there existed groups of people who dedicated their lives to alleviating suffering.

It can be said that in contrast to the Hebrews, Indians and Chinese, the Sumerians and Egyptians left little significant medical legacy other than a corpus of literature that provided evidence of medical care.

Sumer

In Mesopotamian Sumer c. 3500 BCE, medicine was astrologic, numerologic, fatalistic and directed by the interpretation of omens. As a healing craft it relied on deistic intercession, superstition, astrology and practical botanical recipes. Since the liver was considered the source of blood and the seat of the soul, hepatoscopy, an examination of the topical anatomy of an animal liver (generally a sheep) was used for augury or prognosis – much like the reading of tea-leaves or palms.

The Sumerians had specific gods they associated with specific symptoms and organs. Some gods were beneficent and effected cures; others were malevolent and thought to be responsible for maladies. The mother goddess of medicine was the good and beautiful *Ishtar*, invoked during childbirth. *Ninib* and his consort *Gula* were the gods of healing. Gula was the goddess of both death and resurrection often petitioned for a cure. *Nergal*, the god of disease and death, was presciently depicted as a fly. *Labartu* made newborns sick.

The *ashipu* was a spirit doctor who consulted omens for prognostication. The following examples are superstitious – but interesting – twaddle. They are taken from the *Traite Akkadien Diagnostic et Pronostic*, a cuneiform translation by Rene Labat (1951):

> If the *ashipu* sees either a black dog or pig, the
> patient will die.
> If the nipples of a pregnant woman are yellow
> she will miscarry.
> If blood flows out of his penis, it is the hand
> of [the god] *Shamash*.
> If a baby vomits, has diarrhea, if his hands and
> feet are paralyzed: petition [the god] *Sin*.

The clinical doctor or *asu* practiced urinoscopy – an inspection of patient urine – a ritual universally employed for millennia.

Not all medical archeological records from Sumer were clinical references. Several codes – the most famous of which was Hammurabi's (died c. 1750 BCE) – mandated that the asu's remuneration be linked to the patient's means:

> If an *asu* performs an operation on a master
> with a bronze lancet and saves his life, he shall
> receive ten shekels. If he is a freeman, five
> shekels. If he is a slave, two shekels.
> *Code of Hammurabi*, 1728 BCE [215-217]

In Hammurabi's code, clinical lapses, including pharmacologic, were ignored, but surgical failures (the use of a knife) incurred draconian penalties:

> If an *asu* performs an operation on a master
> with a bronze lancet and he dies, they shall
> cut off his hand. If an *asu* performs an opera-

tion on a slave with a bronze lancet and he dies, he shall replace the slave with another slave.
Code of Hammurabi, 1728 BCE [218-219]

Little else is known about early Sumerian medicine and less about the Babylonian culture that followed. Very few medical tablets have survived. Herodotus (484-425? BCE) assumed the Babylonians had no doctors because of a custom peculiar to that culture:

They bring out all their sick into the streets, for they have no regular doctors. People that come along offer the sick man advice...no one is allowed to pass by a sick person without asking what ails him.
Histories, I, 199.

Herodotus mistakenly assumed that the habit of seeking the advice of family, friends and concerned strangers was the only medical intervention. He did not know that, in fact, the Babylonians carried on Sumer's tradition of consulting the *ashipu* and *asu*, and, like the Sumerians, also relied on the gods in matters of health.

Egypt
Ancient Egypt like Sumer had a theurgic pantheon as well as trained medical caretakers. All illness was controlled by *Ra*. Eye diseases were the province of *Thoth*; Epidemics were attributed to *Seth*; near-death was in the hands of *Isis*; childbirth was under the domain of *Neith*; *Sechmet* was the god responsible for disease in women; the survival of a child from illness was attributed to *Seshat*; the intersession of *Meskhenit* was sought for infant health, and that of *Rannut* to assure child nutritional sustenance.

Egyptian medical historiography is evident in papyri, reliefs and murals. Named after owner or location, eight major papyri are known and the most famous is the Smith papyrus with sophisticated modalities of treatment, particularly with respect to the treatment of fractures.

Kahun	1900	women's diseases, pregnancy
Ebers	1550	medical and magical
Hearst	1550	prescriptive
Erman	1550	birth, infant, children
Smith	1500	surgical
Berlin	1350	pregnancy and prescriptive
London	1350	prescriptive and magical
Beatty	1200	proctologic

The polymath, Imhotep (c. 2990), is the first known Egyptian physician (called a *swnw*). During the reign of pharaoh Zoser (2980-2900 BCE) in the 3rd dynasty, he practiced medical arts, served as vizier, and was the architect of the Great Step Pyramid and the temple Edfu. Legendary, he was ultimately deified. Little more is known of him.

Egyptologists have identified two women healers. The tomb of Merit Ptah, who practiced 5,000 years ago, has an inscription that cites her role as "the chief physician;" and Pesehet (c. 2500 BC) bore the title of "lady overseer of the physicians," tantalizingly suggestive that it may not have been an uncommon for a woman to engage in medicine.

Herodotus (c. 484-425 BCE) in *Histories* II, 83 interestingly mentions Egypt had curative specialists who treated diseases of the eyes and stomach and physicians who performed surgeries. Parenthetically, in *Histories* I, 202, he comments on Scythians (ancient Iranian nomads), who burned hemp seed to produce vapors that induced stupor, but there is no data that suggest it was used as surgical sedation.

The Egyptians also had an extensive pharmacopoeia, of which nearly seven hundred were used for matters related to defecation and micturation. The remarkable number of diuretics and cathartics used was grounded in the belief that urine and a fecal contaminant called *ukhedu* or *whdw* had to be eliminated from the human body in order to maintain good health. Many of the purges and clysters used extensively as treatment against *whdw*, themselves incorporated excreta as ingredients, animal dung compounded into prescriptions classified as *Dreckapotheke*.

Whdw was thought to be carried and spread through vessels, called *metw*, that coursed through and around vital organs including the anus and bladder, carrying blood, air, urine, feces and tears. Ancient Egypt considered *whdw* to be an etiologic or causative agent that adhered to feces, precipitating rot. They feared that if absorbed by the gut, it would cause coagulation followed by suppuration and putrefaction. They treated all prodromal stages of disease with purgatives and diuretics, since urine and *whdw* were blamed for putrefaction in the bladder and bowel. Such was the preoccupation with feces that *Iri* was the Keeper of the Royal Rectum.

The Hebrews
Two thousand years of wandering and captivity influenced much of Hebrew culture, and Hebraic medicine reflects how, during that time, healers selectively accepted or rejected concepts and treatment from various places. The theurgic pantheons of Sumer and Egypt were rebuffed, but Egyptian sanitary, dietary and midwifery practices were adopted.

Hebraic medicine reflected the culture's monotheism. It was, moreover, believed that God inflicted disease and God healed. The practice of magic was forbidden, as were the rites and the use of pharmacopoeia of the Euphrates and Nile.

Knowledge of ancient Hebraic medicine derives almost exclusively from the *Torah* (the first five books of the Old Testament – the books of Moses: Genesis, Exodus, Leviticus, Numbers and Deuteronomy) and the *Talmud*. The *Talmud*'s sixty-three tractates are rabbinical opinions and interpretations of the *Torah*. There are two *Talmuds*: the Jerusalem and the Babylonian. The Babylonian is considered the most authoritative. The first part of it was redacted and written in the 2nd century after the time of Christ and was completed by the 5th century.

We learn from these sources that, despite the absence of a professional class of physicians (the practice of medicine was left to empiric priests), few early cultures matched the hygienic public health concerns of the Hebrews. Epidemics in communities were announced by a trumpet blast from the *shofar*. Hand washing was repeatedly emphasized by the *Berakoth* (47b, 53b), *Sotah* (4b) and *Shabbath* (108b), and all were aware of contagion by contact, thus disinfection by boiling water (*Num* 31: 21-24) was the norm. Environmental cleanliness was considered an essential element for community health:

> A permanent threshing-floor may not be erected within fifty cubits of a city. The place for depositing carcasses, a cemetery, and a tannery may not be erected within fifty cubits of a city.
> *Baba Bathra* (II. 8f).

Some important Hebraic dietary admonitions from ancient times remain valid and have been widely adopted, especially in Western societies: children were instructed to eat slowly and chew food well (*Shabbat* 152a), and breakfast was exulted as the most significant meal of the day (*Pesachim* 112a).

Drinking from rivers was forbidden to prevent "the water filament" (*Abodah Zarah* 12b) or *dracunculus*, the guinea worm. Those who were found to harbor the parasite were treated with a castor poultice.

Pregnancy was considered a gift from God, and, significantly, it was understood that the health of a child began *in utero*. Remarkably, biblical writers were aware of the negative effects of alcohol consumption during pregnancy and admonished against imbibing: "Thou shall conceive and bear a son; and now drink no wine nor strong drink." (*Judges* 13:7). This truism, lost for millennia, only in the mid 20th century became a routine admonition to pregnant women. The newborn was washed, salted with natron (sodium bicarbonate decahydrate – an astringent and antibacterial) and then swaddled.

Although human dissection was anathema, studies of animal anatomy and surgical procedures on animals provided insights and skills successfully employed in the treatment of humans. Many observations and treatment of birth anomalies also were based on animal studies. Imperforate anus [no rectal opening], for example, was corrected surgically.

> ...An infant whose anus is not visible should be rubbed with oil and stood in the sun, and where it shows transparent it should be torn crosswise with a barley grain, but not with a metal instrument, because that causes inflammation.
> *Shabbath* (134a)

This example and the descriptions of other congenital anomalies mentioned in the *Talmud* illustrate the level of clinical sophistication of the ancient Hebrews. Cited were head mal-formations (*Bekoroth* 43b), scoliosis (*Sanhedrin* 91a), harelip (*Baba Kamma* 117a), hairy nevi (*Niddah* 46a), congenital deafness (*Hagigah* 2a), and supernumerary digits (*Bekoroth* 45b). Congenital blindness was noted, with the assertion that the infant locates the mother's breast by smell and taste (*Kethuboth* 60a) – a fact confirmed only in the twentieth century (*Lancet* 1994; 344: 989).

Scurvy (*Abodah Zarah* 28a), epistaxis (*Gittin* 69a), trachoma (*Kethuboth* 77b) and epilepsy (*Bekoroth* 44b) were also described in the *Talmud*. Hematemesis was cleverly assessed by dipping a straw into the blood. If clots adhered to the straw it was considered pulmonic in origin; if not, it was deemed to be from the stomach – hepatic portal hypertension varices. (*Gittin* 69a).

The total blood volume of an infant was determined by a dilution technique comparing the color of blood in various solutions (*Pesahim* 19, *Oholath*, III: 2). Fifteen hundred years passed before this technique was duplicated by W.H. Welcker in 1855.

Circumcision of the male was performed on the eighth day after birth (*Leviticus* 12:3), which we now know is about the time the body stabilizes the vitamin K levels that are conducive to the normal coagulation of blood. Originally performed by the mother employing a chipped flint (*Exodus* IV, 25), the rite in time fell to the *mohel*. The serious health risk of a bleeding disorder, (for example hemophilia) was recognized:

> If she circumcised her first child and he died, and the second one who also died, she must not circumcise her third child.
> *Yebamoth* (64b).

The *Talmud* codified hygienic laws asserting the right to health for everyone and the duty of everyone to embrace a commitment to the commonweal. Centuries of captivity and repression instructed the Hebrews that communal survival depended on just such a commitment.

India

The physician in ancient India was called the *vaidya,* who worked in a system of medicine that evolved between 3000 to 5000 years ago. The corpus of Hindu literature pertaining to this system, the *Ayurveda* ("knowledge of life") stems from the four *Vedas* or books of knowledge. The oldest, the *Rigveda,* was redacted from oral tradition about 1500 BCE. Each Veda had two parts: *Mantra* (prayer) and ritual. For example, the mantra, "Giving lifetime, O *Agni,* choosing old age ... having drunk the sweet pleasant ghee of the cow; do afterward defend this boy as a father his sons," was recited at the *Brahma* ritual of placing ghee in the infant's mouth.

Major medical contributions were made during the Brahministic period (800 BCE to 700 CE) when the Brahmin caste of Hindu priests dominated the society. Well trained *vaidyas* introduced hyoscyamus and cannabis as surgical soporifics well before the *spongia somnifera* (see ahead). Most remarkably the glycosuria (sugar in urine) of diabetes, the association of mosquito bites with malaria, and of rats with plague were recognized.

Three major texts evolved during this era: *Susruta* (2nd century BCE), *Charaka* (1st century CE) and the *Vagbhata* (7th century CE). All attributed good health to the balance of seven principles: chyle, fat, blood, flesh, bone, semen and marrow, with prescient recommendations of frequent bathing, mouth care, diet, meditation and the proscription of wine.

Plastic surgery was a surgical skill in ancient India that was not commonly practiced in the West until the 16th century. Harelip, for example, was corrected, but most famously skillful rhinoplasty corrected the disfigurement of those whose noses had been cut off – the penalty exacted for adultery.

The Indian *vaidya* developed general surgical skills and instrumentation to the highest degree in the ancient world, with techniques that would only reach the West with the Translation Movement that coalesced Persian and Greek knowledge (see ahead). The *Susruta* described one hundred and twenty different operative instruments that were used for specialized procedures such as cataract couching, clamping vessels and dental extractions. Incisions were practiced on gourds and cucumbers, venipuncture on cabbage leaves, hydrocele taps on water-filled leather bags and bandaging on dead animals. Bleeding was checked with cautery or pressure. Splints were made of bamboo, and lithotomy and caesarean sections were performed. Ancient India conceived and conducted surgeries that would not be performed in the West for centuries to come.

China

This discussion of ancient China extends into the 16th century of the current era for three reasons: First, it permits elucidation of the Japanese *Ishimpo* written in 982 CE, second, it allows exposition of all the centuries of Chinese wisdom without having to readdress them again in other sections of the text, third, it facilitates an acknowledged and unabashed Eurocentrism in the chapters that follow, a focus that is most germane to the evolution of medicine in the West.

Historiography sources for ancient Chinese medicine are found in oracle-bones, tomb artifacts, and classical texts, the most important of which was the *Huang Ti Nei Ching*. The authorship of the *Nei Ching* is attributed to Huang Ti (c. 2600 BCE). Known as the Yellow Emperor, he may have been only a legendary figure. Scholars place the composition of the *Nei Ching* somewhere between 1000 to 300 BCE. As the example below illustrates, the text takes the form of a dialogue between the Yellow Emperor and one of his ministers, Ch'i Po.

Treatise Seventeen: *On the Essential and Finely Discernible Aspects of the Pulse*

The Yellow Emperor asked: "How is an examination [of the pulse] done?"

Ch'i Po answered: "The examination *zhen fa* [of the pulse] is usually [done] at dawn. The ying *qi* has not yet stirred, the yang *qi* has not yet dispersed, food and drink have not yet been taken, the vessels are not yet overly active, the network vessels are harmonious and stable, and the *qi* and blood are not yet disordered – and for these reasons, an abnormal pulse can be detected. Feel closely the movement of the pulse, then observe the essence brightness *jing ming*. Examine the five colors of the skin, inspect whether the five *zang* organs (internal *ying* organs) are overflowing or insufficient...."

Chinese medicine conjoined extensive pharmacopeia with a cosmic tenet: it was thought that the Creator *Pauku* divided the universe into two complementary principles: *Ying-Yang, a* philosophy founded on two opposing forces, the celestial, and male, *Yang,* which incorporated light, dry, heat, and life, and the female, *Ying,* signifying dark, moist, cold, and death. The energy in Yang was *qi,* an ethereal and intricate force transmitted through the body via intangible meridians or pathways. Blood flowing through anatomical vessels constituted the *Ying*. A disruption in these two "circulations," this balance of forces and elements, resulted in disease – a disharmony of the *qi* and the plasmic energy and vector of life. Several modalities were employed to restore balance, the most dramatic of which is acupuncture. Acupuncture remains a popular form of therapy which aims to control the flow of *qi*. The practice of acupuncture may have holocene roots,* but definitive evidence of it can be found in the Han dynasty (202 BC–220 CE). It is a treatment modality practiced by inserting and manipulating fine needles into specific points (called *xue*) on the body along special meridians for the purpose of pain relief and disease regulation (Fig. 1). Traditional Chinese acupuncture theory holds that special points lay along these meridian lines through which *qi* flows. The meridians are not physical features, but rather functional reference points. Ancient China influenced many cultures in ancient times, and acupuncture, moxibustion, cupping and Ying-Yang concepts of meridians are still employed in many parts of the world. Acupuncture is indisputably a valuable clinical modality, and Western medicine has for some time been studying the practice in an attempt to understand its mechanisms.

Modifying elements and attributes shown in Table 1 influenced the harmony of *qi*. Each viscus had an attribute: the liver stored blood (soul), the heart stored the pulse (spirit), the spleen maintained nutrition (thought), the lungs breath (energy) and the kidneys, germ (will). Circadian rhythms affected the viscera:

> Those who have a disease of the liver are animated and quick-witted in the early morning. Their spirits are heightened in the evening and at midnight they are calm and quiet....
> *The Yellow Emperor's Manual of Corporeal Medicine* (from a 2nd century BCE copy)

---

*Preserved in an alp glacier and found in September 1991, "Ötzi the Iceman" is thought to have lived 3,300 BCE and his body was tattooed with 57 lines, dots and crosses that mark meridian points of acupuncture. Incidentally, he carried in his pouch two lumps of *Piptoporus betulinus* fungus which has purgative and antibiotic properties.

Lancet. 1998; 352: 1864.

Viscera	Season	Element	Taste	Color	Animal	Grain	Emotion	Number	Planet
Liver	Spring	Wood	Sour	Green	Fowl	Wheat	Anger	8	Jupiter
Heart	Summer	Fire	Bitter	Red	Sheep	Gum	Joy	7	Mars
Spleen	Summer	Earth	Sweet	Yellow	Ox	Millet	Sympathy	5	Saturn
Lungs	Fall	Metal	Pungent	White	Horse	Rice	Grief	9	Venus
Kidney	Winter	Water	Salty	Black	Pig	Bean	Fear	6	Mercury

Table 1: Some *Qi* modifying elements and attributes

The belief in cosmic elements did not interfere with the progress of medicine and specialization. The *materia medica* was extensive, with much cupping, massage, acupuncture and moxibustion. China had specialists for diseases of the eye, ear, teeth, abdominal organs and bladder. Some cured defective speech and some, revered as sagacious and perceptive, imparted prudent and far-sighted advice to troubled patients – a form of psychology. There were specialists for women and children. From the Ming period (1368-1644) onwards, doctors used medical dolls – small sculptures of women – as diagnostic aids called a "Doctor's lady." Women pointed to the site of the symptoms and thereby eschewed physical examination by male physicians to preserve modesty (Fig. 2).

During the Chou dynasty (1123-256 BCE) – the era of Lao-Tse (b. 640 BCE), Confucius (551-479 BCE) and Mencius (372-289 BCE) – state medical examinations were introduced for certification. In the Han dynasty (202 BCE-220 CE) clinical cases were recorded on paper and methods of bedside observations became standardized, confirming existing surgical skills, sophisticated instrumentation and surgical methods. As early as the 2nd century, Sanguozhi, the biographer of Hua Tuo (c. 110-207), described how Hua Tuo gave patients a solution of *ma fei* (either opium or hemp boiled with wine) as anesthesia for complex surgeries. Surgical correction of harelip must have been common since it is mentioned in several sources. The Tsin dynasty (263-420) produced *The Handbook of Emergencies*, and Huang Fu (214-282 CE) wrote *Chia-i-ching*, a treatise on acupuncture.

During the T'ang Dynasty (618-970) the Grand (Imperial) College of Medicine functioned with five branches of medical study and required five years of study to qualify for examination.

In the 7th century, Ch'ao Yuan-fang (550-630) wrote *Chu-ping yuan-hou lun* (On the Origins and Symptoms of Various Diseases). In the 8th century, Sun Ssu-Miao (581-682) produced *Ch'ien-chin fang* (A Thousand Golden Recipes) that included treatments for goiter, asthma, jaundice, carbuncles, dysentery, and other maladies. Sung dynasty (906-1280) monograms on specific diseases appeared, such as fevers, diarrhea and asthma. There was an annual statistical record of disease by 1105 that covered the most populated provinces. In 1242, the *His Yuan Lu*

"Instruction to Coroners" was written and has endured as a forensic medical text in China.

During the Ming dynasty (1367-1644), the great herbal formulary *Li Shi Chen* was redacted – compiled from many classic sources. In the same compilation tradition, Chien Lung (1711-1799) wrote the "Encyclopedia of Medicine," a masterful and thorough opus conjoining all classic traditions and *Qi* modulation elements listed in Table one.

Much of the early Imperial period wisdom was lost through destruction of texts, but the *Ishimpo* preserves and provides a window to the ancient medicine of China. The *Ishimpo* was completed by Yasuyori Tamba in 982 and is the oldest medical book in existence in Japan. It consists of thirty scrolls (Table 2), faithfully compiled from Chinese medical works. Of the one hundred and ten classic Chinese documents compiled in the *Ishimpo* only two appear to have survived in China, making the *Ishimpo* an extremely valuable source of ancient Chinese and Japanese medicine, in fact, the major source.

Tamba dedicated his work to the Emperor in 984. A second edition was calligraphed in 1145. Thereafter the scrolls were scattered and hidden away by various noble families, preserved as precious heritage. They were not reassembled again until 1859 when woodblock prints of the thirty scrolls were made available to scholars. A perusal of the table of contents demonstrates the degree of specialization that ancient China had achieved. Scroll 25 of the *Ishimpo* focuses on children and is essentially a pediatric textbook of first millennium China.

The most important Chinese contribution to western medicine was the diversified and comprehensive pharmacopoeia it compiled. The principle work, *Pen Ts'ao Kang Mu* (c.1550), is a fifty-two volume work with nearly two thousand recipes (prescriptions), among them the use of iron for anemia, arsenic for skin disease, mercury for syphilis, rhubarb as a purgative, pomegranate as a vermifuge and opium as soporific and calmative.

New-World
It may appear paradoxical to write of the New World in a chapter on Ancient medicine, but the civilizations of Meso and South America like the preceding ones have paleo-Indian artifact historiography dating back 10,000 BCE, that include obsidian blades, Clovis-like projectiles with bifacial flaking and dated bone fragments. Artifacts from the archaic period (5000-1500 BCE) are richer and include the dietary record of teosinte cobs and early pottery ware dated to 2500 BCE. Yet, with the exception of some Mayan glyphs, there are no written specific records of Aztec, Maya or Inca medicine and nearly all extant sources are secondary, mostly from the

records of Spanish clergymen writing in the 16th century. Since these civilizations were unknown and untouched* until the arrival of Spanish explorers, the assumption is that what was redacted by these early chroniclers and clergymen had not changed in at least five millennia.

Aztec medicine was theurgic attributing illness to divine influences that altered one or more of the three essences: *tonalli* – the vital breath – that resided in the head and collected in the hair; *teyolia* that was kept in the heart and controlled thoughts and emotions, and, *ihiyotl* of hepatic dwelling that governed all instincts. Like the *qi* of the Orient and the *humors* of the West, an equilibrium of these three essences provided for health in conjunction with a balance of "heat" and "cold." Diseases of the head, eyes and heart were related to "heat" and abdominal illness stemmed from "cold" and could be relieved by an offerings to *Tlaloc* – the god of rain. Almost all treatments were by incantation, manipulation, and a rich pharmacopeia, a record of which was redacted in 1552 by Martin de la Cruz (an Aztec convert) from the *Nahuatl* language. The Latin translation *Codex Barberini* was written by Juan Bandiano (1484-c.1552). A later document, the *Florentine Codex,* was written and richly illustrated by a Franciscan friar Bernardo Sahagún (1499-1590), which *inter alia* recorded the treatment of fractures, liquid latex in ear canals for aches, obsidian lancing, and the drainage of abscesses along with other surgical procedures and treatments.

Like the Aztec, Mayan medicine was theurgic and required incantations recited by specialized shamans who possessed significant surgical skills. Wounds were sutured with the patient's own hair, and prosthetic teeth were made from jade, turquoise and iron pyrite. Both the Aztec and Maya used volcanic glass – obsidian – as surgical cutting instruments.

Their botanical medications were prepared for delivery orally, by inhalation, topically and via enema. Treatment often involved the sweat bath in a hot stone "sauna" setting to remove impurities. A form of *similia similubus curantur* was employed, so that yellow fruits were consumed for jaundice and for blood disorders, the feathers of red birds were burned. Their rich pharmacopeia included pain relief from hallucinogenics such a peyote, morning glory seeds and mushrooms. These same substances were also used in rituals to communicate with the spirit world. Cacao was used for various nutritional dysfunctions such as cachexia, diarrhea and gout, while the oil of cacao (butter) was used for skin ailments. Capsicum a topical irritant generated heat and was added to poultices for abscesses.

---

*There is evidence that the fleets of Zheng He (1371-1433) explored the Pacific coast of these cultures (c. 1422), but there is no evidence of botanical or ethnocultural exchange.

Arguably, the most medically sophisticated New World civilization was the Inca which flourished late in the 13th century from Chavin roots (c. 900 BCE). Cuzco was the center of the Incan empire which existed for only four centuries before being extinguished by the Spanish. Like the Aztec, what we know comes from chroniclers like Jesuit Bernabé Cobo (1582-1657) and his *Historia general de la Indias*. Cobo describes healers – *hampicamayoc* – with extraordinary botanical sophistication who knew the properties of hundreds of plants. They fermented maize into alcoholic *chicha,* made different infusions from the Peruvian pepper tree *Schinus molle* against leishmaniasis, dermal ulcers, eczema and gout, and used quinoa for dropsy. Coca was used as an analgesic, as an antidiarrheal and as a poultice for dermal lesions. Asthma was treated with steam inhalations of retama and chamico (*Datura stramonicum*)* and both were used for insomnia and as an analgesic. Tobacco poultices were employed to treat poisonous bites.

But more extraordinary was the sophisticated use of trephination, or the cutting of cranial burr holes to reach the dura and release malignant spirits and perhaps to relieve post-traumatic intracranial pressure. Some trephinations were clearly round and some square indicating a cutting of bone. Based on skeletal evidence of healing and bone re-growth, it is suggested trephination was practiced with a 90% survival rate. A similar form of surgery was practiced in Mesoamerica but employed stone abrasion to grind the skull down to the dura, leaving a beveled bone edge.

The medical heritage of these New World cultures is still with us today in the use of quinine, capsicum, cocaine, ipecac and other botanical products.

Ancient period Summary

This brief glimpse into ancient medicine narrates some strange, bizarre mystical concepts of disease and exotically odd, sometimes odious concoctions used for treatment. Fascinating and often riveting data about curiosities, superstitions and at times frankly ridiculous notions are juxtaposed with genuine pearls of wisdom still recognized as valid and valuable, and reinforce the continuity of medicine's evolution.

---

*During the 1800s and well into the early 1900s, prior to adrenalin vaporizers, asthma cigarettes were sold over the counter made from the leaves of *Datura stramonicum* which delivered by smoke inhalation a bronchodilatory antimuscarinic alkaloid.

William Osler asserted how indispensible knowledge gleaned from the study of the ancients is – especially with reference to Hippocrates (see ahead) and all who followed – in his comments regarding the Four Apostolic Successions of Medicine:

> The critical sense and skeptical attitude of the Hippocratic school laid the foundations of modern medicine on broad lines, and we owe to it: first, the emancipation of medicine from the shackles of priestcraft and caste; secondly, the conception of medicine as an art based on accurate observation and as a science, an integral part of the science of man and of nature; thirdly, the high moral ideals, expressed in...the Hippocratic oath; and fourthly, the conception and realization of medicine as the profession of a cultivated gentleman. No other profession can boast of the same unbroken continuity of methods and of ideals. We may indeed be justly proud of our apostolic succession.
>
> *The Montreal Medical Journal* Vol. XXXI (1902)

Scroll	No. of Pages	Contents
1	148	Disease Treatment, Pharmacology, Posology
2	168	Acupuncture and Moxibustion
3	92	Afflictions of the Nervous System
4	68	Whiskers, Hair, Face, Nose, Body Odors
5	120	Eyes, Ears, Mouth, Tongue, Teeth
6	64	Stomach, Heart, Kidneys, Liver, Lungs
7	52	Genitals, Piles, Intestinal Worms
8	72	Nutritional deficiency, Diseases of Extremities
9	68	Cough, Asthma, Dyspepsia, Nausea
10	88	Hernia, Jaundice, Swelling
11	100	Cholera and Dysentery
12	76	Constipation, Diabetes, Hematuria, Bedwetting
13	68	Consumption, Exhaustion, Insomnia
14	132	Sudden death, Fevers, Drowning, Freezing
15	92	Boils, Growth in Lungs and Intestines
16	100	Carbuncles, Vicious swellings, Varicose veins
17	68	Skin Diseases
18	120	Wounds, Burns, Metal wounds, Arrow wounds, Falls from Horses, Dog bites, Horse bites
19	112	Various Types of Tonics, Mineral Diet
20	72	Antidotes for Mineral Poisoning
21	60	Women's Diseases
22	76	Women's Diseases continued
23	96	Obstetrics
24	72	Conception, Sex prediction, Pregnancy tests
25	184	Pediatrics
26	80	Geriatrics, attaining longevity
27	80	Geriatrics, Mental hygiene, Breathing exercises
28	108	Health principles, Chamber Exercises
29	108	Dietary adjustments
30	104	Materia medica: Cereal, Fruit, Meat, Vegetable

Table 2: *Ishimpo* Table of Contents

II: Classical Period Medicine

Timeline:

    BCE
- 460 Pericles of Athens
- 450 Herodotus histories
- 430 Athenian plague
- 399 Socrates condemned
- 323 Alexander the Great dies
- 305 Ptolemaic Egypt
- 264 First Punic war
-   80 Mithridates' poison experiments
-   55 Lucretius: *De rerum natura*
-   51 Cleopatra becomes queen
-   44 Julius Caesar assassinated

    CE
-   64 Rome burns
-   79 Vesuvius destroys Pompeii
-   98 Trajan becomes Emperor
- 200 Galen dies
- 285 Diocletian divides Roman Empire
- 312 Constantine converted
- 372 Buddhism in Korea
- 476 End of Western Roman Empire
- 571 Birth of Muhammad
- 690 Paulus Aegineta dies

Not to have knowledge of what happened before you were born is to be condemned to live forever a child.

> Cicero: *M. Tulli Ciceronis Orator*
> *Ad M. Brutum* (46 BCE)

The art has three factors, the disease, the patient, the physician. The physician is the servant of the art, and the patient must cooperate with the physician in combating the disease.

> Hippocrates: *Epidemics* I, xi.

I am of the opinion that the art of medicine ought to be rational, but to draw instruction from evident causes, all obscure ones being rejected from the practice of the art, although not from the practitioner's study.

> Celsus: *De Medicina* Prooemium
> (see ahead: Occam's razor)

The brain is the highest of the organs in position and it is protected by the vault of the head; it has no flesh or blood or refuse. It is the citadel of sense-perception.

> Pliny Elder: *Historia Naturalis* XI, 49.

The physician will hardly be thought very careful of the health of others who neglects his own.

> Galen: *Of Protecting the Health* V

Physician heal thyself.

> *Luke*: 4: 23

Classical Period
Reference to the classical world elicits images of the golden age of Greece and the mighty empire of Rome. Not that other cultures were silent or dormant, but the Greek and Roman empires, in the volume of riches their legacies left to the modern world, surpassed all other western cultures combined. The encyclopedic curiosity of Pliny the Elder (23-79) produced a massive work on all aspects of the universe; Tacitus (56-117) recorded history; Emperors such as Trajan (53-117) promoted the social commonweal, funded Roman engineering marvels that still astound us, and formulated principles of urban public health, a bequest the modern world has well utilized. Greece in particular, however, more than 1500 years ago left us the standards of what comprises a civilized world in fields as diverse as philosophy, astronomy, mathematics, art, science and medicine.

Greece
The three most widely known classical Greeks who contributed to healing medicine in varying degrees were Asklepios, Homer, and Hippocrates.

The cult of Asklepios exemplifies the power of psychology and ritual in healing. Its practices likewise strain modern credulity as they exhumed mostly superstitious practices of other, earlier, cultures. As part of the Greek pantheon of gods, the cult of Asklepios (Latinized to Aesculapius) began about 429 BCE when temples were erected as curative sites. These temples often were located near the calming sea and all had fresh water springs (*sanitarias*) at their disposal. The most famous temples were those in Cos, Epidaurus, Cnidus and Pergamum.

Central to the healing process among advocates of the Asklepios cult was to submit to an induced state of unconsciousness with hopes of experiencing a reverie that miraculously restored health. While waiting to be attended by special temple priests, patients spent one to two weeks in residence adhering to a prescription of rest, baths in the *sanitarias* and a dietary regime. Wine was prohibited. This routine in itself would be salubrious and probably restorative. When ready for the temple ritual, at dusk, dressed in a white gown, a patient was led to a temple full of snakes and dogs to witness the sacrifice to the gods of a cock or ram. The patient then lay on a couch to be soporified into a deep sleep. Once unconscious, snakes and puppies licked and dribbled the patient with saliva. Upon awakening, the patient, surrounded by priest, snakes and dogs, bathed in the spring waters. Inunction and massage were the final steps to the ritual, and the patient was discharged with a dietary prescription for purgatives plus an admonishment to avoid wine.

There have been many votive inscriptions uncovered that attest to many purported "cures" from the lick of "sacred" serpents and puppies. Ostensibly it appears to be a ritual devoid of scientific merit until one considers that in fact saliva contains regulatory peptides such as transforming growth factor α-2 and hepatocyte growth factor, as well as antimicrobials such as thiocyanate and lysozymes. (*Lancet.* 349: 1776, 1997). Animals in modern experiments that have had saliadenectomies (removal of salivary glands) are unable to heal skin ulcers by licks in contrast to animals with intact salivary glands. (*Lancet.* 350: 369, 1997). The saliva of two species of sacred serpents (both benign) – *Elaphe longissima* and *quatuorlineata* – have been studied and found to contain active polypeptide epidermal growth factor. Therefore, the ancient rituals of Asklepios may have contributed to the healing of skin lesions, autosuggestion adding to further healing. (*Lancet.* 340: 223, 1992).

In any case, Asklepios belongs in the canon of ancient Greek physicians if only for the following fact: deified images commonly depict him leaning on a staff around which a serpent is entwined – the caduceus (Fig. 3). It famously remains the universally recognized iconographic symbol of medicine.

Greek literature in general played to an audience that was dominated by theurgic beliefs. In Homer's *Iliad* and *Odyssey* the gods, for example, are blamed for disease. Relevant to the study of medical history, however, it is notable that Homer (c. 9th century BCE) described man-made wounds with exceptional precision. Scholarly analysis of the *Iliad* extols the poet's depictions of one hundred and forty-seven wounds and the morbidity and mortality they caused. Aeneas and his femoral fracture in Bk V: 294 and Nestor's arrow wound to his thigh in Bk XI: 754 are examples. The meticulous accuracy of his descriptions has enabled scholars to make a wound by wound analysis that indicates seventy-seven percent died of their injuries. Homer's facility in describing anatomy is apparent in the two examples that follow, one that refers to the cervical trachea and the other to peri-renal fat: "...the point went right through his soft neck; but the ash spear with its weight of bronze did not cut the windpipe, so that he could still speak." (Hector, killed by Achilles, *Iliad* XXII); "And eels and fish were his busy attendants, tearing and nibbling at the fat around his kidneys." (Asteropaios, killed by Achilles and left in the Skamandros River, *Iliad* XXI). A poet, above all, Homer's mention of the wine and vinegar that were used to clean wounds nevertheless presupposes general use by physicians even for non-combat wounds.

With the golden age of Greece (448-404 BCE), crowned by art that sought the perfection of the human form and philosophic expression that aspired to liberate thought, the influence of Greek polytheism gradually waned, as did the cult of Asklepios, until medicine moved from the theurgic to the natural world. One catalyst appears to have been the 5th century BCE sage, Thales (c. 624-547) who, after years of conducting planetary observations in Egypt, returned to his home in Miletus and there accurately predicted an eclipse in 585 after studying the position of the stars, sun and moon. Notably, he did not consult the gods regarding the phenomenon. It marked an enormous shift to the study of the natural world devoid of deistic references, and it altered all scientific – including medical – inquiry and thought forever:

> Day was all of a sudden changed into night. This event had been foretold by Thales, the Milesian, who forewarned the Ionians of it, fixing for it the very year in which it took place. The Medes and Lydians, when they observed the change, ceased fighting, and were alike anxious to have terms of peace agreed on.
>
> Herodotus, *Histories* I, 74

The School of Hippocrates

A striking example of the sophisticated advance in scientific thought in ancient Greece is found in the works of Alcmaeon of Croton (c. 500 BCE). A pupil of Pythagoras (?580-?500 BCE), his theories were later promulgated by the Hippocratic School, whose influence was paramount in medicine for more than a thousand years. Alcmaeon made the original observation that the seat of the senses is in the brain, not the heart. This doctrine was later discussed in Plato's (428-348 BCE) *Phaedo* in which he has Socrates (c. 469-399 BCE) declare that: "The brain furnishes the sensations of hearing, sight and smelling, from which memory and judgment are born, and from these sensations, once established, wisdom is also born." Alcmaeon also subscribed to the belief in humoral qualities described by Anaxagoras (500-428 BCE) that affected the body. Humoral theory in a balanced structure (called *eucrasis*) had elements of two opposites, such as wet-dry, cold-hot, that affected man's healthy nature, thought to be comprised of choleric, phlegmatic, bilious and sanguine humors. Disequilibrium in these elements (called *dyscrasia*), Alcmaeon proposed, produced disease.

Also of the Pythagorean School, Empedocles of Agrigentum (504-443 BCE) in *On Nature* attributed all health to the harmony of the four elements that were identified as earth, water, fire, and air. This theory of harmony was compatible with the thinking applied to the four humors, and both hypotheses gradually melded into a unified premise of disease causation, which – as with Chinese medicine – expanded to include other facets: the visceral attributes of the heart, brain, spleen and liver. However flawed the thinking was in ancient times, the historical significance of these theories pertains, again, to the way in which nature and the natural world irreversibly became the focus for the study of matters concerning life and death, not the gods. This momentous shift paved the way for the natural clinical studies, observations and treatments in the corpus of Hippocrates.

Hippocrates (?460-?377 BCE) lived in the age of Pericles (c. 495-429 BCE), considered the zenith of Athenian democracy and civilization. It was the age of Herodotus (c. 484-425 BCE) and Thucydides (c. 460- 395 BCE) both of whom wrote famous histories, Sophocles (c. 496-406 BCE) and Euripides (c. 480-406 BCE) whose plays still are read and performed, and Phidias (c. 480-430 BCE), Praxiteles (c. 400-330 BCE) and Lysippus (fl. 4th century BCE) who created sculptures of unsurpassed beauty and anatomy.

Hippocrates is renowned for attributing illness to natural causation and for giving the *iatros* – physician – a moral code and purpose. Hippocrates' authoritative voice established what had long been only implied, that the gods did not cause disease, and, in *On the Sacred Disease,* he debunked the thinking of those who continued to attribute disease to deities.

> ...those who first called this disease [epilepsy] "sacred" were the sort of people we now call witch-doctors, faith-healers, quacks and charlatans. These are exactly the people who pretend to be very pious and to be particularly wise. By invoking a divine element they ...conceal their ignorance of its nature.

Much of what is known about Hippocrates is based on legend, and, although no single work can be definitively attributed to him, by tradition the *Hippocratic corpus* consisted of approximately sixty oral treatises assumed to have been redacted by his students between 430 to 330 BCE. Some scholars believe they were collected around 250 BCE for the library at Alexandria. Most famous among these works are *Aphorisms, Epidemics, Airs, Waters, Places, Fractures and Joints* and *Wounds of the Head*, all compiled around 415 BCE.

The Hippocratic *Corpus* judged the four humors as vital fluids to explain health and disease. Blood, phlegm, black bile and yellow bile or choler each served different purposes. Blood sustained vitality, phlegm cooled the spirit, black bile invoked melancholia and yellow bile enhanced digestion. Collectively, the balance of these humors was reflected in body temperature, skin color, somatotype (phlegmatics were stout and cholerics thin) and temperament or disposition (sanguines were warm and bilious thoughtful). As long as these humors were in proper balance and proportion, there was health. A plethora of one or more created imbalance that resulted in illness. Diet, exercise, blood-letting or purgatives were the advised treatments to restore the requisite healthful balance.

Traditionally Hippocrates is credited with the development of case notes and the patient as a teaching model. The *Corpus* reveals his mastery of the art of clinical observation. Hippocrates wrote about medicine, surgery, embryology, nutrition and even about the impact climate has on health. He recorded signs and symptoms. Commonly, causes of diseases remained unknown, but Hippocrates proffered prognoses based on clinical observations, recognizing that when a certain constellation of signs and symptoms appeared, the resultant illness would follow a predictable course. In *Fractures and Joints* (c. 415 BCE) he describes the use of a fracture table, the *scamnum*, which was used for fractures of the thigh and leg. Hippocrates made clear the setting of femoral fractures carried a high risk of deformity. He also recognized that compound fractures were commonly fatal.

Hippocrates used Hebdomadism to define the various periods of life. The Hebdomad divided human life-spans into seven periods of seven years, *infans, puer, adolescens, juvenis, junior, vir* and *senex* – newborn, child, adolescent, young man, man, mature man, old man (Fig. 4). The earliest published hebdomad on human growth and decline, however, was by Solon (c. 595 BCE).

Hippocrates was a keen observer who believed that a physician's knowledge and skills are good and necessary but it is nature that heals or kills. His aphorisms, samples of which follow, best attest to this belief:

I.16   Fluids are beneficial to all who suffer fevers, but it is especially true of children.

II.2   When sleep puts an end to delirium, it is a good sign.

II.33   In disease it is a good sign when the patient's intellect is sound and he enjoys eating; the opposite is bad.

II.40   Those who acquire a gibbous spine with cough and asthma die before puberty.

V.6   Those attacked by tetany either die in four days or recover.

V.14   If diarrhea attacks a consumptive, it is fatal.

I.34   Bubbles in the urine is a sign of kidney disease and a protracted illness.

Hippocrates left a legacy that influenced medical thinking and care for more than fifteen hundred years, despite the lack of a thorough understanding of anatomy, physiology and pathology. His medical construct based on natural science and clinical bedside observation, employed with logical reasoning as to cause and effect, and the ethical concepts he articulated based on moral law continue to be a model in the modern world for the ideal physician. The essence of his ethic is expressed in the Oath encompassed in the *Corpus* (See Appendix A) – an oath which continues to be taken by all those who are accepted into the medical profession

After Hippocrates, the school of Cos thrived under his sons Thessalus and Draco, and then under Crytodemus, physician to Alexander the Great (356-323 BCE) of Macedonia. Little is known of Crytodemus other than he extracted an arrow from a wound Alexander sustained.

The ascendancy of Greek learning and culture was jolted to a near halt by an epidemic, the "Athenian," that appeared to have originated in Ethiopian Africa. Thucydides described a catastrophic illness marked by "violent heat in the head," cough, high fevers, ulcerations, seizures, gangrene and death by day seven or eight. Twenty-five to thirty-five percent of the population died, and Greece had difficulty sustaining the manpower needed for crucial battles of the Peloponnesian war. Scholars have speculated on the nature of this epidemic, citing over thirty possible causes, most prominently typhus, influenza and even Ebola fever, but, nothing more is known about it.

Aristotle

Before the Greek apotheosis faded, Aristotle (384-322 BCE), pupil of Plato and teacher to Alexander the Great, left his seismic imprint on the world. He wrote on physics, metaphysics, poetry, theater, music, logic, rhetoric, politics, government, ethics, biology, and zoology. Aristotle descended from three generations of physicians who espoused the idea of observing and exploring nature. Aristotle studied the teleology – the origins and purpose of nature – and produced a great work, the *De Generatione Animalium* that prefigured what would evolve as botany, zoology, comparative anatomy, embryology, taxonomy, teratology and physiology.

Aristotle's physiology was cardiocentric. He noted that death came with cardiac standstill and that, in the embryo, the first motion came from the heart: *primum oriens et ultimum moriens* (the first to be born and the last to die). Among his clinical observations are:

> Frequently the child appears to be born dead, when it is feeble and when, before the tying of the cord, a flux of blood occurs into the cord and adjacent parts.

> Some nurses who have already acquired skill, squeeze [blood] back out of the cord [to the baby] and at once the baby, who had previously been as if drained of blood, comes to life again.
> *De Generatione Animalium*, Bk.vii

> There is evacuation of excrement sometimes at once, sometimes soon, but always within the day, and this excrement is more than accords with the bulk of the child. Women call it meconium; its color is like blood and it is extremely black and like pitch but after this it already assumes the milk-like character for the infant draws the breast at once.
> *De Generatione Animalium*, Bk. vii

> All children directly they are born have their eyes bluish, but afterwards these change to the sort they are destined to remain.
> *De Generatione Animalium*, Bk. v,1

> In man the male is more often born with deformity than the female.
> *De Generatione Animalium*, Bk. vi,6

Alexander's defeat of Darius III (c. 380-330 BCE) had brought Egypt into the Grecian realm and, after his death in 323, Ptolemy (c. 367-283 BCE) ruled Egypt until 282. Ptolemy turned Alexandria and its famous library into a center for science, attracting Archimedes (287-212 BCE), Euclid (fl. 300 BCE), Herophilus of Chalcedon (c. 330-260 BCE), and Erasistratus of Chios (c. 330-255 BCE) as prominent teachers. The dissection writings of Herophilus and Erasistratus (c. 280), were lamentably lost, but what is known of their work and study are known through the writings of Cornelius Celsus (see ahead) and Quintus Tertullian (163-220), both of whom allude that Herophilus and Erasistratus performed vivisection on prisoners.

Herophilus, a student of Praxagoras of Cos (fl. 350), was a notable anatomist who through his dissections differentiated the cerebrum, cerebellum, meninges, and the 4th ventricle. He described the parotid, pulmonary artery, duodenum, ovaries, prostate and the anatomy of the eye, and analyzed the pulse using a water-clock. Agnodice (fl. 340), midwife and gynecologist, is said to have studied anatomy with Herophilus.

Erasistratus' dissections described the aortic and pulmonary valves, chordae tendinae, analyzed cardiac and digestive physiology, and formulated early metabolic concepts. He placed hens in jars, weighed them before and after feeding and weighed their excreta. He associated ascites with cirrhosis and, remarkably, conceived of *pneuma* [blood] passing from veins to arteries through tiny connections, a concept lost to medicine until Malpighi's observations in the 17th century (see ahead). Ignoring the humoral theory, Erasistratos turned his attention to organs and tissues as the site of disease.

These dissections could only have occurred in the atmosphere of a newly governed Alexandria, in which scientific inquiry was encouraged, and which eschewed the proscriptions of Greece where dissection was frowned upon. The anatomical studies of Herophilus and Erasistratos invited critical attention, both positive and negative, in the centuries that followed. Those opposed to their study came to be known as Empiricists who opined that theoretical conjecture and further human dissection were futile. A physician, they contended, should focus on signs and symptoms and follow known successful modalities of treatment – a restoration of the Hippocratic model. Rationalists or Dogmatists held that experimentation, dissection and the application of natural philosophy to the study of medicine generated new understanding of disease.

While these contrary schools of thought engaged in dispute, from 250 BCE on the power of the Greek kingdom declined and the ascent of Roman power and influence began. By 80 BCE Greek physicians were under Roman domination. The Greek Empirical and Rational Schools of thought, however, were rejected by the Romans as too convoluted and replaced them with Methodism (see ahead).

The importance of the Greek empire in the history of medicine, despite Roman opinion to the contrary, cannot be underestimated. The resplendent minds that invoked nature as causative and defining and devised essential precepts in science, medicine and philosophy all ensured, despite the polytheism of conquering Rome, that Greek thought would influence the course for science and medicine in the centuries that followed.

Rome

The roots of Rome and its empire lay in antecedent cultures, particularly those of the Etruscans and Greeks. In medicine for instance hepatoscopy was adapted from the Etruscans. Rome's greatest influence, culturally and in medicine, however, derived from the Greeks. Its pantheon, certainly – including gods of healing and medicine – was Greek, although the Romans supplemented the roster with minor gods of health of their own minting, such as *Carna*, who safeguarded vital functions, *Carmenta*, who watched over pregnant women, *Lucina*, who protected parturition, and *Cunina*, who looked after babes in cribs. The Greek language was the Roman scientific *lingua franca,* and commonly, Greek physicians were the predominant deliverers of health care; although the citizenry also consulted midwives, herbalists, bone-setters and faith-healers. Interestingly, Pliny's *Historia Naturalis,* XXIX, cites monuments in Rome that had accusatory inscriptions that suggest there were Greek doctors with tarnished reputations. One such reads: "It was the crowd of [Greek] physicians that killed me."

Three philosophies of healing prevailed in Rome – Solidism, Pneumatism and, most importantly, the Humoralism of Greek derivation. The Greek concept of humors formed a numerological schemata of "four," considered an equilibrious awareness of order in nature. The concept four, such as in the four humors, also referenced and studied the four seasons, four winds and the then known four gustatory tastes, and balance in all elements and qualities were key. Good health was determined by a balance of humors and any "excess" or imbalance of a particular quality was treated by bleeding. Fasting prevented the formation of any new excess and purges diluted any threatening excesses, thus keeping the humors in salubrious balance (Fig. 5).

Solidism was based on the work of Asclepiades of Bithynia (c 120 BCE), a friend of Cicero (106-43 BCE), Crassus (115-53 BCE) and Mark Antony (83-30 BCE). Asclepiades opposed humoral causes of disease. His theory was Atomistic and claimed that health depended on the normal movement of atoms (indivisible particles as defined by Democritus (460-370 BCE) in body pores.

Themison of Laodicea (fl. 1st century BCE) modified the theory as Methodism that posited disease is due to one extreme or another of atom movement; it is the result of imbalance between atoms of rigidity and flaccidity, and that treatment should aim to restore a proper balance of constricted or relaxed solid body particles (*strictum et laxum corpus*). Treatment was fresh air, light, diet, massage, hydrotherapy, clysters and sparing doses of oral medication.

Pneumatism was based on the action and status of *pneuma* (vital air) which when inhaled cooled the inner heat of the heart. Early anatomists had noted that arteries are empty after death (blood drains back into veins) and mislabeled the artery as the "air duct" that carried *pneuma*. It was believed there was perfect health when *pneuma* maintained tonus and this could be determined by the quality of the pulse.

The eventual transition of Greek medicine into Roman is best recounted by Aurelius Cornelius Celsus (c. 30 BC- 45 CE) in his classic Latin work, *De medicina,* that consisted of eight tomes. Books one through four discuss diseases treated by diet and regimens. Books five to eight focus on drugs and surgery. Book four describes the four classical signs of inflammation, *calor, dolor, rubor, tumor*. Book seven is surgical and indicative that under the Romans, it would appear, surgery achieved the highest standards for the times. Lithotomy, herniotomy, plastic surgery, cataract couching (dislodging the lens out of place to fall to the bottom of the eye), and Caesarean sections were well practiced. Celsus was a great encyclopedist best remembered for the validity of his dictum *"Ex toto non sic pueri ut viri curari debent"* – children should be treated differently than adults.

Medicine in the Patristic Period

Pedanius Dioscorides (fl.1st century CE) of Anazarbus, was a Greek surgeon in Nero's army who originated the Western pharmacopoeia of over six hundred plants. Travelling with the army allowed him to collect medicinal specimens across the extensive Roman Empire. Around 50 to 70 CE he wrote his major *De materia medica* that contained five volumes arranged according to therapeutic groupings: Aromatics – oils, ointments, trees; Unmutated – milk, cereals, herbs; Plant – roots and herbs; Vine plants – wines and poultice vines – and Metallic ores. For sixteen hundred years, the work was reproduced and its precepts followed.

Aretaeus of Cappodocia (fl. 55-80 CE) in his major work *De Causis et Signis Morborum* rendered classical accounts of pneumonia, pleurisy, empyema, diabetes, tetanus, aura of epilepsy, elephantiasis and diphtheria. He differentiated the insanity of melancholia from maniacal-circular-depressive disorder. He was a proponent of uterine wandering as a cause of suffocation and neurologic symptoms in women (etymology of hysteria).

Books twenty-two through thirty-three of Pliny the Elder's (23-79 CE) encyclopedic *Historia Naturalis* touched on medicine. It was read steadily throughout the middle ages in eighty editions as the printing press made the work widely available. Pliny was a strong believer in dietetic and botanical medicine and low strength dosages. Ironically, Pliny, who was distrustful of physicians, bequeathed them a memorable maxim about child growth, the validity of which has not diminished with time: "At the age of three years, the body of each person is one half the length that it will ever attain."

Soranus of Ephesus (fl. 98-138) wrote during the reigns of Trajan (98-117) and Hadrian (117-138), and was the first male western authority on the subjects of gynecology, obstetrics, newborns and children. In his *Gynecologia* 1:61 he gave excellent descriptions of contemporaneous contraceptives: pessaries of fine wool with old olive oil or honey or cedar resin alone or with white lead. The sap of silphion,* an extinct genus of *Ferula* which grew only in Cyrene, was considered the best contraceptive. Soranus had several recipes for "cyrenaic juice" to be taken orally to prevent pregnancies. Soranus recognized gymnasia suppressed menses. His pediatric section is the finest in antiquity, devoted to neonatal care,

---

*Hippocrates used it for rectal prolapse: "When the gut protrudes and will not remain in its place, scrape the finest and most compact silphium into small pieces and apply as a cataplasm."

nutrition, and rearing. Chapter titles exhibit the extent of his pediatric acumen: "How to know what is capable of being reared," "How to divide the cord," "Inunction," "Swaddling," "Feeding," "Choice of a wet-nurse," "Cord separation," "Teething," "Rashes," "Wheezing and cough," "Seiriasis" and "Flux of the belly."

Artemidorus of Ephesus (fl. 2nd century CE) wrote *Oneirocritica*, a work dedicated to the interpretation of dreams. It consisted of five volumes, the first three encyclopedic on the nature of dreams and the last two devoted to the interpretation of dreams. The opus, thought for centuries to pertain to divination, was in the past century revitalized by Sigmund Freud (1856-1939) in his development of psychoanalysis (see ahead).

In the history of medicine there are personages that evoke strong and contrary opinions. Most historians would agree that Galen, Paracelsus, Trotula, Descartes and Hahnemann are among those in that circle, and most would agree that it was the first of them, Clarissimus or Claudius Galen of Pergamon (129-216) who historically was the most influential.

Galen wrote nine books on anatomy, seventeen on physiology, six on pathology, sixteen essays on the pulse, fourteen books on therapeutics, and thirty books on pharmacology. His concept of good health as expressed in *On Hygiene* was premeditated on controlling six environmental factors to maintain humoral balance: air and temperature, diet and fluids, sleep cycles, exercise, evacuation and emotions. He established the principle that a lesion in an organ changes its function and thereby identified some pathogonomic sequences – *e.g.* tenesmus led to urgency and severing the spinal cord led to paralysis. At Pergamom he was physician to the gladiators and learned wound-exposed anatomy from still-living bodies.*

Between 200 to 600, the canons of Galen and Hippocrates were a highly regarded part of medical pedagogy that continued to be cited in books for over a millennium. None were more impressed with his theories than Galen himself:

> Never as yet have I gone astray, whether in treatment or in prognosis, as have so many other physicians of great reputation. If anyone wishes to gain fame…all that he needs is to accept what I have been able to establish.

---

*Gladiatorial contests would not end until 326 AD, when banned by Emperor Constantine.

Galen studied functional human anatomy based on dissections of apes and pigs and arrived at flawed conclusions. His teachings were responsible for anatomical and physiological misconceptions that persisted for over a millennium. He performed no human dissections, and freely assigned to human anatomy his observations about animal anatomy however mistaken. Since the writings on anatomy based on human dissection by Herophilus and Erasistratos had been lost, the medical world inherited Galen's faulty anatomy. Galen modified physiology to fit Aristotelian concepts and insisted for example that the heart ventricles communicated through pores, a view that was readily accepted.

Since Galen was a monotheist who believed the body was an instrument of the soul his teachings, including his tenets on physiology based on the theory of humors, were embraced by the new Christianity. His medical doctrine was unchallenged by church and Christian society and his works were even admired by Hebrews and Arabic writers of medicine. The theories of Galen and his followers retarded western medicine's informed evolution for fifteen hundred years.

It should be noted that Roman medicine excelled in two particular and interconnected areas – public health and military medicine. The avant-garde measures common to urban areas were employed to protect the Roman army, estimated to number over three hundred thousand men. To maintain a healthy fighting force at their postings capable of patrolling the many borders of the Roman Empire, clean water, sanitary toiletry conditions and uncontaminated food were assured by Roman engineers who drained swamps for encampments and thereby reduced malaria and other insect-borne diseases. They built aqueducts to assure copious amounts of clean water, constructed sewer conduits and erected baths and gymnasia.

In addition to these public health measures that sustained a trim, strong body of men, able and experienced surgeons were dispatched to serve the army's needs. As a generalization and not surprisingly, in the battlefield those who suffered penetrating injuries of the abdomen or chest, shattered skulls or severed major arteries perished. Those with clean cuts or simple fractures, conversely, were commonly successfully treated. To this end Roman innovations included the training of "medics" who provided bandaging, hemostasis and splinting and established special evacuation units to take the wounded to field hospitals or *valetudiariums*. There, vinegar was employed for wound washing and bleeding vessels were ligated. Hypnotics were administered to minimize the trauma of amputations.

The *Pax Romana* finally collapsed in the reign of Marcus Aurelius (121-180) as the empire's frontiers intermittently were violated by Goths and other barbaric tribes, and epidemics rampaged across the continent. Small pox and measles from the East decimated populations between 165 to

180 and from 251 to 266. Galen described what has come down to us as the Antonine plague. Roman Empire troops returning from Asia minor campaigns in 165 started the pandemic strongly believed to be small pox. Galen records victims with fever, diarrhea, pharyngitis and skin eruption, both dry and pustular, appearing on the ninth day of illness. Roman Emperor Lucius Verus (130-169) died and his co-regent Marcus Aurelius Antoninus (121-180) survived and lent his name to the plague. Over the next twenty years, it spread along the Rhine valley killing an estimated five million and decimating the Roman army and irreparably weakened the Empire.

There were periods of crop failure and famine as well as of disease that exacerbated suffering and poverty in the provinces, while in Rome, rich from the crippling and ever increasing taxes collected from the outlying regions, depraved behavior increased, eroding the social order of what had been a great civilization. In 193 Emperor Commodus (161-193) was assassinated and a period of social instability ensued that lasted seventy-five years, during which twenty-seven emperors ruled, twenty-three of whom died violently. Under the auspices of Augustus Diocletian (284-305) the Empire was divided into East and West and, while sustaining his own position as *augustus*, Diocletian appointed supreme leaders in each (a *caesar* and an *augustus*), that formed a tetrarch of rulers, and thereby affected a short-lived stability.

In 305 Diocletian and his co-augustus Maximian (c. 250-310) resigned their offices, and Roman society reverted to its chaotic state and civil war. In 312 Constantine (272-337) ended the civil war, established Christian suffrage, reunited East and West and established his Holy Roman Empire's capital in Byzantium (later, Constantinople). This history is significant since, with the ascendancy of the Byzantine Empire, Constantinople became the seat of medicine, the "depository" of knowledge. Four prominent compilers, encyclopedists Oribasius, Aetius of Amida, Alexander of Tralles, and Paul of Aegina, preserved the precepts of Western medicine in Greek that would make their way to the West.

Oribasius of Constantinople (325-405) compiled the encyclopedic *Synagoge* in seventy volumes. Although only one third survives, scholars value this work for its exact quotes and attributions, and credit Oribasius for having preserved the works of many ancients. He interestingly observed that endomorphic girls mature early and the ectomorphic late – a prevailing axiom. He is best remembered for his pioneering pedagogy and his belief that children should be confided to humane and gentle teachers.

Nemesius, bishop of Emesa (Syria) (c. 390), wrote *On the Nature of Man* in which he originally presented the concept of the localization of mental functions. To the "frontal cavities" he assigned sensation and imagination, to the "central," intellectual thought, and to the "posterior," memory:

> If the central cavities are damaged in any way, the senses are impaired but thought remains unharmed. If the central cavity alone suffers, thought is overthrown but the sense-organs continue ... [if] the cerebellum suffers, memory alone is lost without sensation or thought being harmed ....

The works of Aetius and Tralles were encyclopedic compendiums that were referenced until the 16th century. Aetius of Amida (fl. early 6th century) was from Mesopotamia and studied at Alexandria. He was the royal physician to Justinian I (482-565). His *Tetrabiblion* reflects the many works he studied in the Alexandrian library. He carefully described many uterine disorders based on the observations of Soranus. Alexander of Tralles (525?-605?) wrote *Libri duodecim de re medica*. He was a fastidious observer of clinical situations and rendered accurate descriptions of chest conditions, including pleurisy.

Paul of Aegina (625-690) wrote the final compilation of the era, the *Epitome*, in seven comprehensive volumes. The first dealt with dietetics, the second pathology, and the third diseases of brain, nerves, ear, nose and throat. Volume four focused on skin and burns, five, on poisons, six described surgery, and seven, pharmacology.

Volume six was the most valuable since it illustrates the commendable surgical skills of the 7th century. Paul described the removal of foreign bodies from the nasopharynx and esophagus, tonsillectomy, tracheotomy, mastectomy, hysterectomy and even abdominal trocar insertion. To even contemplate such procedures at the time suggests that he likely had reasonable success.

During this period the Church solemnly affirmed Canon law as the final arbiter of faith, morals and science, and clerics initiated a tradition in which they devoted themselves to the ministry of the sick. They established treatment centers – *xenodochion* (shelters), *nosokomium* (hospital archetypes) and *brephotrophium* (children's hostels). Actual hospitals were not instituted until several centuries later. In 325 the Council of Nicaea ordered a *xenodochion* built in every town. The first office created by the new church in Jerusalem was the Deaconate to care for the sick. In 390 Roman noble woman Fabiola (?-400) opened the first Christian *nosokomium* in Ostia, the port city of Rome. Merovingian queen, Radegonde (525-587), founded a convent/hospital in Poitiers for lepers and the poor.

Classical medicine summary

The entire Mediterranean basin experienced profound cultural, social and moral upheavals in the tumultuous centuries following the reign of Hadrian. The erosion of culture and power was slow and protracted (it took over five hundred years) as Roman society mutated into an amalgam of pagan and Christian, Eastern and Western cultures. Natural catastrophes strained the Empire's resources and contributed to decline. In 512 the volcanic eruption of Vesuvius caused earthquakes that destroyed Aegean islands. In 526 another earthquake destroyed Antioch. Justinian's (527-565) plague began around 541 and decimated entire cities, killing over twenty-five million people. It ravished Constantinople, where half the population died. It can be said that the course and vector of modern European history were launched by this plague, as it made possible Arabia's ascendancy to power, a seismic societal shift from west to the Arab world that was to endure for centuries. Arabia conquered Egypt, Palestine, Syria, Libya, Persia, Mesopotamia, Barbary Africa and Spain. The Western Empire was in disarray, the Eastern was battered by forces of nature and contagion, and the Byzantine civilization whimpered further to the East, into Syria, seeking refuge and help, thereby shifting its political identity and allegiance. The Roman Empire's ebbing glow finally was extinguished with the death, in 565, of Justinian the Great, its last emperor.

III: Medieval Medicine

Timeline:

- 552 Buddhism in Japan
- 625 Muhammad dictates the *Koran*
- 711 Moorish invasion of Spain – al Andalus
- 800 Charlemagne crowned
- 910 Cluny Abbey founded
- 1066 Battle of Hastings
- 1085 Moors defeated at Toledo
- 1131 Council of Rheims forbids clerics medical practice
- 1163 Construction of Notre Dame begins
- 1215 Magna Carta
- 1271 Marco Polo sets off
- 1291 End of the Crusades
- 1309 Papal See moved to Avignon
- 1336 Start of the Hundred Years War
- 1347 Black Death
- 1387 *The Canterbury Tales*
- 1434 Cosimo de Medici in Florence
- 1453 End of the Byzantine Empire
- 1454 Gutenberg's press
- 1478 Spanish Inquisition

Honey and wine are bad for children but salutary for the elderly.
>	Maimonides: *Mishna Torah* IV, 12

From Earth's dark center unto Saturn's gate I've solved all Problems of this World's Estate,
From every Snare of Plot and Guile set free each Bond resolved – saving alone Death's Fate.
>	Avicenna: *The Canon*

Pluratitas non est ponenda sine necessitate. (Occam's razor) – Do not posit plurality unless necessary.*
>	William of Occam (c. 1285-c. 1349):
>	*Quodlibeta Septem*

With us ther was a doctour of phisik;
In al this world ne was the noon hym lik,
To speke of phisik and of surgerye
For he was grounded in astronomye.
He kepte his pacient a ful greet deel
In houres by his magyk natureel.
Wel koude he fortunen the ascendent
Of his ymages for his pacient.
He knew the cause of everich maladye,
Were it of hoot, or coold, or moyste, or drye,
And where they engendred, and of what humour.
He was a verray, parfit praktisour.**
>	Chaucer: *The Canterbury Tales* (c. 1400)

*A universal and still relevant truth in science – and in life – that the simplest is usually the wisest supposition. In medical school students always are advised, "when you hear hoof beats don't think of zebras," or "the bird you hear outside your window may be a canary but it is most likely a sparrow."

**With us there was a doctor of medicine; There was none like him in all this world when speaking of medicine and surgery; Because he was knowledgeable in astronomy. He kept his patient healthy for hours with his natural magic. He could determine by the planets the talismanic figures of his patient. He knew the cause of every illness, whether it be hot or cold, or wet or dry, And where it began, and of what humour; He was a true good practitioner.

Arab-Influences
The debt to the Arab world in preserving classic Greek and Roman knowledge is inestimable, and it is historically helpful to comment on how this transpired. In the 5th century, the residue of Roman power was centered in Constantinople, but the focus by that time was on Christian themes, and pagans and all of their beliefs and knowledge, legends and writings, including that of the scholarly Greeks, defiled. Paradoxically, disinherited Christians were to be a significant link in preserving Greek wisdom. Nestorius (c.386-c.451) the Christian patriarch of Constantinople (428) was deemed a heretic because he taught Mary was the mother of Christ, not God. Emperor Justinian I expelled him, his followers and important pagan philosophers who had been intellectually formed by the works of Greek civilization. The exiles went to Persia, and the pagans took with them all of the classic Greek scholarship in their possession. Once the School of Plato in Athens collapsed a century later in 529, theirs was the only remaining source of Greek erudition, and, by that time in the Arab world, medical influences gleaned from Greek writings had been become well established. The influence in medicine was so strong that a great medical school and hospital were operant around 560 in Jundishapur, Iran, under the Persian leader, Khosru I (531 to 579). Medicine in the Western world was bankrupt, its foundations shattered, cut off as it was from the ancient classical bounty of learning that had informed it. It was to remain so for centuries. In parts of Persia, Egypt and Syria, Syriac, a late dialect of Aramaic, was the *lingua franca* of pedagogy, and initially the writings of Greece and Rome were translated into Syriac. The Arab conquest of the 7th century engulfed the Syriac speaking world, and absolute power and an Arabic Empire emerged, and its capital in time was moved from Damascus to Baghdad in 762. Eastern scholars flourished under the Caliphs (c.749-1258) who sanctioned the translation, from Syriac into Arabic, of the Greek canon. An arbitrary decree, made for political expediency, the edict empowered the preservation of Greek knowledge for all time, and the Arabic Empire became the caretaker of the classics that eventually were reintroduced into Western cultures: the works of Galen and the wisdom of Hippocrates, the philosophy and teleology of Aristotle, the dramas of Euripides, Aeschylus and Aristophanes, the poetry of Homer and others, the astronomy of Thales and Apollonius and the mathematics of Pythagoras, Archimedes and Euclid. The Aristotelian belief in a purposeful divine creator – Aristotelian philosophy in general – was but one aspect of learning these monarchs encouraged as new science and all of Greek classic works were promoted and studied, with scholars clamoring for more Greek knowledge.

The great Translation Movement that began in the 8th century continued for centuries. Initially concentration was on the transcription of the Greek canon from Greek into Syriac and then Greek and Syriac into

Arabic. In time the Translation Movement would refer to the translation of texts from Arabic into Latin that reintroduced classical wisdom to the Western world. Jewish physician Maser Djwawah ibn Djeldjal of Basra (fl. late 7th century) prevailed on his patient Caliph Moawia I (602-680) to sponsor translations of Greek classics. Djeldjal himself translated the *Pandects* of Haroun of Alexandria (c. 800). (It was on this work that Rhazes would base his work on smallpox. See ahead). Abbasid caliphs Harun al-Rashid (764?-809) and his son al-Ma'mum (786-833) opened a translation bureau in Baghdad called the *Bayt al-Hikmah* that sought scholarly works in every language for translation into Arabic. (By the ascendency of al-Ma'mum, pharmacists (*Saydalani*) were required to pass examinations for licensure).

Three great periods of Arabic medicine were launched that spanned a millennium and occurred in the East and the West. In the first period (750-900) the illustrious Greek to Arabic translators Yuhanna ibn Masawayn (Johannes Mesue of Damascus (777-857), Hunayn ibn Ishaq al-Ibadi (Johannitius 809-873) and Yuhanna ibn Arabi or Serapion (fl. 9th century) were most productive. Mesue, who wrote a compilation of twelve volumes entitled *Aphorisms*, was a Christian physician who wrote in Syriac and Arabic. In 830, Caliph al-Mu'tasim (794-842) named Mesue the director of a school for the translation of Greek classics into Arabic. The Caliph also provided him with apes for dissection that resulted in the writing of several anatomical works. Of medical writings, "Disorders of the Eye" ("Daghal al-ain") is the earliest ophthalmology extant treatise in Arabic. (See appendix G).

Mesue's pupil, Johannitius, a Nestorian, translated more than two hundred works into Arabic, including Hippocrates' *Aphorisms* and *Prognostics* and Galen's *Techneiatrike*. They were in time coalesced and translated into Latin as the *Isagoge Johannitii in Tegni Galeni*, and popularly as the *Ars Medica* – the "Art of Medicine" – and then as the *Ars Parva*, or the "Little Art." To the work were added short complementary treatises on the pulse and urine – in all a mini-handbook of medicine. Johannitius had been the original catalyst for what was, for a period of two hundred years, a practical *vademecum*. With the importance of Salerno and other universities in Italy, the *Ars Parva* became popular as the *Articella*, and the work decisively enshrined Hippocrates and Galen that ensured their place in the medical curriculum of the West.

Serapion is remembered for two works, *Aphorismi Magni Momenti de Medicina Practica* and *al-Kunnash*, both compilations of the writings of Greek and Arabic physicians. He appears to be the sole Arabic translator of Alexander of Tralles.

Essential to the academic ascendancy of Arabic science and medicine was the dissemination of information. Producing books was a slow and tedious exercise, as parchment was labor intensive to make and costly. The Chinese had been making paper since the 2nd century BCE, but the secret of the process remained in China. At the battle of Talas (c.751) the Abbasid Caliphate fought the Tang dynasty in Kyrgyzstan for control of Syr Darya. Chinese paper makers were captured and taken to Baghdad, where they demonstrated the process to receptive audiences. Harun al-Rashid (763-809) founded Baghdad's first paper shop. By the end of the 12th century, over four hundred paper-making shops existed in the Middle East. Paper, a superior technology than the tediously prepared and expensive parchment that continued to be used in Europe, greatly facilitated the publication of books.

The second period of Arabic medicine (900 to 1100) produced great Persian physicians renowned in the West. The works of Rhazes, Haly Abas, Avicenna, Isaac Judaeus, Jazzar Abulcasis and others spread across the Arabic Empire, Alexandria and the cities of the Barbary States, Sicily and Provence, where Moorish influences were prominent, and Spain (Cordova, Seville, Toledo, Granada, and Saragossa). They were translated into Latin, as were their Arabic texts, and all were disseminated to all of Europe's universities in what was a continuation of the Translation Movement. The movement, as noted, had spanned hundreds of years, with the conversions from Greek into Syriac, then into Arabic and finally, into Latin.

At this point, Cordova had 70 libraries and a university with 225,000 volumes, while in contrast the University of Paris had 400 tomes. The city attracted scholars from all of Europe, among them Gerbert of Aurillac (946-1003) who replaced the cumbersome and limiting Roman numerals with the Arabic system. (Leonardo Fibonacci, (c. 1170-1240), more successfully promulgated the Hindu/Arabic numerical system in 1202 through his book *Liber Abaci*). However, eventually Toledo, having fallen into Christian hands in 1085, became the center for scholarly translations because of its rich stores of Arabic manuscripts.

The first of the Islamic writers to have had works translated into Latin from the Arabic was Rhazes (865-925) – Abu Bakr Muhammad ibn Zakariya al-Razi. Several hundred years after his death, his *Book on Medicine Dedicated to Mansur* (c. 903) was translated into Latin by Gerard of Cremona as *Liber ad Almansoris* in 1187, and, his major work, the *Kitab al-Hawi fi al-tibb,* or the *Comprehensive Book on Medicine*, was published in Latin under the title *Liber Continens* in 1279. It contained aphorisms of ageless wisdom such as:

> At the beginning of a disease choose such remedies as will not lessen the patient's strength.

> When you can heal by diet, prescribe no other remedy, and, where simple remedies suffice, do not take complicated ones.

> Physicians ought to console their patients even if the signs of impending death seem to be present. For the bodies of men are dependent on their spirits.

Rhazes' major contributions were small treatises: diseases of children, smallpox and measles. He noted the frequency of smallpox in children and its differentiation from measles, the various presentations of both diseases and the complications in children. The material was appended to his *Almansoris,* which totaled twenty-three chapters detailing major known illnesses of children, and translated into Latin under the title *De Aegritudinibus Puerorum et Earum Cura.* It was published in Europe multiple times from the 10th to the 16th century. The chapters discussed epilepsy, eye diseases, dental problems, vomiting, dysentery, otitis, cough, constipation, itching, worms, fissures, bladder stones, strabismus and other ailments.

A curious condition called *mater puerorum*, marked by crying, nocturnal restlessness, insomnia and fever, was discussed and apparently was – uselessly – treated with Theriac magna. The nature of this ailment remains a mystery to medical scholars, but is mentioned here since Theriac magna had general credence as a "wonder drug." Originally, the compound was formulated by the Greeks to treat the bites of wild animals (*Theria*). Gradually the legendary poison antidote, Mithridatum (probably grounded goat bezoar) used for over a millennium, was added to the compound, rendering it an "all-purpose" drug. Over time, sixty-four ingredients enhanced the mix, including the flesh of viper and opium. It was used for all manner of illnesses, in all manner of patients including children. It remained in use until 1884. There is general agreement that it was ineffective, as were various elixirs peddled throughout history both by earnest physicians and clever quacks.

Isaac Judaeus (?880-?932) of Tunisia was a renowned Jewish scholar and philosopher who was physician to the Fatimid caliph Ubaid Allah al-Mahdi (909 to 934). He wrote many medical works in Arabic that were translated into Latin in 1087 by Constantine the African (c. 1020-1087). *De febribus, De urina, De Dieta* and a guide of comportment for physicians were his major works. The Arabic version of the guide has been lost, but it has survived in Hebrew, entitled *Manhag*.

Ibn al-Haytham – Latinized Alhazen (c 965-1039) – from Iraq, described the physics of vision and demonstrated that vision resulted from light entering the eye, rather than the eye sending out detection rays.

Constantinus Africanus also translated The *Almaleki* of Haly Abbas al-Majusi (930-994) into Latin as *Liber Regius* in 1080. It contained twenty chapters, many of which were devoted to surgical treatment and other procedures such as trocar insertion for ascites, cauterization methods, and ligature of arteries.

The most famous of all the medieval Arab physicians was Abu Ali al Husayn ibn Abd Allah ibn Sina, known in the western world by his Latinized name Avicenna (980-1037). He was a prodigy who could recite the entire Koran by ten years of age. He mastered dialectics and the *trivium* (grammar, rhetoric, logic) and the *quadrivium* (arithmetic, geometry, astronomy and music). Avicenna was a skilled surgeon and physician of great fame who, during internecine wars, studied injuries and devised innovative therapies for bone trauma. He was particularly skilled in performing tracheotomy, and described the procedure with great detail. He was a keen observer who for example noted that before the advent of a plague, rats and mice come out of their burrows and stagger about until they die. Unfortunately the prescient and practical epidemiological significance of this observation eluded him and others for centuries.

Avicenna's best known works are *Canticum de Medicina*, numbered aphorisms in the tradition of Hippocrates, and an encyclopedic work, *Canonis Medicinae*. His Canon is an integration of the concepts of Hippocrates, Galen and Aristotle that was translated by Gerald of Cremona (1114-1187) into Latin one hundred and fifty years after his death and divided into five books organized as follows: book one covers theoretical medicine; book two discusses treatments; book three describes diseases *a capite ad calcem* – from head to foot; book four analyzes systemic diseases and book five reviews drugs and their use. Avicenna's method, *a capite ad calcem,* became the core clinical methodology of the School of Salerno, and his entire canon was a major source for medical students for centuries (see ahead). His widespread influence continues in Unani medicine, which as practiced today traces its roots to the healing system elucidated by Avicenna in the *Canonis*. Written in Persia, the Unani method contains elements of Islamic medicine as well as Indian from the *Sushruta* and *Charaka*. Modern India has some one hundred Unani schools where the six year course in the Unani method of medicine is taught.

In Spanish Cordova, Khalaf ibn al-Abbas al-Zahrawi – Abulcasis (fl. 936-1013) – was as famous for surgery as Avicenna was for general medicine. His three volume *Kitab al-Tasrif* remained a leading text in surgery until the 17th century. Mostly based on the works of Paul of Aegina, it was rich in personal observations and experience. Volume one focused on cautery and instruments. Volume two described lithotomy, amputation and wounds. Volume three discussed fractures and dislocations. Abulcasis preoperatively inked incision marks on his patients. He used catgut as absorbable sutures, silk sutures for plastic incisions and described the plaster and egg white poultice for fractures applied before splints. The *Kitab al-Tasrif*, translated into Latin as *Concessio ei data qui componere haud valet*, was studied thoroughly by medieval surgeons, and Guy de Chauliac quoted him over two hundred times in his *Chirurgia Magna*. Even in the 16th century, Fabricius de Acquapendente would admit to his influence. Fabricius acknowledged that he owed the most to three great medical figures, Celsus of the 1st century, Paul of Aegina from the 7th century and Abulcasis of the 10th century. Fabricius, notably, was the teacher of William Harvey (see ahead).

The third great period of Arabic medicine (1100-1300) coincides with both internecine Arab strife in Spanish al-Andalus, and the growing political power of Christianity there. In the midst of considerable civil unrest, three great physicians emerged – Avenzoar, Averroës and Maimonides.

Avenzoar (1113-1162) and his pupil Averroës (1126-1198), both from Cordova, began to challenge Galen and Plato. They advanced Aristotelian naturalism and belief in the healing powers of nature, which in turn convinced ibn Zuhr – Avenzoar – that surgery was inferior to the practice of the medical arts and that surgeons were unworthy of the status of physicians. As far back as the Greeks a bias against surgery had been articulated: in his physician's oath, the immortal Hippocrates admonished physicians to leave the lancet to those who lance. When medieval Church councils, theologians, scholars and canon lawyers issued edicts of interdiction, the most authoritative was that of the Fourth Lateran Council of 1215 that in constitution number 18 prohibited deacons, priests and clerics from performing surgeries. It was a setback to progress in surgical medicine. For centuries, surgery divorced and isolated from the medical mainstream, became the provenance of barbers, quacks, mountebanks and gelders.

Ibn Rushd – Averroës – wrote commentaries on Aristotle and Plato and therefore was instrumental in the West's rediscovery of Greek thought. He wrote thirty-three works, of which only three concerned medicine. His *Kulliyat*, or Colliget, later translated as the *Compendium of Medical Knowledge* conjoined Greek and Islamic traditions of medicine, and seven sections on anatomy, physiology, pathology, diagnostics, materia medica, hygiene and therapy. His other two books on medicine were *Cantica of Avicenna* and a treatise on Theriac magna. The *Compendium* remained popular for centuries and was on medical reading lists as late as 1900.

Polymath Abu Imram Musa ibn Maimun (1135-1204) – Maimonides – was born and educated in Cordova and studied law, philosophy, theology and medicine. When he was twenty years of age he traveled east and settled in Cairo where he became a student of Averroës and eventually court physician to Saladin (1138-1193), Sultan of Egypt and Syria. (In Saladin's court, Richard the Lion Hearted (1157-1199) learned of Maimonides and his skills and spread his fame to England, where he was known as "Moses Aegyptaeus"). Maimonides wrote ten medical treatises in which he described, among many things, asthma, diabetes, pneumonia and hepatitis. His most famous medical work was *Tractus de Regimine Sanitatis* (on personal hygiene) written for the son of Saladin. It was the model on the subject until the 17th century. In it he advocated a warm bath at least weekly, instructed on nutrition, proper evacuation habits, and eschewed venesection unless the illness was serious. As a celebrated philosopher and Talmudist, he was quoted often by Albertus Magnus, Thomas Aquinas, Alexander of Hales and Duns Scotus, and referred to as Rabbi Moses ben Maimon. His medical writings are extensive and reveal original thought that challenged some of Galen's conclusions.

Jewish physicians did not consistently command respect. The Castilian code, *Las Siete Partidas* admonished "we forbid any Christian from receiving medicine or cathartics made by a Jew..." In 1397, in Aragona, Queen Maria decreed "we ordain and establish that no Jew in any case of a Christian's infirmity should dare to exercise his office of medicine unless a Christian doctor will take part in the cure." Various councils, Treves (1227), Beziers (1246), Albi (1254) and Vienna (1267) all proscribed Christians from seeking medical care from a Jew. The Provence edict of 1306 stated "we order that no one...should turn to a Jewish doctor...[nor] will any license to practice among the faithful be awarded to any Jew..." But, the "scarcity of Christian doctors" forced King Charles to annul the edict. Additionally, the Popes and Kings themselves favored Jewish doctors, keeping them on retainers and Arnold of Villanova (1235-1315) observed "we see that the custom is for no other physician to enter cloisters unless he is Jewish."

The Corpus of Simples was written by ibn al-Baitar (1197-1248) of Malaga. It is a complete *materia medica* that contained the *materia* of Dioscorides and Galen and botanicals introduced by Arabs that included amber, musk, cloves, peppers, ginger, betel nut, sandalwood, rhubarb, nutmeg, tamarind, camphor, senna and cassia that were all used for medicinal purposes. Many of these botanicals found use as culinary ingredients, and are still used pharmaceutically and in the perfume industry (see Appendix H).

Until the 8th century only the aforementioned proto types, the shelter *xenodochion,* the hospital *nosokomium* and *brephotrophium*, rendered institutional medical care. Hospitals as we know them were established in Damascus in 707 and in Baghdad in 918. They were called *bimaristan.*

The medieval Islamic hospital emerged both from religion and compassion. The teaching of the Prophet called for helping the sick and caring for them was perceived as religious duty in the *Ayat Ash-Shifa*: "Mankind, there has come to you a guidance from the Lord and a healing in your hearts, and for those who believe a guidance and a mercy. Yunus 10:57" The charity took the form of a *waqf*, an endowment set aside by a wealthy believer for humanitarian projects, fulfilling the Islamic commandment for charity. During the Abbasid Caliphate, the government used these *waqf*, plus government revenues to build and sustain hospitals. Under Caliph al-Muqtadir (895-932) physicians were tested and licensed and medical records were kept within the institution.

The hospital attached to the Pantocrator Monastery (today known as Zeyrek Camii) in Constantinople is a good example of a medieval facility. Built by John Komnenos II (1087-1143) in 1136, the hospital maintained an outpatient clinic, medical school and library. The Pantocrator's administration provided proper heating, lighting, bed linens, bathing facilities and latrines. The Pantocrator's patients were fed a carefully planned vegetarian diet, and received pocket money for purchasing additional food or drink. Medical care was supplied by a large and specialized staff of physicians, medical assistants and orderlies. It had fifty hospital beds and an attached *lazaretto*. There was a home for the aged that provided for twenty-four people at a time, and a general pharmacy.

Historians speculate that the crusaders who conquered and occupied Constantinople in 1204, impressed by the region's hospitals, took the Arab concept of hospitals to the West, and, by 1250, England, France and Italy had hospital institutions similar to those in the East. The largest hospital in the middle ages, however, was built in Cairo in 1276. There was no charge for treatment. As per the charitable tenets of Islam, the State assumed the cost. There were separate wards for potentially mortal diseases, women's wards, surgical and convalescent wards. Music was played for insomniacs. There were storytellers, a library for patients, and upon discharge, transition funds were given to the indigent. There were asylums for the insane (*mauristans*) and for orphans (*brephotrophia*). These medieval models differed from the Patristic period's *xenodochion* and *nosokomium* in that they were larger, specialized, and contained cells that separated patients. Both the sick and the wounded were cared for. Early examples of Western hospitals are London's St. Bartholomew, founded in 1123, the renowned 13th century St. Thomas hospital, founded in 1215. In 1423 Venice transformed the island of Santa Maria di Nazaret into an isolation hospital. Florence boasted thirty-three hospitals by the end of the 15th century.

In the West, in 1236, Cordova fell to Ferdinand II (1452-1516) and, in the East, in 1258, the Mongols destroyed Baghdad. The medieval

Arabic civilization collapsed but not before, it unified the *materia medica* of East and West and restored medicine to the laity.

Western Medieval Medicine
Western medieval medicine can be studied through four phases: the golden era of monasticism, which extended from the 5th through the 10th centuries, the Salernian period of the 10th through 13th centuries, the al Andalus during the 13th century and the pre-Renaissance phase of the 14th century.

Following the collapse of the Roman Empire and the ascendancy of Byzantium in the East, Germanic conquerors in the West fell under the sway of Christianity. Among other things, Latin became the official language of learning, and monasticism became the dominant pedagogical element in Western society, with powerful influences, therefore, that were ecclesiastic. In fact, most medicine was practiced and studied in monasteries and for several major reasons. During periods of famine, war and pestilence, only the Church, powerful and organized, had the means to offer scholars asylum and stability. All of the "literature of medicine" made its way to the scriptorium, where monastery scribes conserved and copied existing works, and produced new "textbooks" from scholarly data entrusted to their calligraphic skills. About one hundred and fifty manuscripts survive from the period 800 to 1000, a time when probably some one thousand medical texts existed in all centers. Like the Egyptian *swnw* or the Greek *iatros* who trained in the temples, the medieval physic trained in the "temple" of the Church. Importantly too, hospitals were built in monasteries, and flourished with the strong support of chivalric orders: Knights Templar, Knights of St John, Knights of Malta, Knights of the Holy Sepulcher etc., who, when the occasion arose, also defended these institutions against all adversaries.

In sum, physicians practiced in monastery hospitals, their works and that of their antecedents were inscribed by monks in the scriptoriums, and, in monastic cloisters, extensive gardens of medical botanicals kept a ready supply of medicinals available, and were classified and recorded for the edification of those involved in medical care.

The monastic rules of Benedict of Nursia (480-547) mandated the care of the sick be a *prime* duty of the monks, an obligation rigorously enforced. Under Cassiodorus (485-575), the Benedictine Abbey of Montecassino became the most famous medical center of the medieval period. In many regards, the medieval cleric/physician brings to mind the ancient model of high priest and healer, a conjoined profession that would endure, particularly among Protestants, into the 18th century. This era of a monastic and medical partnership, however, did not endure. It began to dissolve after the millennium when the Church decided that care of the sick distracted monks from monastic contemplation, which was considered the foundation of their vocations. New monastic branches and orders, such as the Cistercians, Dominicans and Franciscans, agreed with this assessment, and forbade their monks from activities related to science and medicine. When Church Councils in Clemont in 1130, Rheims in 1131 and Lateran in 1139 issued proscriptive edicts regarding medical care in monasteries, the responsibility for the administration of hospital facilities and care fell to municipal authorities. Pope Honorius III (1148-1227) enforced this interdict in 1216, but the ecclesiastic orders managed to govern and administer many hospitals for some time after. The long tradition of administering to the sick, a mandate imbedded in scripture (Matthew 25:36) – "I was naked and you clothed me; I was sick and you took care of me" – resisted church suppression vigorously. But as cathedral schools and universities began to expand their curriculums and grow in numbers, the study of medicine inevitably became concentrated in those institutions and away from the monastery.

An important phase of medieval medicine began with the founding of the School at Salerno in the 10th century. It was the first European School of Medicine, and for nearly three hundred years the most important medical center in the West. Its founding owes a debt to Constantine of Africa, Adelard of Bath and Gerald of Cremona, all of whom took the entire Muslim cornucopia of medical literature to Salerno. Constantine of Africa (c.1020-1087), a Benedictine from Carthage, had translated into Latin the works of Haly Abbas, Isaac Judaeus, and the Arabic translations of Galen and Hippocrates. English scholar, Adelard of Bath (c.1080-1152), is known both for his original works, and for his Arabic to Latin translations of scientific works in astrology, astronomy, philosophy and mathematics. Gerald of Cremona (1114-1187) took his translation of Rhazes and his translation of the entire *Canon* of Avicenna to Salerno.

Studies at Salerno in human anatomy were based on Galen's swine and ape dissections, and examinations for diagnosis emphasized interpreting the qualities of the pulse and urinoscopy. Lessons in general treatment, however, were dietetic and rational. The culture of the school blended the Greek, Latin, Jewish and Arabic influences instrumental in the establishment of the university. For centuries the curriculum at Salerno required a three year study of the *trivium* and *quadrivium* followed by five years of medicine and a one year internship. A final examination was mandatory. The school's fame was such that German Holy Roman Emperor Frederick II (1194-1250) ruled that no physician could be licensed except by Salerno. Frederick's law also regulated medical fees, required free treatment for the poor and mandated that apothecaries control the purity and price of drugs. With respect to drugs, Salerno introduced therapeutic innovations, among them the use of sea sponge for goiter and mineral iron for hypersplenism.

Presbyter Gariopontus (d. ca. 1050) of early Salerno wrote *Passionarius* – a compendium of practical treatments which illustrated the manner of cauterization. Arranging matters *a capite ad calcem*, Gariopontus' redaction was original in that he borrowed from well-known manuscript chapters then arranged them in useful and facile therapeutics and coherent anatomical groupings.

The most famous manuscript written at Salerno was the anonymous *Regimen Sanitatis Salernitanum* (c.1260) that consisted of dietetic and hygienic precepts. It was written for Robert Curthose (1053-1134), son of William the Conqueror (1027-1087), in Latin leonine hexameter, and was committed to memory by thousands of physicians until the 15th century.

A notable member of the Salerno School from the 12th century is Nicolaus Salernitanus (sometimes called Nicolaus Praepositus) (fl. 1140) who wrote the *Antidotarium,* a major formulary of prescriptions. Probably based on the anonymous *Antidotarius magnus* (composed between 1087 and 1100), it contained one hundred and thirty-nine complex recipes in alphabetical order, including the original recipe for the *spongia somnifera* and a table of weights and measures.

The principle contribution to advances in medicine from the School of Salerno was the work of two surgeons, Roger of Palermo (fl. 12th cent.), who wrote *Practica* in 1170, and his student Roland of Parma, who re-edited the work about 1230. *Practica* included data on the treatment of cancer, goiter, scrofula, styptics, sutures and ligature. The work was arranged, as with Avicenna, *a capite ad calcem* and contained some remarkable and original concepts. For example, for the patient with exposed viscera he recommended opening the abdomen of an animal and placing it over the exposed viscera of the patient to keep it moist and clean until repair could be attempted. For suspected bladder stone he advocated bimanual exam to distinguish between stone and a "soft and fleshy" mass, such as benign prostatic hyperplasia that obstructed urine flow.

Salerno's Trota or Trotula (?-1097), a member of the noble di Ruggiero family and one of two famous women of medieval medicine, wrote exclusively about women's ailments. Her major work is *De curis mulierum.* The work known as *The Trotula* is a compendium of three separate works most likely authored by three physicians: *Liber de sinthomatibus mulierum, De curis mulierum* and *De ornatu mulierum. Liber de sinthomatibus mulierum* is based on the *Viaticum* of Ibn al-Jazzar.

Trota combined her knowledge of folk-medicine practice, traditional midwifery and her own medical acumen and practice in her writing (which was widely plagiarized by others). For example, on pregnancy:

When a woman is first pregnant care must be taken that nothing be named in her presence which cannot be had because if she shall ask for it and it not be given to her she has occasion for miscarrying. If she craves strange foods, like potter's earth, coal or chalk, let her be given beans cooked with sugar. As the time of birth nears, let her bathe often and her abdomen be massaged with oil of violets. Give her light, easily digestible food, like oranges and pomgranates. If her ankles swell, massage them with oil of roses and vinegar. If she suffers from wind, give her mint, mastic, cardamom and carrot.

De curis mulierum

With respect to contraception Trota had a wide array of botanicals as her disposal. Many of them had been recorded by both Soranus and Dioscorides. *Artemisia* species (wormwood) was considered both a contraceptive and abortifacient – depending on the dosage. Because of its potential toxicity Soranus recommended that it be taken with myrrh and ruta. Peter Hispanus in his *Treasury of the Poor* also described the use of *Artemisia* as a contraceptive. Myrrh, the resin of *Commiphora africans*, was frequently prescribed with an infusion (tea) of pennyroyal or *Mentha pulegium*. Pulegone, the active contraceptive constituent of pennyroyal is also a strong abortifacient and modern study now reveals it is very hepatotoxic. The seeds of the wild carrot *Daucus carota* or Queen Anne's lace were known to Dioscorides as an abortifacient, as was rue or *Ruta graveolens*. Both, when used as a weak tea, were effective as a contraceptive. *Ecballium elaterium* or the squirting cucumber was considered the abortifacient of choice by the Greeks and this botanical along with all that been mentioned would have been well known to midwives and Trota. How often they were prescribed or used is unknown because their use was proscribed by the Church. In the confessional, the priest would ask: "Have you drunk any *maleficium* ...so that you could have no children?"

Of the infant she says:

> Let there be in front of him varied pictures, cloths of various colors, and pearls. In his presence one should employ songs and gentle voices and no one should sing with a harsh voice. Nor should there be noisy persons about....Frequent and gentle words spoken...
> *De curis mulierum*

Although not trained at the University of Salerno, it is worth mentioning here that the second woman of medieval medical fame was Abbess of Rupertsberg, Hildegarde von Bingen (c. 1099-1179), who was oblated to a Benedictine abbey at eight years of age. Hildegarde became a very influential figure, was the intimate friend of Bernard of Clairvaux (1090-1153), and corresponded with four Popes as well as with Emperors Conrad (c. 990-1039) and Frederick I Barbarossa (1122-1190). She wrote a series of books, most of them on mysticism and meditation, but two books were on medicine intended for the nuns who ran the Benedictine infirmaries: *Liber Simplicis Medicinae*, later called the poem *Physica* (a botanical), which was to have a great influence on the German botanists of the 16th century, and *Causae et Curae*, a catalogue of over fifty diseases.

Urso of Salerno (fl. 1160-1200) was the last of the great Salernian physicians who wrote a famous book of aphorisms in which he expressed his belief that incantations recited with medication would enhance the effect of treatment.

Salerno laid the educational foundation for secular Renaissance physicians. The University flourished until the 1300s, after which its prominence diminished. Napoleon's suppression of the institution in 1811 was its death knell. It may be that, with the establishment in Europe from 1200 to 1400 of multiple universities with medical curriculum, Salerno's importance waned. The University of Montpellier, for example, was founded shortly after Salerno along Salernian lines and became itself a model for a *Universitas*. There were twenty universities built in Italy, nineteen in France, fourteen in Germany, five in Britain, four in Spain and two in Portugal during this period.

The medical program of each followed the Salernian model that consisted of the *trivium*, *quadrivium*, philosophy, law, and theology. For *physica* – medicine – they studied Avicenna's *Canonis*, Hippocrates-Galen's *Ars Parva*, Hippocrates' *Aphorisms, Dietetics and Prognostics*, Rhazes' *Liber Medicinalis* and the works of Soranus, Paulus Aegineta, Aetius, Alexander of Tralles and Dioscorides. Additionally, the medieval physician learned bedside manner and comportment, as exemplified by Archimathasus of Salerno (Appendix-B).

The growth and influence of great medical universities in Paris (1110), Bologna (1113), Oxford (1167), Montpellier (1181), Padua (1222) and Naples (1224) contributed to an intellectual milieu receptive to new and original ideas. The Rational Surgery Movement was the first attempt to reinstate surgery as a legitimate and respected aspect of medical education in universities. Between 1240 to1320 four surgeons, Guglielmo da Saliceto, Lanfranchi of Milan, Teodorico Borgognoni and Henri de Mondeville, were major proponents of the movement. They emphasized in their writings the science of anatomy. Their approach was attractively conservative; for example they recommended noninvasive treatment of chronic conditions such as inguinal hernia or nasal polyps before any operative procedures be attempted.

The School of Bologna produced Guglielmo Salicetti – Saliceto (c. 1210-1277) – and his pupil Lanfranchi of Milan (d. c. 1306) who, as mentioned, were among those who attempted to enhance the status of surgery. They wryly posited persuasive syllogistic logic to advance their academic cause such as:

> *Omnis practicus est theoricus;*
> *Omnis cyrurgicus est practicus;*
> *Ergo, omnis cyrurgicus est theoricus.*

Initially Lanfranchi's *Cyrugia Parva* made an attempt to align surgery with medicine. He was the foremost cranial surgeon in Bologna and presented guidelines for trephination and irrigation of the dura insisting that the procedure be used only when absolutely essential. Despite efforts such as Lanfranchi's to reinstate surgery as part of the study and practice of medicine, the process took eighty additional years.

In Bologna, Theodorico Borgognoni (1205-1298) propagated the work of his father, Hugh of Lucca (c.1190). Borgognoni challenged the practice of healing by coction: "For it is not necessary…that pus be generated in wounds. Such a practice prolongs the disease and prevents conglutination of the wound" (*Cyrugia* II, 27). This thinking contradicted the teachings of Hippocrates, who in *Places in Man* held that suppuration was essential to healing, but the weight of Hippocrates' reputation sustained his theory to the detriment of patient care.

It is evident that Borgognoni and his father before him were original in their thinking. Both Borgognoni and Lucca treated lesions with mercurial salve – *unguentum saracenicum* – sparing patients painful cautery. In surgery they used botanical anesthesia in the form of *spongia somnifera* (the soporific sponge). These little pieces of sponge were steeped in a mixture of opium, hyoscyamus, mulberry juice, lettuce, hemlock and mandragora and then dried to preserve their potency. Held in reserve for future use, the dried sponges were portable; physicians carried them in pouches to the bedside of a surgical patient where, moistened with a liquid, the sponge was placed in the nostril to sedate the patient. Following the procedure, the sponge was removed and the patient awakened by dripping fennel juice into the same nostril. Although the medieval recipe for the sponge was published by Nicolaus Salernitanus, this sleeping potion had ancient origins: Dioscorides in second century Rome used a similar compound.* Today scholars question its efficacy for prolonged or highly invasive surgery.

Opium of itself has a rich history. The Sumerians cultivated the poppy as "the plant of happiness." The Egyptians used it for infant colic and the Greeks used it for analgesia. Dioscorides, Galen and Celsus all used it preoperatively. Avicenna additionally used it for diarrhea. Paracelsus called it "the stone of immortality." In 1805, the active ingredient of opium was isolated by Friedrich Sertürner (1783-1841) and named after the Greek god of dreams, *Morpheus* – morphine.

From Padua, Leonardo Bertapalia (?1380-1460) practiced in Venice and studied head injuries. Little is known about him other than he taught anatomy and had a strong interest in head injuries. His observations regarding the art of surgery merit attention since more than any other surgeon of the period he humanized the discipline and placed emphasis on the importance of anatomical knowledge:

> The perfect surgeon must always bear in mind these eight notations...[First] to become a good surgeon should be to use his eyes....[Second] accompany and observe the qualified physician, seeing him work before you yourself practice....[Third] command the most gentle touch in operating....[Fourth] assure your instruments be sharp....[Fifth] be courageous in operating and cutting but timid to cut in the vicinity of nerves, sinews and arteries, and, so as not to commit error, study anatomy, which is the mother of this art. [Sixth] be kind and sympathetic.... [Seventh] never refuse anything brought you as a fee, for the sick will respect you more.... [Eighth] never argue about a fee...for avarice is the most ignoble vice....
>
> *On Nerve Injuries and Skull Fractures* (1519)

---

*A famous reference to it as part of the plot can be found in Shakespeare's (1564-1616) *Romeo and Juliet* (Act IV: i).

The famed university of Montpellier flourished in the 13th and 14th centuries and produced celebrated scholars Gilbertus Anglicus, Arnald of Villanova, Bernard of Gordon, Henri de Mondeville, John of Gaddesden, John of Arderne and Guy de Chauliac.

Henri de Mondeville (1260-1320) was a pupil of Saliceto and friend to Lanfranchi. Like Lanfranchi, he rejected the notion of "laudable pus" as necessary to healing and emphasized the importance of washing and drying wounds. There are several axioms associated with his name. Some are based on clinical observations such as "Wounds dry much better before suppuration than after it." Other dictums reveal a man endowed with an acerbic, droll wit:

> Many more surgeons know how to cause
> suppuration than to heal a wound.
>
> God did not exhaust all His creative power
> in making Galen.
>
> Never dine with a patient who is in your
> debt. *Dum dolet accipe* – (while he is in
> pain, take your fee).

In 1230, Gilbertus Anglicus (c. 1180-1250) wrote a Latin compendium, *Laurea*, that conjoined original medical work from Salerno and Arabic medicine. It consisted of seven volumes that quoted extensively from the works of Roger of Palma, Galen, Hippocrates, Theophilus Philaretes, Averroës and Avicenna. Gilbert's fame was such that Chaucer included him in his bead-roll of great physicians:

> Wel knew he the olde Esculapius
> And Deyscorides and eek Rufus,
> Olde Ypocras, Haly and Galyen,
> Serapion, Razis and Avycen,
> Averrois, Damascien and Constantyn,
> Bernard and Gatesden and Gilbertyn.

Bernard of Gordon (1260-c.1320) wrote *Lilium medicinae*, a popular manual that had seven incunabula editions. It contains the earliest Western reference to spectacles made from beryllium that were called *oculus berellinus.* He believed that talismans (amulets with written parchment) when worn around the neck could prevent epileptic attacks.

The most common writing was the palindromic SATOR-AREPO which dates back to the first century.

SATOR
AREPO
TENET
OPERA
ROTAS

English Franciscan Roger Bacon (1214-1292) was a polymath – a philologist, mathematician, astronomer, chemist and physician who suggested in his *Opus Majus* of 1268 that ground lenses could correct poor eyesight. However, there is no evidence he ever pursued the experiment. Some scholars credit Dominican Alessandro di Spina (d. 1313) with inventing eyeglasses in Venice in 1282.

Catalan Arnald of Villanova (1235-1315) was a theologian, lawyer, philosopher and physician, as well as counselor to Peter III of Aragona (1239-1285). He studied in Paris, Montpellier and Salerno, and wrote over sixty treatises. Best known are the *Regimen sanitatis* and *Parabolae medicationis*. The former was a commentary on the famous Salernian publication and the latter a collection of three hundred and forty-five aphorisms published in 1300. He is credited with introducing brandy – *aurum potabile* – into the pharmacopeia.

Salernian John of Gaddesden (1280-1361) was physician to Edward II (1284-1327). He wrote the first printed medical book by an English author: *Rosa anglica practica medicine a capita ad pedes* which loosely translates to "The English Rose of the practice of medicine from head to toe." It was divided into five parts that concerned fevers, injuries, hygiene, diet and drugs. Commonly referred to as *Rosa Anglica* or *Rosa Medicinae*, it was compiled around 1314 and circulated in manuscript form before its first printing in 1492, more than a century after being written. Of scrofula he wrote: "If this does not suffice, go to the King that he may touch and bless you; because this disease is called the royal disease and the touch of the most serene King is valuable." This superstitious belief persisted for centuries. Charles II (R. 1660-1685) was said to have touched over 96,000 during his reign. Gaddesden is believed to have been the model for Chaucer's "doctor of phisik," cited above as one of Chaucer's famous physicians.

During the 14th century, dissections, generally performed on executed criminals, became a fixed part of the medical curriculum in most universities. Special amphitheaters were designed for the events which occurred only four to five times per year. One medieval surgeon who achieved prominence in this discipline was Guy de Chauliac of Bologna (1300-1360), a cleric/physician who was skilled in the resection of cancers and the reduction of fractures with the use of pulleys for traction. He was physician to three popes in Avignon.

During Guy's tenure in Avignon, there were two epidemics of plague. While other physicians fled, he remained in Avignon to care for the thousands afflicted and to make observations about the disease, which he recorded in *The Great Mortality of 1348 and 1360*. Guy himself contracted the plague but recovered after a grim six weeks. His great work was *Chirurgia magna* which taught that a surgeon should be a man of letters who was intelligent, of good habits, well experienced and who knew anatomy thoroughly. Guy's was a popular book that was published in Latin, English, French, Italian, Dutch and Hebrew. In fact the *Chirurgia magna* remained the premier surgical text for over two hundred years until it was superseded by Paré (see ahead).

The Rational Surgery Movement in France was stalled by Guy de Chauliac when, in 1311, French king Philip IV (1268-1314) repealed the regulation that surgeons be trained at a university. He assigned the responsibility for surgical training to the surgical guild, and once the guilds resumed schooling surgeons, books of surgery began to appear in the vernacular. Latin, however, persisted as the language used to teach academic medicine. Sadly, economic and political power ploys by guilds, barbers, gelders and dentists widely abased the practice of surgery.

In England John of Arderne (1306-1390?), an exceptional surgeon, learned his skills during service in the One Hundred Years' War. As a medical student at Montpellier, he devised the *fistula in ano* operation described in his text, *Fistula in the Fundamenti*, an operation that is still in use today. Arderne used opium to soporify so that the patient, in his words, "schal slepe so that he schal fele no kuttyng." This use of sedation and his original procedure must have earned him a great reputation, for he is said to have received a considerable sum (one hundred gold sols) for his fistula in ano repair.

In Antwerp Jean Yperman (1295-1351), student of Lanfranchi, mastered harelip surgery nearly a thousand years after such correction was introduced in China's Tsin dynasty. In his work, *Chirurgie*, he describes how fresh edges of incision were necessary for a good plastic finish and a minimal scar. He employed special delicate sutures and innovatively fed the patient via a small silver tube. Skeptical that a royal touch effectively healed anyone of anything, he perceptively commented that curable cases would resolve themselves without the royal laying of hands.

Mondino de Luzzi (Latinized name Mundinus) (1270?-1326) was a surgeon whose most prominent opus was from his work in anatomy. He was assisted by Alessandra Giliani (c.1307-1326) who injected colored solutions into the vessels of cadavers to study the anatomy of veins and arteries so as to trace their origins and ends. In 1316 Mundinus wrote the first genuine book of dissection, *Anathomia*, which was not published until 1478 in Padua. It was more a hornbook-like manual of dissection rather than a formal text of anatomy. He adhered to Galen's anatomical principles, and thereby helped to perpetuate Galen's anatomical errors. For example, he, like Galen, claimed that yellow bile from the gall bladder and black bile from the spleen reached the stomach via canals that were in fact non-existent and, like Galen, stated that the heart had three chambers. For three centuries his popular work was required reading that hindered advances in anatomy study.

One hundred and fifty years before Giovanni Morgagni (see ahead) enhanced the understanding and study of pathology, Florentine Antonio Benivieni (1443-1502) routinely performed autopsies to uncover the "hidden causes of disease." He kept meticulous records of his dissections, and his findings were published posthumously as *De Adbitis Morborum Causis* in 1507. It was only fifty-four pages in length but, in contrast to the work of Morgagni, it recorded autopsies conducted solely by him.

The most learned man of the Middle Ages was considered to be the Dominican priest from the school of Paris, Albert von Bollstaedt – Albertus Magnus (1193-1280). Most of his writings were philosophical, but he also wrote a great deal about natural science. As a Dominican priest, medical study was anathema. Yet he was a famed teacher who influenced his students to pursue original studies in the spirit of Aristotle, and he counted the philosophers Thomas Aquinas (c.1225-1274) and Roger Bacon (1214-1292) among his students.

The final phase of medieval dialectical medicine was a movement that attempted to meld the Arabic tradition as disseminated in Europe with Aristotelian naturalism. Prominent in the movement was Florentine Taddeo Alderotti (1223-1303), founder of medical dialectics in Bologna, and an early proponent of the *Consilia* or medical case book. Dialectics sought to pursue truth through debate and Aristotelian naturalism, and espoused truth as observed in nature. It eschewed mystic revelation. Alderotti's colleague in dialectics was Peter of Abano (1250-1315) from Padua, whose *Conciliator differentiarum* consisted of two hundred and ten moot points, two examples of which are: "Do nerves originate in the brain or not?" "Is medicine a science or not?" (*"Utrum nervi oriantur a cerebro necne?" "Utrum medicina sit scientia necne?"*) It was a very influential work that advanced the prominence of Padua and became the model for dissertations well into the 17th century. The nature of pain was disputed. Aristotle and

Hippocrates both considered pain a defining human conceit and as a medical issue it came to be accepted as a humoral disharmony and the nature, location, duration and intensity were considered diagnostic aids. In the dialectical exercise Alderotti asked "do the mentally ill suffer pain" and "can a larger pain obscure a lesser pain?" Peter of Abano even classified pain qualities as throbbing, dull, stabbing, pressing, piercing, gnawing, freezing, itchy, etc. To the medieval physician the challenge was to balance the humors by bleeding, purgatives, clysters, astrological seals and dietary alterations in tandem with his pharmacopeia of opium, mandrake, hyoscyamine and local measures such as poultices, heat and ice.

Abano's teaching methodology was adopted by many disciplines. His calculation of a calendar year of three hundred and sixty-five days, six hours and four minutes was an extraordinary achievement.

Dialectical medicine was a short-lived movement, as practical knowledge was valued and needed in the exercise of medicine. It was more important to define medicine as a curative pursuit than medicine as a science. Even more crucial to late medieval medicine was the shift of hospitals from ecclesiastic authority to that of municipalities. Famous examples of secularly administered hospitals, some of which are still active, are the *Hôtel Dieu* of Paris (Fig. 6), founded c. 650 by Landry Bishop of Paris, the *Santo Spiritu* of Rome (founded 727, reconstructed 1204) and *Santa Maria Novella* in Florence (1286), built by Folco Portinari (parenthetically, the father of Beatrice, Bice di Folco (1266–1290), Dante Alighieri's (c.1265-1321) great legendary muse and love).

Despite several insightful challenges to Galen over the centuries, and after finding contrary evidence from human dissections, Galenic principles prevailed until the 17th century. Medieval diagnostics and treatments reflect Galen's precepts in their entirety. Moreover, urinoscopy remained a prime diagnostic modality and the *matula*, a transparent bulbous flask in which a physician swirled and observed urine, became the physician's symbol. Urinoscopy was based on humoral pathology that assumes urine is produced in the liver which in turn transforms chyle into a mixture of blood and humors. It was thought that urine, excreted by the kidneys, could by color, smell, clarity, taste and viscosity proffer information about the state of the humors which in turn enabled speculation about the condition of the individual's health and suggested a course of treatment (Fig. 7).

Throughout the middle ages and up to at least the 19th century bleeding remained a primary modality of treatment with very specific determinants. Bleeding could be performed by lancing, cupping, via leeches (hirudotherapy), blistering, or scarifying. The procedure had to be performed on favorable days, on a specific vein for a specific purpose, with the number of bleedings based on age and temperament. *Vademecums* provided these guidelines as well as those for frequency and quantity of blood to be let, but many physicians simply followed skin color and pulse as indicators. Guy Patin (1601-1672) for example seems to have used bloodletting extensively as a general cure-all. Age was no hindrance: he bled his father-in-law at the age of eighty and his young son twenty times for a fever. He boasted, "We also bleed very fortunately children of two to three months...." Equally aggressive – perhaps more so – was Benjamin Rush of Philadelphia (1745-1813) who advocated bleeding to a point of syncope.* Clysters, purgatives and bleeding were the major treatment alternatives employed by physicians. The first and second medical texts produced by Johann Gutenberg's (?1400-?1468) revolutionary printing press were related to these modalities: *Purgation Calendar* (1457) and *Bloodletting Calendar* (1462) (Fig. 8). It should be noted that not all physicians favored bleeding. John Radcliff (1652-1714) of London, for example, preferred applying blisters and Pierre Louis (see ahead) would provide statistical evidence against the practice.

When treatment modalities such as Rush used failed, physicians had long opted for a procedure known as revulsives to vent wounds, a surgery particularly popular in the 15th-16th centuries. The belief was that by keeping a wound open and allowing it to vent, the "miasma" would escape the body and the patient would be restored to health. Physicians made incisions on the opposite side of the site where the focus of the disease was thought to be. Salernians used an incision called a fontanelle or "little window" kept open by inserting a bean, pea or other foreign body until removed. The seton followed the same principle, but required two parallel incisions, usually made at the neck. A thread was inserted to prevent closure.**

The faculty at the University of Paris followed the Salernian "Revulsionism." "Derivationists" advocated bleeding or venting on the same side of the body. Amazingly, this became a contentious subject for dispute so intense that the derivationists appealed to Emperor Charles the V (1500-1558) who, with Pope Clement VII (1478-1534), ruled in their favor. There is no evidence that either of these two procedures produced positive results and general treatment for most diseases continued to be supportive with the use of diet, herbals and poultices, abstinence from wine and the ubiquitous bleeding.

*Federalist William Cobbett (1763-1835) writing in his *Porcupine Gazette* (1797) referred to Benjamin Rush as "Doctor Sangrado" – the bloody doctor.

**The seton, which remains in use by modern surgeons who have a comprehensive understanding of modern pathophysiology, is performed to prevent fistulas from closing and forming abscesses, particularly in perianal Crohn's. A thread is still employed.

Childbirth continued to be hazardous for mother and baby. In addition to the absence of knowledge of anatomy and ignorance of asepsis, there were no forceps or anesthesia, although soporifics were used during parturition. At best midwives tried to ensure a good fetal position. Mortality, as may be expected, was high and would remain so until the 19th century when the great debate regarding the cause of puerperal fever was settled by Semmelweis and Osler (see ahead).

Although concepts of contagion were for the most part ill-informed, Bernard de Gordon (1307) inspired by Rhazes, indentified eight infectious diseases: *febris acuta* (plague), *phthisis* (tuberculosis), *pedicon* (epilepsy), *scabies, anthrax, lippa* (trachoma), *lepra nobis contagia praestant* (leprosy) and *sacer ignis* – now ergotism.*

There was a resurgence of leprosy carried to Europe by afflicted crusaders, foot-soldiers and pilgrims, and incidences of the disease reached their height in the 13th century. By then Europe had 19,000 leprosaria. France itself had over two thousand leprosaria or lazarettos. (Current research indicates that c. 1300, twenty-five percent of adult Scandinavians died with skeletal evidence of leprosy). As in the ancient Levant, fear of contagion was great and lepers were pariahs who had to wear a black robe with two white bands across the chest, a hat with a white ribbon, and a clapper or bell to warn all around them of presence or their approach.

Epidemics-Pandemics
When Dante (1265-1321), Giovanni Boccaccio (1323-1375), Geoffrey Chaucer (1343-1400) and Giotto di Bondone (1269-1337) were creating their masterful works in literature and art, catastrophic epidemics of small pox, measles, influenza, diphtheria, and plague were simultaneously devastating Europe and all semblance of governance.

Small pox was a pervasive scourge that erupted into epidemic form unpredictably. It ravaged towns, killing nearly a quarter of the population from vasculitic hemorrhages or secondary bacterial pneumonias. Measles also flared sporadically, skipping generations and thereby afflicting children with no acquired antibodies from prior epidemics. Diphtheria was ever-present, perniciously asphyxiating children with malignant membranes, biofilms fueled with toxins that formed on tonsillar beds. Influenza of severity appeared in the average of thirty-five year cycles. It is now known that annual influenza epidemics are due to antigenic drift and that those occurring in prolonged intervals are due to mutations and subtypes.

---

*Ergotism, caused by the contaminant fungus on rye, *Claviceps purpurea*, often led to gangrene, that was called *sacer ignis* or sacred fire (St. Anthony's Fire) because of the burning peripheral neuropathy it occasioned.

In medieval times, influenza – as were almost all illnesses – was attributed to supernatural powers. In Italy it was called *influentia coeli* or *influentia del diavolo*. Like epidemics today, symptoms varied widely from mild catarrh to hemorrhagic disease to secondary bacterial pneumonia. It is probable that the epidemic recorded by Hippocrates in 412 BCE and the epidemics of "sweating sickness" in 15th century England were due to some form of a malignant influenza.

These diseases materialized in siderated blankets of death, and mortality was redoubled by internecine wars and periodic droughts with parched land that yielded no crops, which produced widespread malnutrition and starvation. The most malignant infectious villain of the medieval period was the plague. There were several pandemics that had catastrophic consequences, depicted for posterity and *memento mori* in Church *transi* effigies, apocalyptic paintings and the fear inspiring murals of the *Totentanz, Danza de Muerte* or *Danse Macabre*.

Of the three forms of plague – pneumonic, bubonic and septicemic – the septicemic was the most virulent and could kill in a matter of hours. The pneumonic form generally killed in three days and the bubonic form in five. The earliest recorded major epidemic of plague occurred in China in 224 BCE. In Europe the disease was recorded in three long-lasting pandemics. The first was the so called Justinian plague of 541-750 that decimated nearly a third the population. In Constantinople alone, three to five thousand per day became infected. (Researchers have identified eleven strains during the Justinian outbreak of the 6th to the 8th centuries). The second began in Asia in 1333, migrated to India in 1340, to Constantinople in 1343, Egypt 1346, and to Messina on the Island of Sicily and to all of Europe in 1347. In two years (1347-1349), the now known deadly bacteria *Yersina pestis* killed nearly sixty percent of the European population.

People called the apocalyptic devastation that incited terror, panic and general despair the Great Pestilence or the Black Death. Cities and towns barred travelers from entering their gates, but the disease ravished those populations anyway. Half of the victims who died were children. In 1348 travelers to Venice were isolated for forty days (*quaranta giorni*, from which derives the word quarantine). With no known cause or treatment doctors were completely ineffective. They bravely walked among the sick (and themselves died as a consequence) administering anti-miasmics in a costume of a long leather coat and a bird-like mask. The beak of the mask held a sponge soaked in vinegar with dissolved cloves, cinnamon and other ingredients believed to obfuscate and disable the miasma they opined was responsible for the disease (see cover). The only truly effective recourse was the recommendation: *fugo cito, vade longe, rede tarde* – flee quickly, go far, return slowly. Much of what we know about this epidemic comes from journals and woeful diaries. They say little about treatment, but a great deal about the toll of human suffering.

Although the virulence of plague ebbed in 1349, it migrated eastward to Russia in 1351. By 1353 the severity of the pandemic had run its course despite sporadic local outbreaks that erupted throughout Europe in 1357, 1359, 1362, 1363 and 1364. The outbreak of 1363 was called the "children's plague" because it struck infants and toddlers with particular virulence. Perhaps it was a second round of a strain for which older children and adults still had circulating antibodies and therefore affected the more susceptible of the population, or perhaps that particular strain of plague had a propensity to strike immature immune systems. Whatever the reason, it robbed the populace of most of its very young. Children who survived found themselves in decimated, economically devastated communities faced with hunger and starvation, all vulnerable to other diseases. Europe's population continued to decrease for the next hundred years, a bleak reminder of almost three generations of the young eliminated by disease.

For the next three centuries, the plague reoccurred at intervals throughout Europe, but with a relative diminished intensity and virulence. In 1599, Valladolid, Spain, lost twenty percent of its population. London suffered three epidemics in 1603, 1625 and, in 1664-1665, lost twenty-five percent of its inhabitants. After London's Great Fire of 1666, with extensive rebuilding and improved sanitation, the plague, along with the conflagration, died out. The last great epidemics of the 18th century were in Marseilles, France, in eastern Europe and in Russia. A third pandemic began in China in the mid 19th century that spread westward leaving ten million dead in India alone, after which it disappeared in epidemic form. Today, *Yersina pestis* infects 1000 to 3000 persons yearly.

Medieval medicine summary

With Europe in ruins, medicine made little progress. At the end of the 15th century Galen's premises remained essentially unchallenged and the belief in the humors and urinoscopy persisted. Phlebotomy and balneology were universal. The disciplined study of anatomy was in its infancy. Methodical dissection was just evolving and, since only executed criminals could be dissected, there was a dearth of bodies for anatomical study that was a perennial problem until the 19th century so called "resurrection men" and grave robbers developed a defiling and scandalous industry (see ahead). Some medieval municipalities even forbad dissection of the head.

Still reeling from the aftershock of plague, every major city nevertheless endeavored to have a university that taught medicine. Training became structured and systematic, and hospitals and foundling homes became commonplace. Medical practice for most of the impoverished population, however, was probably an adjunct to the universal reliance on theurgic forces – a link with ancient beliefs and petitions to Greek and Roman gods.

Throughout the medieval period in Europe there was active reliance on saints and relics. Petitions for protection against diseases were made to saints designated as having the power to heal specific afflictions and even organs. The examples are inexhaustible: St. Blaise (d. 316) safeguarded the throat, (and the blessing of throats by priests in Christian churches on the saint's feast, February 2nd, continues to be practiced). St. Lucy (283-304) is the patron saint of eyes (and several major artists painted depictions of her with eyes prominently featured). St Agatha (d. 251) is considered the saint who protects women from breast diseases and St. Apollonia (d. 249) is the saint who looks after the teeth. In medieval times, humble St. Fiacre (d. 670) was prayed to for hemorrhoids, St. Dymphna (c. 7th cent.) protected the mind and St. Anthony (d. 1231) prevented leprosy. Both the Breton St. Roch (c.1295-1327) and Roman St. Sebastian (d. 288) shielded supplicants against the plague. St. Dionysius (c. 3rd cent.) was invoked against syphilis and St. Hubert (c. 657-727) for dog bites and rabies. Roman physician saints Cosmas and Damian (both beheaded c. 287 CE) were called the *anargiri* because they rejected remuneration. They became the patron saints of the Medici. They are most famous for allegedly performing a miracle in which the leg of a man's cadaver was successfully grafted to the fresh stump of a church sacristan whose gangrenous leg had been amputated. The subject has been depicted in many paintings. Cosmas and Damian in our day are the saintly patrons of transplant surgeons.

IV: Renaissance Medicine

Timeline:

1503 Leonardo finishes the *Mona Lisa*
1508 Michelangelo paints the Sistine Chapel
1511 Erasmus *In Praise of Folly*
1513 Ponce de León in St. Augustine, Florida
      Machiavelli begins *The Prince*
1517 The Reformation
1520 Süleyman "the Magnificent" and the Ottoman Empire.
1521 Cortes conquers the Aztecs
1530 Pope Clement VII crowns HRE Charles V
1534 Jesuit Order is founded
1535 Thomas More executed
1543 Copernicus' heliocentric theory
      Vesalius' *De Fabrica*
1547 Henry VIII of England dies
1553 Servetus describes pulmonary circulation
1556 Tartaglia *A Treatise on Numbers and Measurement*
1558 Elizabeth I ascends the throne
1564 Death of Michelangelo
      Birth of Galileo
1569 Mercator *World Map* projection

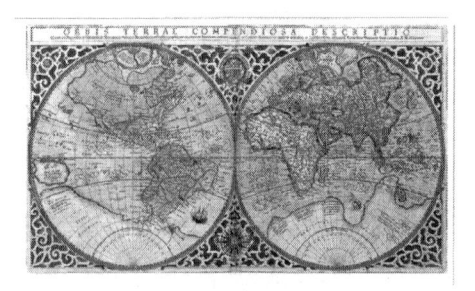

1588 Spanish armada is defeated
1597 Shakespeare *Romeo and Juliet*

[On the printing press] He who first shortened the labor of copyists by device of moveable types was disbanding hired armies, and cashiering most kings and senates, and creating a whole new democrate world: he had invented the art of printing.
        Thomas Carlyle (1795- 1881) *Sartor Resartus* I:4

This is my vow: To perfect my medical art and never to swerve from it so long as God grants me my office, and to oppose all false medicine and teachings. Then, to love the sick, each and all of them, more than if my own body were at stake. Not to judge anything superficially, but by symptoms, not to administer any medicine without understanding, nor to collect any money without earning it. Not to trust any apothecary, nor to do violence to any child. Not to guess, but to know.
        Paracelsus *Sketches Notes and Revisions* (1577)

Five things are proper to the duty of a Chirurgian; To take away that which is superfluous; to restore to their places such things as are displaced; to separate those things which are joined together; to join those that are separated; and to supply the defects of nature.
        Paré: *Works* I, 2. (1575)

To begin with, there was this strange fact; though the infection was there, the moon had often four times circled the earth before clear symptoms of the disease appeared. For when it has once been received into the body it does not immediately declare itself....
        Fracastoro: *Syphilis* I (1530)

Health is a precious thing, and the only one, in truth, which deserves that we employ in its pursuit not only time, sweat, trouble and worldly goods, but even life….
        Michel de Montaigne (1533-1592): *Essays* II, 37.

Renaissance

Irrefutably the period we call the Renaissance altered Western history and ushered in the modern era. In every instance of human endeavor there were astounding achievements in just a few hundred years: da Vinci's innumerable inventions, Gutenberg's printing press, the circumnavigation of the globe, the discovery of the Americas and passages to the East.* New concepts such as the helio-centricity of Copernicus that affirmed the earth rotated around the sun emerged. In the Renaissance works of great beauty were created in art, architecture, literature and music. Inevitably the momentous advances in these fields had favorable influences on medicine directly and indirectly.

The key factor to the rapidity with which ideas took hold was the invention of the printing press that rendered scriptorium produced calligraphic texts obsolete, facilitated wide distribution of texts and, in medicine, reproducible illustrated teaching aids, such as the bleeding points man that mapped out sites for venipuncture, the astrologic man that depicted the zodiac-anatomic conjunctions** and the wound man that illustrated the type of injuries a body could sustain (Figs. 8, 9, 10). The consistency with which the printing press reproduced texts eliminated the possibility of errors in transcription that in fact had been made over centuries by scribes. For example, in 1443 a copy of Celsus' ancient *De Medicina* was found in the church of St. Ambrose in Milan. It had been lost for centuries. The dusty treasure was immediately printed and widely circulated. Comparing the newly printed version to several other inscribed copies revealed conflicting passages and recopied errors that deformed Celsus' prime thinking.

The use of gunpowder in armed conflicts resulted in new kinds of wounds that challenged surgical skills of the times and obliged the development of innovative procedures in the treatment of injuries.

The circumnavigation of the globe had unanticipated impact on the field of medicine as ships took to Europe cargos of goods that enriched the *materia medica.* There were cloves from Moluccas, cinnamon from Ceylon, aloes and pepper from Cochin China, ginger and benzoin from Sumatra, nutmeg and mace from Banda, camphor, musk and rhubarb from China, all of which were used for old and rediscovered medicinal formulae.

---

*Gunpowder, invented in China, reached Europe (c. 13th century) with portentous ramifications and repercussions. Some scholars believe that the ideas for numerous mechanical devices attributed to da Vinci were actually taken to Venice by the expeditionary forces of Chinese Zheng He during 1421-23.

**Aries-head, Taurus-neck and shoulders, Gemini-arms and hands, Cancer-chest, Leo-heart, Virgo-stomach and bowels, Libra-kidneys, Scorpio-genitals, Sagittarius-thighs, Capricorn-knees, Aquarius-lower legs, Pisces-feet.

Heated debates about helio-centricity promoted an atmosphere of question and challenge: no longer, as the Church had insisted, was the earth the center of our galaxy, but the sun. The logical inference was that if Church authority was wrong in this respect, it could be wrong about other assertions. Renaissance philosophy and thinking, which embraced humanistic ideas handed down by the Greeks, enthusiastically stimulated originality, independence and a new intellectual energy – a monumental shift that breached man's relationship with the Church.

During the Renaissance, just as Plato and Hippocrates displaced the dialectics of Aristotle and Galen, medical humanists, many of whom were cleric/physicians, abandoned the encyclopedic compilations that had to that point been the stylistic norm for texts and began to record original and innovative ideas that contributed to a new era of critical thought. Universities flourished, and humanism advanced with the writings of poet-philosophers such as Petrarch (1304-1374), Erasmus (c. 1466-1536), Boccaccio (c.1313-1375), Marsilio Ficino (1433-1499) and Thomas More (1478-1535). Ficino was the son of Cosimos de Medici's physician and was himself a physician. Although nearly all his writings were philosophical, he did publish a practical treatise on the plague during the Florence epidemic of 1478. Other science luminaries and enthusiasts published pioneering, landmark scholarship.

One of these was Niccolo Leoniceno (1428-1524), professor at the University of Padua, who corrected the botanical errors of Pliny and Galen. He touched on holy ground. Pliny and Galen's writings in the medical world were considered sacrosanct and unimpeachable. Leoniceno was excoriated by his colleagues and the ensuing furor forced him to resign his professorship. His pronouncements at a later time were completely vindicated. Leoniceno is best remembered for *Libellus de epidemia qual vulgo morbum gallicum vocant* (1497), the earliest text to describe an epidemic of syphilis, and as a distinguished neo-Platonist who taught Paracelsus (see ahead).

François Rabelais (1483-1553) established a revised and innovative medical curriculum at Montpellier, enlivened teaching methodology and discarded faulty texts. A Benedictine, satirist and physician, he published novel translations of Hippocrates and Galen but his memorable writings, among them *Gargantia, Pantagruel* and *Laughter is the proper function of man*, were social and political satirical commentaries. In the words of historian Arturo Castiglioni (1874-1952), Rabelais "ridicules the charlatanesque forms of treatment" which certainly abounded, and mocks prevailing superstitions. He was an exemplar of Renaissance humanism who cherished "the Greek ideals of developing all aspects of man."

The consummate humanist in medicine, Jean Fernel (1497-1588), was an astronomer, mathematician and physician who systematized medical thought in his *Medicina* (1554), which was divided into three parts: physiology, pathology and therapeutics. Fernel drew attention to many Galenic errors. He opposed severe blood-letting, and correlated the respiratory and gastrointestinal manifestations of the influenza as one disease. His description of iliac passion – "passion" as a term to express exquisite pain – is the earliest recorded diagnosis of pre-mortem appendicitis. He was physician to France's Henry II (1519-1559), his wife Catherine d' Medici (1519-1589) and his mistress Diane de Poitiers (1499-1566). He apparently cured Catherine's sterility by suggesting the excision of psychosomatic "demons." Fernel attended all ten of her accouchements.

Geronimo Cardano (1501-1576) was a teacher of medicine at the University of Pavia, but is best known as a mathematician noted for his contributions to algebraic solutions in cubic and quartic equations published in his *Ars Magna* (1545). In *De utilitate ex adversis capienda* he presciently anticipated psychiatry when describing immorality as a disease of the spirit and distinguished between the truly wicked and wrongs committed through passion (*perfidi*). Cardano described typhus as *morbus pulicaris* in 1536 and, in *De subtilitate rerum* (1550), wrote about a device to teach the blind to read by touch. As an advocate for the education of the deaf and blind he belongs in the pantheon of giants of social evolution.

In England the spirit of the Renaissance was embodied by Thomas Linacre (1460-1524) who travelled to Bologna and studied alongside the sons of Lorenzo d'Medici. He was awarded a degree in medicine with distinction from Padua and returned to Oxford University to teach. In 1509 he was appointed court physician to Cardinal Wolsey (1471-1530), Henry VII (1457-1509) and Henry VIII (1491-1547). Linacre persuaded Henry VIII to enact a law that only those approved by the Bishop of London could practice medicine (Act of 1511). In 1518, at the behest of Linacre, the King granted a charter to the Company of Physicians (renamed the Royal College of Physicians in 1551) to regulate all persons "practising physic" in greater London. In his later years, Linacre designed and implemented the medical curriculums of Cambridge and Oxford. As an academic he must have been aware of the challenges to Galen being raised, but nevertheless rendered a new translation of Galen's major works into Latin. In 1520 he became an ordained Anglican priest.

German authors began publishing in the vernacular beginning in the late 15th century. Four great medical treatises on children's diseases were written, collectively referred to as the *Pediatric Incunabula*. Attesting to Europe's increasing attention to children's growth and development, they were widely consulted in their time and influenced in a major way the proliferation of pediatric manuscripts of subsequent centuries. The incunabula were written by Heinrich von Louffenburg (1391-1460), Bartolomaeus Metlinger (?-1491), Paulus Bagellardus a Flumine (?-1492) and Cornelius Roelans (1450-1525). These works primarily focused on the newborn and toddler, expounding on teething, fluxes, rashes and the fevers of childhood. However, they had chapters dedicated to the prevention of accidents, nurturing and appropriate comportment.

Jakob Rueff (1500-1558) wrote an obstetric book in rhymed couplets, *Hebammen Buch*, that was translated into Latin as *De conceptu et generatione hominis*. It was one of a series of medical "poems" that were the fashion for nearly three centuries (see appendix C). The text contained chapters devoted to conception, prenatal care, the birthing stool, management of a frank breech, embryotomy and congenital anomalies. Harshly judgmental, he was philosophic about the latter, stating "God doth permit for the punishment and admonition of men...yet afterward also the corruption and fault of the seed is to be acknowledged, to wit, which was either too much, or too little, or corrupted, from whence those monsters are engendered...."

The Renaissance in medicine reached its apex with the emergence of three great names of the 16th century: Paracelsus (1493-1541), Vesalius (1514-1564), and Paré (1510-1590). Of the three, only Paracelsus remains controversial and his dictums still fiercely debated because of his views on surgery, alchemical opinions and occasional expression of eccentric ideas.

The son of a physician, Paracelsus' birthname was Theophrastus after the botanist pupil of Aristotle.* Because Paracelsus questioned and challenged medical authority he has been referred to as the Luther of medicine, but despite some inconsistencies he remains a major force in the evolution of medicine that challenged the common and often erroneous convention and wisdom.

Following medical studies, he studied botany in Switzerland. When his family moved to the mining region in Austria, he learned metallurgy. While at the University of Ferrara he attended the lectures of Leoniceno and absorbed the neo-Platonism of Marsilio Ficino. Thereafter he began to publically challenge Galen and traditional medicine, and he burned the books of Avicenna, among others, for having integrated the precepts of Hippocrates, Galen and Aristotle. His impulsive and vitriolic personality made a post in academic medicine impossible. He renounced scholastic medicine and traveled extensively in Italy to learn folklore. In many towns he used what he knew of treatments favored by miners – Fe, S, Hg and mineral waters instead of traditional Galenic herbals.

Despite prodigious scientific curiosity and acumen, he embraced a curious notion that, by applying a specially prepared ointment or salve to a weapon, the wound would heal, the premise being there were vital spirits

---

*His full name was Aureolus Theophrastus Bombastus von Hohenheim. Endowed with a strong and clever ego, he called himself Paracelsus (equal to or greater than the Roman Celsus).

that adhered to the blood on the weapon that the salve – somehow – reunited with the spirit in the victim. Amazingly, it was a widely held conviction: Shakespeare referred to "weapon salve" in *The Tempest*.* Belief in weapon salve persisted as late as 1630 when Englishman William Foster (1591-1643) disproved the remedy and labeled it witchcraft in *Hoplocrisma-spongus*.

In *Archidoxa* (1569) Paracelsus discredited Galen's humors and uromancy and replaced alchemy with chemistry. In his major work *Opus Paramirum I-II*, he also disavowed Galenic theories, urinoscopy, humoral medicine and healing by coction. He promoted the concept of occupational diseases, advocated minimal surgical intervention and espoused natural wound healing and balneology (therapeutic thermal baths). In his mineral pharmacopoeia he tried to expunge all animal and vegetable concoctions, but he was inconsistent. He devised for example dreckapotheke (*zebethum occidentale*) from dung, and weapon salve from human skull, fat and blood, desiccated mummy, oil of rose, bole and linseed oil. His disregard for the emerging discipline of anatomy can be inferred by the following, which seems to express a notion of the psycho-somatic:

> ...the more essential Anatomy is the Anatomy of the living inner man. The latter is the kind of Anatomy which is the most important for the physician to know. If we know the Anatomy of the inner man, we know the Prima Materia, and may see the nature of the disease as well as the remedy.

He was certainly maverick enough to believe in psychosomatic illness. Despite inconsistent and at times erroneous assumptions, Paracelsus is a major force in the evolution of medicine because he astutely and judiciously challenged prevailing wisdom and modalities of treatment.

Paracelsus gradually embraced alchemy, but not as a hermetic science that sought merely to transmutate base metal to gold. He, like Roger Bacon, Newton, Boyle, Hooke, Leibnitz and others, believed alchemical studies would unravel many mysteries of nature and medicine. Alchemy obfuscation by enciphered recipes employing numerology and Decknamen contributed to the perception that it was akin to magic and witchcraft.

The singular value of Paracelsian medicine comes from his observations in *Die grosse Wundartzney* (The Great Surgery Book) (1536)

---

*Spirit Ariel says "Anoint the sword which pierc'd him [Hippolito] with this weapon salve, and wrap it close from air till I have time to visit him again." V:i in which he underscores the stunning principle that less is more, an admonition that continues to be a well advised dictum. "Surgery consists in protecting Nature from suffering and accident from without, that she may proceed unchecked in her operations." He viewed the surgeon's role as primarily to create the best conditions for the healing powers of nature, which may be nothing more than to keep the wound clean and free from infectious matter.

In this work Paracelsus was logical and insightful, but, paradoxically, he accepted the popular Doctrine of Signatures (*similia similubus curantur*) that subscribed to the notion that the use of a drug must resemble the disease. Thus walnut shells were used for injuries of the head, bear's grease for baldness, turmeric or saffron for jaundice, powdered mummy for aging, thistle for a stitch and rust or red wine for anemia. He also believed in an oppositional theory of treatment – *contraria contrariis curantur*. Fever was treated by drafts of cold beer and bleeding to remove hot blood and cool the body. Conversely, chilblains were treated with warm-blooded mice applied directly and delicately to the skin.

Paracelsus astutely observed that dust caused miner's disease. He also opined that goiter was related to some missing element in water and noted that cretins often were born to goiterous mothers. He believed that the physician should begin his diagnostic exercise from observation of the presumed causes rather than from the signs of disease or the body, thinking that was contrary to the hollowed teaching of Hippocrates' clinical bedside medicine.

Art and the Great Anatomists
Although old masters had surpassed the medieval illuminated and woodcut homunculi that passed for anatomical drawings, progress in art as well as in science was hindered by Church belief that the body was the "temple of the soul." Dissection was considered a desecration and consequently was discouraged. This prevented artists, not to mention physicians, from learning human anatomy. Artists such as Leonardo da Vinci and Michelangelo defied Church sentiment and performed surreptitious dissections for the purpose of learning with exactitude the topography and plasticity of the body. Italian anatomists, schooled in the new humanistic thinking, also violated Church dictum with secretly performed dissections that yielded vital information about the body. In 1482 papal permission by Sixtus IV (1414-1484) – a della Rovere – finally allowed dissection, but only on executed criminals and unidentifiable corpses and the Bull specifically excluded study of the head.

The importance of dissection became clear in art when the life affirming humanistic philosophy of artists like Leonardo da Vinci (1452-1519) was given expression as a result of firsthand knowledge of anatomy that enabled them to depict the human form in anatomical sketches that are without equal. Leonardo dissected thirty males and females of varying ages, injected veins with colored solutions and infused liquid wax in body cavities to better understand visceral space and anatomy. Remarkably, Leonardo was the first to depict a gravid unilocular uterus with fetal membranes (Fig. 11). He produced over 750 anatomical sketches.

Michelangelo's (1475-1564) understanding of body musculature rendered sinewy tone and *contraposto* tension in paintings, frescos and sculpture that continue to inspire wonder in all who see and study them.

By 1537 when a Church edict allowed dissection of the human body for the purpose of teaching students, Renaissance art, with its heady accomplishments in all artistic conceits – perspective, composition, chiaroscuro, contraposto, accurate depictions of the human form – had already been securely established. Less dramatic but none the less evolutionary progress began in western medicine as scientists, having kept apace with artists regarding the importance of anatomical studies, were quick to grasp the relevance of dissection as essential to progress in medical and surgical understanding and treatment. Dissection of the normal and abnormal in time became an indispensible component of medical study everywhere (see ahead).

Several Renaissance medical practitioners worked directly with artistic giants of the period. Anatomists Berengario da Carpi (1470-1530) and Marco Antonio della Torre (1478-1511) were friends and colleagues of Leonardo da Vinci, and all performed dissections together. Della Torre's trained medical eye is reflected in the details of Leonardo's exquisite drawings of the uterus, fetus and heart. Michelangelo was the pupil of anatomist Realdo Colombo (1510-1559). Colombo wrote *De re anatomica* and succeeded his colleague Vesalius at the University of Padua. John Stephen of Kalcar (1500-1546), a pupil of the artist Titian (1485-1576), etched Vesalius' anatomical plates. Dürer (1471-1528), Holbein (1497-1543) and Cranach (1472-1553) studied topographical anatomy. Albrecht Durer's work on human proportions, *De Symmetria* (1532), gave a mathematical blueprint of human body proportions. Piero della Francesca (c.1412-1492) in his *De Perspectiva Pingendi* (c.1470) illustrated orthogonal head projections – images that would find expression in the CAT and MRI of the 20th century. Peter Paul Rubens' (1577-1640) *Théorie de la figure humaine* (1773) contained beautiful anatomical plates. There was a strong societal revulsion about depicting human dissections and also some ambivalence, as the public's aversion was mixed with great deal of curiosity.

Artists attempted to reconcile the conflicting mind-set by "humanizing" anatomical studies. They portrayed skeletal structures and musculature in whimsical postures and in varied ludic and animated poses that registered live emotions (Fig. 12). They painted colorful landscape backgrounds to diminish the impact of the *écorché* (flayed bodies), exploited religious themes such as *memento mori* ("you know not the moment of death") that reminded all that mortality was inevitable and they embellished skeletal drawings with *banderlinos* or inscriptions that echoed Christian reminders of death: *pulvis eris et in pulverem revertis* – dust thou art and to dust thou shalt return. It was a clever conceit that incorporated morality lessons for the general public and at the same time depicted detailed images of the human body important to both artists and anatomists.

One of the effects of the iconoclastic Reformation was that it produced a more secular art. Although the *memento mori* was as powerful as ever, Reformation iconography discarded Catholic imagery and associations and replaced them with worldly references. Skeletons and flayed bodies now held aloft shrouds, hourglasses and flowers, still all suggestive of an inescapable fate, the passing of time and matter that decayed. Later, and in a secure secular environment, hand-colored plates of the 17th and 18th centuries appeared that rendered more accurate anatomical depictions without a presumed need to make iconographic references. Importantly, honorific paintings of anatomists with their cadavers, such as Rembrandt van Rijn's (1606-1669) *The Anatomy Lesson of Nicholas Tulp* (1632) and *The Anatomy Lesson of Dr. Jan Deijman* (1656) became popular, increasing further secular acceptance of dissection in addition to elevating the importance of the anatomists in medicine.* By the 19th century anatomical illustrations lost any pretense of polite or softened images and frank – sometimes gruesome – images of dissected bodies were made. The artistic conceits and flummery ended in art, and true depictions became essential in medical and surgical studies, evident in the exceptional yet straight-forward clinical depictions in *Gray's Anatomy* (see ahead).

Anatomy and Surgery
In France Charles Etienne (1503-1564) was an early exponent of anatomical study who is credited with demonstrating that a canal runs the entire length of the spinal cord. He produced a series of anatomical and obstetrical plates to illustrate his dissections, but lamentably died in obscurity in a dungeon, a victim of internecine religious conflict. His work was soon forgotten and in any case was overshadowed by the exceptional work of his contemporary Vesalius.

---

*These paintings romanticized and sanitized the actual environment of the dissection theater which, in the absence of proper embalming, was suffused with the prodigious stench of putrefaction. Dissections were conducted in the cold months of the year and over three to four days before the decay became intolerable. Evacuated stomach contents, feces and other body fluids encountered during a dissection were emptied into a large tub, while pans of deboning solutions with disarticulated body parts boiled away over open fires – all contributing to the overall penetrating stench of decomposition. Rats stealthily hovered, eager to scarf dropped bits. William Hogarth (1697-1764) in his satiric and contumelious cartoon, *The Rewards of Cruelty* (1750), came closer to the truth of the circus that was the dissection theater (Fig. 13).

Dissection was introduced in England by John Caius (1510-1573), a medical graduate of Padua and founder of Caius College in Cambridge. He was physician to Edward VI (1537-1553) and Queens Mary (1516-1558) and Elizabeth (1533-1603) and was able to secure permission for the college to dissect two bodies a year.

Fleming Andreas Vesalius (1514-1564) trained in and taught medicine in Italy. The human dissections he performed gave him original insights into the best ways to learn and teach anatomy. He was able to produce accurate anatomical charts of the circulatory and nervous system as student aids. His *Tabulae Sex* containing six images with description in Greek, Latin and Hebrew was published five years before the *Fabrica* and was phenomenally popular with students. Additionally, his study of blood vessels resulted in the publication of a more visually accurate guide for blood-letting.

Vesalius was physician to the Holy Roman Emperor Charles V (1500-1558) and to King Philip II of Spain (1527-1598). In 1543, at the age of twenty-eight, he wrote his incomparable classic seven volume *De Humani Corporis Fabrica*. *De Fabrica* described many new observations: the sphenoid, the three parts of the sternum and the five portions of the sacrum, the relationship of the omentum to the visceral organs, the space of the mediastinum and pleura, hepatic vein valves, the vena azygos and, importantly (although the physiologic role remained unknown), the fetal ductus venosus. This anatomic work completely discarded Galenic osteology, muscular anatomy and visceral anomalies, but not without a price: Vesalius' challenge to Galen resulted in the loss of his post in Padua. For unknown reasons Vesalius traveled to Jerusalem, although it has been suggested he went there as a penance imposed on him by the Inquisition. On the way back to Italy he was shipwrecked and died in obscurity on the isle of Zante.

Giovanni Canano (1515-1579) in Ferrara in 1541 had published only the first part of *Musculorum humani corporis picturata dissection*. The entire work had been conceived and planned before Vesalius' opus *De Fabrica*, but Vesalius finished and published his complete work in 1543 before Canano completed his study. Demoralized by the superiority of Vesalius's plates, Canano abandoned the project. The work he published in 1541, however, originally includes the first description of vein valves that would prove critical to the development of Harvey's theory of circulation (see ahead). In his time, Canano's work was ignored. In 1603, however, Fabrizio ab Acquapendente (1533-1619), known as Fabricius, in *De venarum ostiolis*, acknowledged Canano's contributions. There are now only eleven known copies of *Musculorum.*

Another contemporary of Vesalius was Bartolomeo Eustachio (1520-1574) who studied the structures of the ear, evolution of teeth, thoracic duct, kidneys, the adrenal glands and cranial nerves. He is best remembered for describing the eustachian tube. His master work, *Tabulae Anatomicae* (Anatomical Drawings), was completed in 1552 but remained unpublished until 1714. In the wake of excitement that swept scientific Europe over the extraordinary findings of anatomists, acclaim eluded him and instead was accorded to his able and observant student, Falloppio.

Gabriele Falloppio (1523-1562) succeeded Vesalius as Professor of Anatomy at Padua. His *Observationes anatomicae* (1561) also challenged Galen, and Vesalius understandably admired his work. Falloppio originally noticed that the umbilical cord of the fetus has two umbilical arteries and one vein, insight important to the understanding of fetal circulation.

It was the originality and comprehensiveness of Vesalius' *De Fabrica*, however, which would inspire the next generation of anatomists such as Valverde, Gautier d'Agoty, Albinus and Fabricius ab Acquapendente. Juan Valverde de Amusco (1525-1587) published *Anatomia del corpo humano,* best remembered for a famous illustration of a cadaver holding his own flayed skin – a motif perhaps inspired by the portrayal of St. Bartholomew in Michelangelo's *The Last Judgment*. Gautier d'Agoty (1717-1785) did mezzotints of dissected bodies in fanciful poses – a style and conceit that disappeared by the end of the 18th century when anatomy became part of the core curriculum in medical schools. The same fanciful conceits were to be found in *Tabulae sceleti et musculorum corporis humani* (1747) by Bernhard Siegried Albinus (Weiss) (1697-1770). The engravings were done by Jan Wandelaar (1690-1759) who placed the anatomical figures in whimsical postures and backgrounds.

Fabricius (1533-1619) succeeded Falloppio as professor at Padua, where he taught anatomy and surgery, and designed and built the first anatomical theater in circular form. He also wrote *Pentateuchos chirurgicum* (1592) in which he illustrated his *oplomoclion*, a figure composed of prostethic parts which illustrated the manner of healing fractures and dislocations. However, he is mostly remembered now as the teacher of William Harvey, and undoubtedly Harvey's inspired discovery regarding circulation – that valves facing toward the heart prevented flow of blood backwards and that the arteries carried blood in one direction and the veins in another – first germinated in Fabricius' anatomical theater (see ahead).

In Germany prominent surgeon Wilhelm Fabry von Hilden (1560-1624) published a series of six hundred case reports entitled *Observationen, oder Wahrnehmungen in der Wundartzney* (Observations in Wound Surgery). He became skilled in treating gangrene, and noted that when necessary, amputation should be through healthy tissue above the level of necrosis. Von Hilden addressed causes of bowel disease such as parasites, trauma, foreign bodies, polyps, etc. He designed an instrument for placing deep sutures after removal of polyps that was widely adopted. Importantly, von Hilden emphasized that localized, limited inflammation did not necessarily result in systemic disease. Von Hilden worked with his wife Marie Colinet (c. 1560-c. 1640) who trained as a midwife and surgeon and perfected techniques for caesarean delivery. She was an ingenious and observant practitioner who often looked after patients when her husband was travelling. In 1624, after von Hilden had failed to remove a metal foreign body from a patient's eye, Colinet suggested he use a magnet, which successfully removed the object. Colinet was justly credited with the procedure in von Hilden's *Centuriae* (c. 1640).

Also from Germany was Johannes Scultetus (1595-1645) whose posthumous book *Armamentarium Chirurgicum* (1653) became one of the most famous surgical documents of the time. It contained a complete catalogue of known surgical instruments and forty-three pages of superbly detailed plates depicting surgical procedures, many of which were reproduced in texts in subsequent centuries, and many of which were excruciatingly painful. His depictions of mastectomy and applied cautery causes wonder that any patient survived – or indeed endured – the treatment (Fig. 14).

During the 14th and 15th centuries, dissections as we have observed, were few and performed on executed criminals. Cancer was occasionally encountered during the course of anatomization, but the correlation with signs and symptoms or the mechanisms of disease generally escaped the anatomist. Cancer was more often associated with external signs such as ulceration, foul smell or palpable tumor – all considered reflections of a grossly imbalanced humoral system – heavily tilted towards melancholia, the black bile. Humoral flow could be obstructed by a hardening "scirrhus" mass which could grow slowly over months or years until it turned into *cancri venenum* – a cancerous poison. Cancers were seen to spread into the flesh like the legs of crabs and crayfish* and following the precept of *similia similubus curantur* a crayfish was often bound to the tumor. With the increasing sophistication of dissection and microscopy would come the early concepts of cancerous metastasis or "seeding" – the *semina cancri* – which both le Dran and Paget would appreciate. Henri François le Dran (1685-1770) who worked at the Charité alongside Jean Louis Petit (1674-1750) recognized that cancer progressed in stages and advocated surgery before lymphatic spread, while Stephen Paget elaborated on the metastasis theory. (See ahead).

Ambroise Paré (1510-1590) is one of the leviathans of Renaissance medicine. His influence, particularly in the discipline of surgery, was far-reaching. A Huguenot, he was a friend to the kings of France, and physician to the court of Henry II (1519-1559). Although renowned for his battle-field surgical skills, he unsuccessfully attended the king after a jousting

---

*Hippocrates called cancer "*karkinos.*"

accident in which a lance mortally penetrated Henry's eye and brain. Despite the outcome, somewhat ironically, Paré's prominent role in the matter made him widely sought after in several court circles. His medical acumen was extensive, and Charles IX (1550-1574) consulted him, for example, about the powers of the bezoar against poisons. Paré counseled against its use to the monarch, but the practice continued nevertheless until the end of the 17th century.

Paré made Vesalius' Latin *De Fabrica* accessible by writing a vernacular epitome, thereby ensuring its far-reaching popularity. In 1582 he published *Discourse, a scavoir, de la mumie, des venins, de la licorne et de la peste* in which he categorically debunked the absurdity of mummy and unicorn horn for medicinal use.

Paré experimented with wounds that resulted from newly invented armaments. He reintroduced ligation for amputations and discarded the use of hot oil in favor of warm egg white, oil of roses and turpentine for wounds. The harquebus fired a ball the size of a walnut with bits of cloth and gun powder detritus that caused horrendous wounds. The customary approach to treatment, established by Juan de Vigo (c.1450-c.1520) in his *Practica Copiosa*, was to cauterize these gun wounds – considered poisonous – with scalding hot oil of elder which caused excruciating pain. Paré had no reason to challenge the treatment until a campaign in Piedmont when, by happenstance, he used a non-invasive therapeutic remedy as an alternative to cautery. He never used hot oil again:

> "At last my oil lacked and I was constrained to apply in its place a digestive made of the yolks of eggs, oil of roses, and turpentine. That night I could not sleep, fearing that by lack of cauterization I should find the wounded upon whom I have failed to put the oil, dead or poisoned…[Rising] early to visit them, where beyond my hope I found those upon whom I had not put the oil feeling little pain, their wounds without inflammation, having rested fairly well during the night. The others, to whom I had applied the boiling oil, I found feverish, with great pain and swelling about their wounds. Then I resolved with myself never more to burn thus cruelly poor men wounded with gunshot."
> Paré: *Ten Books of Surgery*

Paré advocated experimentation by trial and error rather than adhering to prevailing theories and systems he viewed were ineffective or harmful. His dictum was: *Je le pansay, et Dieu le guérit* – I dress the wounds and God heals them.

The extant wisdom of "wet" wound healing was challenged by Bartolomé Hidalgo de Agüero (1531-1597) from Seville. He performed controlled studies between 1580 to 1583 among 456 patients admitted with wounds. The wet method applied emollients to open wounds to encourage "laudable pus" and drainage. The dry method first cleaned the wound with white wine, cut away damaged tissue, approximated the wound edges, applied astringent and finally bandaged the wound. Hidalgo noted a 3% mortality with the dry method vs. a 50% for the wet. His work was published posthumously in 1604.

Another surgeon whose skills were acquired on the battlefield was Fabricius Hildanus (1560-1634) from Germany, who, unlike many of his fellow surgeons, knew Latin and Greek. He studied all available anatomical books with the deep-seated belief that a surgeon should have a strong grounding in anatomy. The ongoing Thirty Years' War had enveloped almost all of Germany with marauding and foraging armies armed with harquebuses. Hildanus designed novel surgical instruments to probe, locate and extract the missiles.

Although used in Roman times for battleground transport to field hospitals, the ambulance was reintroduced only in 1492 in Spain as a then considered innovation, apparently as the result of an order by Queen Isabella of Castile (1451-1504) to send a veritable field hospital to the siege of Granada where the Spanish army endeavored to oust the Arabs who had flourished there for centuries. There were four hundred *ambulancias*, wagons that transported physicians, attendants, bandages, surgical equipment and medicines to the battlefield and the wounded to safety.

French military surgeon Dominique Jean Larrey (1766-1842) in 1792 designed a special horse-drawn two wheel carriage to transport the wounded from the battlefield. It was equipped with small pockets and cupboards to hold dressings, instruments and medication. Napoleon himself ordered Larrey to implement his *ambulances volantes* throughout the army. Larrey incidentally, packed extremities to be amputated in snow and ice for the numbing effect.

Not until the high Renaissance did surgery become a respected profession, largely the consequence of outstanding academic texts published by insightful anatomists throughout Europe, particularly those of Vesalius and Paré. Venetian Andrea della Croce (1514-1624) wrote one of the early specifically surgical works – *Chirurgiae* (1573). He was the first to introduce synonyms for Greek, Arabic and Latin terms and to coalesce medical terminology recognizable in the vernacular. Croce was particularly interested in head trauma, and volume VII of his work devotes more than seventy pages to skull fractures, simple and complex, and their repair.

Anatomist and surgeon Giulio Cesare Arantius (1530-1589) practiced rhinoplasty in Bologna and provided Gaspare Tagliacozzi (1545-1599) the basic principles he used in his modifications. Tagliacozzi was known for plastic surgery techniques on the lips, ears and nose. His rhinoplasty procedure described in *Chirurgia curtorum per insitionem* (1597) was based on sound anatomy, a significant improvement from the ancient "Indian method" described in the *Susrata* that employed a cut-graft taken down from the forehead. Tagliacozzi used a brachial flap of skin, a pedicle taken from the upper arm kept viable until healed, thus sparing the patient an unsightly scar on the forehead (Fig. 15).

Andrea Cesalpino (?1519-1603) of Arezzo shattered another major Galenic concept by rejecting the view that the liver was part of the circulatory system, and, like Vesalius and others, was reviled by his contemporaries for challenging and discrediting Galen. Cesalpino, who was physician to Pope Clement VIII (1536-1605), grasped the concept of systemic and pulmonary circulation before Harvey, but failed to prove it experimentally.

Mateo Realdo Colombo's (1516-1559) description of ventricular and valvular action facilitated an understanding of pulmonary circulation. The results of his investigation were published as *De Re Anatomicâ Libri XV* (Venice, 1559). The most important feature of the book is a rudimentary elucidation of pulmonary circulation: "The blood is carried by the artery-like vein to the lungs, and being there made thin, is brought back thence together with air by the vein-like artery to the left ventricle of the heart."

Modern physiology, history makes clear, had a lot of catching up to do on the subject of pulmonary circulation of the blood. In China circulation was first described during the Tsin dynasty (264-419) and, in the Arab world, Ibn al-Nafis (1213-1288) wrote about both pulmonary and coronary circulation in *Commentary on Anatomy in the Canon of Avicenna*. This work and *Commentary on Compound Drugs* were finally translated into Latin by Andrea Alpago (d. 1522). In Europe in 1559, Cesalpino was the first to use the term "circulation." This reference preceded Harvey's description by thirty years.

Theologian physician Miguel Servede (1509-1553), best known by his Latinized name of Servetus, studied at Montpellier. Although he gave no name to the physiologic phenomenon of blood circulation, he did explain pulmonary circulation, albeit with imbued mystic comments. In *Restitutio Christianismi,* published in 1553, he wrote, "The divine spirit is not in the walls of the heart or brain or liver – but in the blood as taught by God himself.* He correctly posited that blood in the right ventricle passed into

---

*Quia anima carnis in sanguine est. *Leviticus* 17:11.

the left ventricle, not through the septum (as Galen would have it, through "pores"), but through the lungs mixed with air, so that "the vital spirit is transformed from the left ventricle into the arteries of the whole body." However, Servetus was a controversial figure in the Catholic and Protestant worlds – an anti-Trinitarian and an opponent of infant baptism – and therefore his published observations on circulation were immediately denounced as heretical by the Catholic Church and he was condemned by John Calvin (1509-1564). In Geneva, all but two copies of his *Resitutio* were conflagrated with him at the stake in 1553.

A common belief that syphilis originated in the western hemisphere is based on the evidence Seville physician Ruy Diaz (c. 1539), who treated Columbus' (c. 1451-1506) sailors for the disease in 1493. A reasonable conclusion was they had contracted the disease in Haiti and introduced the disease in Europe. Renaissance documents, however, refer to the malady in Europe as early as 1440. Germans called it the French disease; in France it was the Spanish pox; to the Turks it was the Christian disease. The name, syphilis, derives from Girolamo Fracastoro's (1478-1553), *Syphilis siva morbus gallicus* (1530).* Geographer, astronomer, poet, musician, mathematician, geologist and biologist, he recognized the nature of fossils and the existence of the magnetic poles.

Fracastoro's greatest contribution to medicine was his *De contagione* published in 1546 in which he theorized on micro-organisms. He studied epidemics of his time and distinguished three types of spread: simple contact, as with scabies or leprosy, indirect contact, such as with small pox fomites, and distant unexplained transmission via *seminaria prima* – seeds of contagion.

In a short but prolific life – dead at 29 – Prussian botanist Valerus Cordus (1515-1544) described the synthesis of sulfuric ether in 1540, added 500 new plants to the pharmacopoeia, and, on Dioscorides wrote several commentaries. His *Dispensatorium* (1535) published in Nürnberg, was the first of the great pharmacopoeias of the millennium. The cities of Basel and Antwerp published their own versions that set a trend to provide pharmacopoeias provincially, a practice that persisted into the 20th century. A standardized municipal pharmacopoeia started to appear in the 17th century: in London in 1618, Brandenburg in 1698, Edinburgh in 1699, Russia in 1778, Portugal in 1794, and, in 1820, the first in the United States of America.

---

*In five volumes, the poem whimsically narrates the tale of a shepherd who complained to the sun god, Apollo, about the pitiless heat, and in protest worships a mere and mortal king. The sun's retribution was to afflict the shepherd, named Syphilis, with "buboes dreadful to the sight."

The first quasi-pediatric work of the 16th century was the *Rosegarten*, a manual of midwifery, written by Eucharius Roesslin (?-1526) and published in 1512 in Strassburg as *Der Swangern frawen und hebammen Rosengarten*. It contained a large section devoted to the care of the newborn. It was popular with the public for two centuries (Fig. 16).

Thomas Phaer (1510-1560), called by some the "Father of English Pediatrics," in 1544 published in English a genuinely comprehensive text of pediatrics named the *Boke of Children.* The table of contents conveys its scope: Aposteme of the brayne [meningitis], Watryng eyes [tearing], Swellyng of the heed [hydrocephaly], Scabbynesse and ytche, Scalles of the heed, Diseases in the eares, Watchyng out of measure [insomnia], Pyssyng out of measure [polyuria], Terrible dreames, Bredying of teeth, The fallyng evill, Canker in the mouth, The palseye, Quynsye or swellyng throte, Crampe, Coughe, Styfnesse of lymmes, Straytness of wynde, Bloodshotten eyes, Feblenesse of stomacke, Yeaxyng or hycket, Colyke, Fluxe of the bellye, Worms, Stoppyng of the bellye, Fallyng of fundament, Chafyng of skynne, Small pockes-measels, Fevers and Leanenesse.

In 1577 in Verona Italy Ognibene Ferrari, known by his Latinized name Omnibonus Ferrarius, published an innovative illustrated book *De arte medica infantium* that, in addition to discussing diseases of childhood, described how to "baby-proof" homes to minimize the all too common dangers of accidents. He was a strong advocate of developmental and safety apparatus for children, such as walkers, potty chairs and a "helmet" to prevent head-injury (Fig. 17).

Renaissance medicine summary

In the Renaissance the collaborative and parallel work of art and medicine resulted in stunning representations of the human body based on careful and accurate anatomical studies. At the same time an extraordinary punctilious Vesalius turned the world of anatomy upside-down with new and astounding observations that exposed the shibboleths of Galen. Others, such as Paré and Fracastoro, contributed to a critical reexamination of Galen and sparked new venues of research for surgery and infectious diseases. Provocative Paracelsus thrust aside Galen, humors, and uromancy, espoused balneology, chemical pharmacology and introduced the concept of occupational medicine. The first standardized municipal pharmacopoeia appeared. Phaer rekindled interest in child health. The printing press facilitated the wide distribution of great texts that reproduced new learning and did so in an economic fashion. Emphasis was given to the natural universe and man's role in it, further secularizing society and enabling additional exploration of the human animal through dissection. Church control of Western medicine was at its nadir as Humanism melded into the age of Enlightenment.

V: Seventeenth Century Medicine

Timeline:

1601 Astronomer Tycho Brahe dies
1603 Elizabeth I dies
1604 Polymath Kepler describes inverted retinal image
1607 Henry Hudson sails into New York
1608 Galileo invents the telescope
1611 King James Bible
1617 Woodall: lemon juice for scurvy
1620 Pilgrims arrive in Plymouth
1622 Moliere is born
1625 Harvey publishes *De motu cordis*
1630 Malaria treated with cinchona
1637 Descartes' *Geometrie*
1642 English civil war begins
1653 Cromwell takes the title Lord Protector
1654 Louis XIV enthroned in France
1660 English restoration of monarchy
1666 Great London fire
       Newton describes gravity
1673 Leeuwenhoek's microscope
1679 *Habeas corpus*
1685 J.S. Bach is born
1692 Salem witch trials
1694 Birth of Voltaire
1696 Death of Peter the Great

The mind is so intimately dependent upon the condition and relation of the organs of the body that if any means can ever be found to render men wiser and more ingenious than hitherto, I believe that it is in Medicine they must be sought for.
>   Descartes: *Discours de la Méthode* VI

When I first gave my mind to vivisection as a means of discovering the motion and uses of the heart, and sought to discover these from actual inspection, and not from the writing of others, I found the task so truly arduous, so full of difficulties, that I was almost tempted to think with Fracastorius, that the motion of the heart was only to be comprehended by God.
>   Harvey: *De motu Cordis* I

...the blood passes through the lungs, and heart by the force of the ventricles, and is sent for distribution to all parts of the body, where it makes its way into the veins and porosities of the flesh, and then flows by the veins from the circumference on every side to the centre, from the lesser to the greater veins, and is by them finally discharged into the vena cava and right auricle of the heart, and...it is absolutely necessary to conclude that the blood in the animal body is impelled in a circle, and is in a state of ceaseless motion; that this is the act or function which the heart performs by means of its pulse; and that it is the sole and only end of the motion and contraction of the heart.
>   Harvey: *De motu Cordis* XIV

I watched what method Nature might take, with the intention of subduing the symptoms by treading in her footsteps.
>   Sydenham: *Medical Observations* V: 2

Bachelierus: Cysterium donare, postea seignare, ensuita purgare.
Chorus: Bene, bene, bene, bene respondero. Dignum, dignus est intrare in nostro docto corpora.*
>   Moliere: *Le Malade Imaginaire* Act III

---

*[On being asked how to treat the patient] Bachelierus: First I administer a clyster, then I bleed him, followed by purgation. Chorus: Good, good, good, well said. Worthy, you are worthy to enter our profession of medicine.

Seventeenth Century

Galileo Galilei's (1564-1642) studies of the known planets, using the telescope he developed, confirmed Nicolaus Copernicus' (1473-1543) heliocentric view of the cosmos (1543). In 1610 Galileo began to annote his observations and finally published, in 1632, *Dialogue Concerning the Two Chief World Systems – Ptolemaic and Copernican*, which was immediately condemned and banned by the church. On 22 June 1633, an elderly and frail Galileo appeared before the Inquisition Council clad in a white shirt that signified contrition. The council charged Galileo with writing a heretical work and sentenced him to perpetual house arrest. His ideas, however, and those fomented by the power of the Reformation undermined papal and Church authority, liberating inquisitive minds engaged with newfound vigor in all aspects of human intellectual endeavors, experimentation, dissection and writing.

Tremendous scientific advances were occurring in medicine, the most important of which were the results of the ongoing anatomical studies in the dissection theaters and William Harvey's cardiocentric discoveries.

Englishman William Harvey (1578-1657), as noted a student of Fabricius, received his MD in Padua in 1602. Examination of his *Praelectiones Anatomicae* (1616) reveals he was lecturing about circulation at least twelve years before *De Motu* was published in 1625. *De motu cordis*, was a stellar work that also (and finally) totally discredited all of Galen's concepts about the heart and circulation, and pioneered the anlagen of physiology. Over a period of twenty years Harvey's animal experiments consistently demonstrated the function of systole and diastole and the resultant pulse associated with circulation. The description, finally, of circulation was a seminal one in the history of medicine. Nevertheless, there were dissenters and when Harvey's work was criticized and challenged, George Ent (1604-1689) wrote a defense *Apologia pro circulations sanguinis*.

The work of Colombo, Servetus, Canano and Fabricius greatly benefited Harvey in his investigations, but all constructed incomplete models of circulation, whereas Harvey's epic insights are thorough, completely original in Western medicine and based on sound animal experimentation. Harvey revolutionized medical understanding of cardiologic function and elegantly provided a virtually complete model of the circulation of the blood.

There was one gap in his theory of circulation. He did not describe the capillary, the terminal juncture of arterioles and venules. By 1661 Marcello Malpighi (1628-1694) augmented Harvey's monumental work with microscope studies that enabled him to see capillaries and provide a more complete understanding of capillary function, thereby making possible a complete cardiovascular construct: blood passes through terminal arterioles directly to venules that sustain a circulatory continuum. Malpighi also proved lingual papillae were organs of taste, and in *De Pulmonibus* (1661), demonstrated the lungs to be a spongy "vascular organ."

Harvey's methods produced a clutch of young English researchers – "Harveians" – who followed his blueprint for animal experimentation and documentation. Among them were Thomas Willis, Richard Lower and Robert Hooke. Willis pioneered the study of brain anatomy; Lower and Hooke collaborated in experiments on how the lungs changed dark blood to bright red (see ahead).

Dissection and anatomy commanded newfound respect in academic medicine and a cadre of fresh anatomists reported novel findings and original conclusions that contributed significantly to clinical understanding and practice. Thomas Wharton (1614-1673) discovered the duct of the submaxillary salivary gland, now called Wharton's duct, and the gelatinous matrix of the umbilical cord (Wharton's jelly). He made a special study of pancreatic anatomy and concluded that all glands have ducts by which to discharge their products.

Johan Wirsung (1600-1643) illustrated the pancreatic duct in 1642 (Wirsung's duct). The insights of how the duct functions, however, were made by Regner de Graaf (1641-1673), who conducted studies using parotid, biliary and pancreatic fistulae that complemented Wharton's work on pancreatic anatomy. He published these findings in 1664 in *De Succi Panreatici Natra.* In 1668 he wrote a remarkable account of how, when the testis is stripped of its capsule and the specimen teased out anatomically, it reveals an organ composed of tubules. His most famous work was *De Mulierum Organis Generatione* (1672) in which he gave a thorough description of what was then called the female testis and its follicles and proposed the name ovary for the organ.

Niels Stensen (1638-1686) was an Enlightenment polymath proficient in geology, theology and medicine who studied anatomy with Bartholin (see ahead). He confirmed Wharton's findings and additionally described the parotid and lachrymal ducts. In his Paris lectures on anatomy of the brain (1669) he corrected Willis' contentions that common sense resides in the corpus striata, memory in the cortex and imagination in the corpus collosum. In later years he became a Roman Catholic priest, then bishop, and a powerful force in the Counter-Reformation movement.

Francis Glisson (1597-1677) was Regius Professor of Physic at Cambridge and one of the founders of the Royal Society, serving as president from 1667 to 1669. Glisson rendered the first thorough account of infantile rickets (1650), therapeutically employed suspension to relieve spinal deformities and elaborated on liver anatomy. He boiled livers until their substance almost sloughed off and exposed ducts, vessels and the fibrous cover now called Glisson's-capsule.

The most important contributions on the lymphatic system are the works of Gaspare Aselli (1581-1625) of Cremona who, in performing dog dissections, discovered the lacteals. In *De lactibus sive Lacteis venis* (1627) he described what he called *venae albae et lacteae* (white and lacteal veins), chyliferous vessels that become evident after the animals have been fed. Aselli's work was replicated and advanced by Frenchman Jean Pecquet (1622-1674), who studied at Montpellier, where his dog dissections ascertained the course of the lacteal vessels, including the receptaculum chyli and the termination of the major lacteal vessel – the thoracic duct – into the left subclavian vein. His work was replicated by Danish physician Thomas Bartholin (1616-1680) from the dissection of two human cadavers, criminals donated by the King. He found the duct and reported his findings in *De lacteis thoracis in homine brutisque nuperrime observatis* (1652).

Swiss Johann Conrad Peyer (1653-1712) in 1677 published a work on enlarged intestinal lymph nodules in typhoid patients, now called Peyer's patches. Peyer collaborated with Jakob Wepfer (see ahead) and Wepfer's son-in-law Johann Conrad Brunner (1653-1727). Brunner described duodenal glands. Their work contributed to appreciating the gut as both a secretory digestive organ and an organ reactive to infection.

At the age of twenty Lorenzo Bellini (1643-1704), pupil of Redi and Borelli, began his studies on the structure of the kidney. His description of the papillary ducts was published in *Exercitatio Anatomica de Structura Usu Renum* (1662). Bellini also conducted microanatomy study of the tongue and the taste organs as well as elegant microdissections of the tonsils, their fauces, and adenoids.

Another Italian anatomist given eponymous tribute is Antonio Valsalva (1666-1723), usually remembered for the Valsalva maneuver, forcible exhalation against a closed airway to equalize pressure in ears and sinuses. His detailed study of the anatomy, physiology and pathology of the ear, published in 1704 as *De aure humana tractatus* is his major work, and remained the principle work of reference on the subject for several generations. Parenthetically, Valsalva advocated and implemented humane treatment of the mentally ill.

Advances in gross anatomy set the stage for a higher level of examination – microscopic dissection of human tissue. It began with tradesman Anton van Leeuwenhoek (1632-1723) from Delft, a self-taught microscopist. All of his studies were made using a simple handmade biconvex instrument capable of two hundred fold magnification with which he described red blood cells, spermatozoa, protozoa, striped muscle, capillaries and even organisms in dental detritus. His findings were translated into Latin and published in the *Philosophical Transactions* of the Royal Society in London in 1673.

The development and evolution of the compound microscope was a revolutionary step forward. It made possible the visualization of histopathology and the understanding of disease at the cellular level. Around 1590 the compound microscope was made by Zacharias Janssen (1580–1638). A weak instrument, Galileo's experiments with lenses strengthened the instrument's power and, with enhanced optical magnification, the number of original observations increased exponentially.

Extraordinary German polymath Athanasius Kircher (1602-1680) was a Jesuit priest, an archaeologist, biologist, mathematician, philologist, astronomer, musicologist, physicist and volcanologist who even once had himself lowered into the then dormant Mt. Etna. He knew Hebrew, Aramaic, Coptic, Persian, Latin and Greek in addition to several modern languages. Kircher wrote *Scrutinium pestis* (1658) in which he described his microscope experiments. Using a 32x scope he placed putrefied meats, milk and cheese under the microscope and noted tiny organisms which he called *contagium animatum*. It was an original observation from which he construed that minute, as yet unidentified bodies, were the cause of the plague.

Francesco Redi (1626-1668), poet and physician in Pisa, in 1664 wrote a thesis that disproved the commonly held belief of the spontaneous generation of maggots. He described over one hundred different parasites and the reproductive organs of many species. Some consider him the "Father of Helminthology."

Dutch microscopist Jan Swammerdam (1637-1680) studied medicine in Leiden with de Graff, Stensen and Ruysch. He described the red blood cell, lymphatic valves, and observed that fetal lungs float after respiration (1667).* Swammerdam advanced de Graff's work and confirmed that ovarian follicles contained eggs. Significantly, he pioneered specimen preparations for anatomical and physiological experimentation. He preserved anatomical specimens with paraffin injection and devised a novel dissection of frog leg muscle and nerve exposure for contraction studies. There is a poignant irony that the microscopist who first described red blood cells prematurely died at the age of forty-three of tertian fever malaria and the hemolytic destruction of red cells it produces.

Medicine in the 17th century, as a result of direct observations in the dissection theaters and microscopic analysis, finally began a comprehensive repudiation of Galen, humorism and urinoscopy, and, by so

---

*This observation was used by Johann Schreyer in defense of a 15 year old girl accused of infanticide. When the infant's uninflated lungs sank in a vessel of water, it indicated a stillborn birth, and the girl was acquitted by the examining judges.

doing, made possible substantial advances in clinical insights. Multiple and sometimes conflicting theories, however, frustrated the development of what most was needed – a unified system of medicine that was scientifically unimpeachable. New and sometimes erroneous movements purported to disclose a unified, cohesive concept of the cause of disease, but in fact thwarted aggregate progress in medicine.

New schools of theory began to evolve that centered around the natural sciences of mathematics and physics. Inspired by Robert Recorde's (1510-1558) catalytic work *The Grounde of Artes* (1540), in which he introduced and standardized mathematical language, symbols and numerical systems, the basis for *iatromechanical, iatrochemical* and *iatromathematical* medical theories followed.

In 1662 Rene Descartes (1596-1650) published *De Homine*, the first book of physiology. Cartesian philosophy reasoned that the activity of the organism could be measured precisely, thinking that gave rise to iatrophysics. The iatrophysicists believed all phenomena of life and disease could be explained by the laws of physics like locomotion, respiration and digestion, etc. The leading advocates of the *iatrikos* ("healing") schools were Borelli, Baglivi and Santorio. Radical as the iatromathematical and iatrophysical schools of thought were, their approach was initially popular and was followed by like minded iatromechanics who also examined physiology with the rigid laws of physics. Avant-garde but otiose, it was nevertheless the beginning of modern physiologic research.

In Italy Giovanni Borelli (1608-1679) from Pisa was a proponent of "mechanical medicine." A pupil of Galileo and teacher of Malpighi, he wrote *De motu animalium*. The book's unique thrust was based on his observations of muscle motor forces. There were detailed notes on muscle contractions, the movements of breathing, the gallop of a horse, how fish swam, birds flew and how a human stood from a sitting position (Fig. 18).

His younger compatriot Giorgio Baglivi (1668-1706) took the iatrophysical concept to absurd extremes, comparing teeth to scissors, stomach to a flask, blood vessels to hydraulics and the thorax to a bellows – in effect reducing the body to a complex of small machines. He made at least one substantive observation regarding the distinction between smooth and striped or striated muscle.

Paduan Santorio Santorius (1561-1636) experimented with a clinical thermometer of his devising and a pulse clock to determine temperature changes and its influence on circulation. The thermometer was a long twisted glass tube with a bulb the size of a small egg at the top. The open end of the tube was placed in water. The patient held the bulb in the mouth and body heat expanded air that escaped through water. On cooling, the air contracted and water rose into the line-gauged tube, thus measuring the change in temperature. His *Ars de statica medicina* in 1614 described metabolic experiments. He checked his body weight after meals, toiletry, and measured the amount of his perspiration. He coined the classic physiology term "insensible perspiration."

The last significant writer to expound on iatromechanics did so, not so much from a medical perspective, as from a philosophical discourse. Julien Offray de La Mettrie (1709-1751) received his medical degree in Rheims in 1728 and in 1742 while serving as military surgeon during the war of Austrian succession he developed a prolonged fever and noted how it disturbed his thought process – concluding that organic changes in the body affected his brain – the seat of his soul. This resulted in works called *Histoire Naturelle de L'âme* (1745) and *L'Homme Machine* (1747). The analysis of man as a machine for La Mettrie was not a medical systematic but an acceptance man as a pure biologic entity. The works were perceived as atheistic – burned, and La Mettrie was forced to flee.

The iatrochemical school, inspired by the nosology of iconoclastic Paracelsus, was embraced by the Capuchin friar and physician Jan Baptist van Helmont (1577-1644), who believed that each physiological process was caused by a special ferment (gas) presided over by a particular spirit (blas). He believed each organ had its own "blas" that was controlled by the soul and was capable of producing six types of digestion that converted food into flesh. He believed body secretions were the byproducts of this digestion and thus he measured various excretions of the body. He was the first to measure 24 hour urine outputs.

The genuine founder of the iatrochemical school was Leyden professor Franciscus de le Boe (Latinized to Sylvius) (1614-1672) who stripped all of the mysticism from the work of van Helmont, but validated his studies of digestion, saliva and pancreatic secretions. Sylvius also studied the anatomy of the brain and discovered the cleft in the brain now known as Sylvian fissure. Among his pupils were Swammerdam, de Graaf, Stensen and Thomas Willis.

Diehard reactionaries rejected the interpretation of a purely mechanistic and/or chemical nature of the body that ignored the soul, in their view the body's essence. Furthermore, for want of a unified medical system, the iatrikos schools imploded, their glaring deficiencies all too obvious. The iatrikos schools, however, were the forerunners of an embarrassing succession of useless movements in vogue for a short period of the 18th century – Animism, Phlogistics, Tonics, Brunonism, Vitalism, Magnetism – all of which, like the iatrikos, searched for a "System" of medicine (see ahead).

Although Thomas Willis (1621-1675) was a student of Sylvius and led the iatrochemical school in England, his research findings were well-grounded in observation. Willis studied the qualities of urine, but he is best remembered for his study of neuroanatomy and the book it spawned: *Cerebri anatome* (1664). Illustrated by the notable polymath architect, Christopher Wren (1632-1723), it was the best and most accurate account of its time of the central nervous system, particularly the brain and its vessels.

A small group of Englishmen engaged in the study of physiological chemistry, an emerging discipline, to unravel ancient mysteries of respiration. Understanding evolved in stages with the coordinated efforts of Robert Boyle, Richard Lower, Robert Hooke and John Mayow.

Robert Boyle's (1627-1691) experiments with flames, animals and vacuums demonstrated that air was necessary not only for combustion, but for life. In *The Spring and Weight of the Air* (1662) he defined the inverse relationship between pressure and volume, now known as Boyle's law. His experimental apparatus were made for him by Cornishman Robert Hooke (1635-1703), curator of the Royal Society (whose motto was *Nullius in Verba*).* Hooke, who served under Thomas Willis at Oxford, enlisted the interest of the general public with eye-catching demonstrations and experiments, some romantically depicted by artist Joseph Wright of Derby (1734-1797). A microscopist, he authored *Micrographia*, an exquisitely illustrated book of the microscopic kingdom of "vinegar eels, cheese mites, and the blue of plums."

Richard Lower (1631-1691) wrote *Tractus de Corde* (1669), a physiology text that described his experiments on congestive heart failure, heart muscle fibers, and clot formation in the heart. He performed the first dog to dog transfusion. In 1672, Lower disproved Galen's belief that nasal secretions originated in the pituitary. The most astute of his findings derived from an experiment in which he injected dark blood into insufflated lungs and recognized that the brightened color of the blood was due to absorbed air through the lungs. (Hemoglobin oxygenation of Bohr). (See ahead).

John Mayow (1643-1679) from Cornwall repeated Lower's experiments and concluded that the change in blood color was due to the absorption of what he referred to as "spiritus igneo-aereus," a substance that supported combustion and was essential to respiration. When he placed a small animal and a lit candle in a closed vessel full of air, he noted the flame expired, followed shortly thereafter by the animal; but if the candle was not lit the animal lived twice as long. He concluded that spiritus igneo-aereus was a constituent of the air vital to sustain life and he assumed the lungs extracted and passed this substance into the circulation. Lavoisier in the 18th century called it oxygen (see ahead). The scheme below summarizes each man's experimental contributions towards an understanding of respiration.

---

*Nullius addictus jurare in verba magister – There is no master in whose words I am bound to take an oath. Horace (65-8 BCE), *Epistulae* (c. 15 BCE).

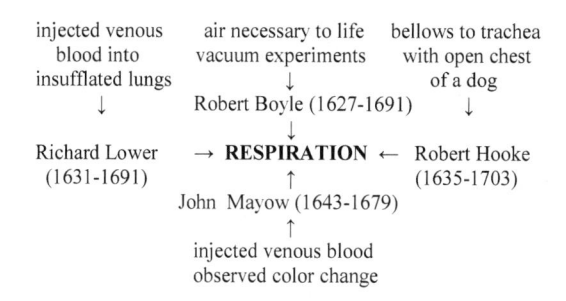

```
injected venous      air necessary to life    bellows to trachea
  blood into         vacuum experiments       with open chest
insufflated lungs             ↓                   of a dog
       ↓             Robert Boyle (1627-1691)        ↓
                              ↓
Richard Lower   →    RESPIRATION    ←      Robert Hooke
 (1631-1691)                ↑                (1635-1703)
                  John Mayow (1643-1679)
                            ↑
                    injected venous blood
                    observed color change
```

In a movement led by Thomas Sydenham (1624-1689) the time honored diagnostic approach of clinical bedside observations formed by Hippocrates in *Prognostics* was reintroduced after nearly two thousand years. Sydenham was called "opiophilus" because of his casual use of laudanum, but he was also called the "English Hippocrates" because of his caring manner with patients and the simple and clear language he used when discussing their condition with them.

The scope and significance of Sydenham's inquiries have had enduring relevance. He made epidemiological observations related to weather, geography and periodicity. He wrote about gout and influenza. He differentiated scarletina from measles and used iron tonics for chlorosis (anemia). His impressive description of St. Vitus dance is now referenced as the eponymous Sydenham's chorea. He treated malarial fever and published on the subject, popularizing the use of chinchona or Peruvian bark in its treatment.

As an aside, Peruvian bark – quinine – was introduced in Europe by missionary Jesuits in 1632. Legend has it that in 1638 the wife of Count Chinchon, Viceroy of Peru, was cured of her tertian fever by the bark. She took with her to Europe a supply of the powdered bark – *pulvis comitissae*. The powder, an effective oral treatment, indirectly further contributed to the diminution of Galenism because it was not a purgative, one of the hallmarks of Galenic treatment. At about the same time, the root of ipecachuanha, also from the new world (Brazil), was introduced in Europe by Willem Piso (1611-1678) and successfully used to treat dysentery.

Sydenham's descriptions of measles, small pox, and gout are classic. He used only treatments that he had personally observed as valuable, such as Fe for anemia and quinine for malaria. A prominent figure in his time, he is a truly seminal figure whose legacy to clinical medicine was far reaching. His *Processus integri* (1695) was the favorite therapeutic vademecum in England until the 19th century.

Ironically, given the arcane and sometimes bizarre ideas and treatment modalities developed as a consequence of a quest for a coherent system of medicine, it was the simplicity of Thomas Sydenham's classical clinical approach that held the key to defining the illusive system. He emphasized how to make diagnoses and offer treatment by studying a disease from first to last through signs and symptoms and by thoughtful consideration of the origins of a disease and its clinical course in order to arrive at a diagnosis and prognosis – a system still in force.

Sydenham was a hands-on physician. In Europe, a genre of medical practice called *consultationes* was conducted by university professors, in which the patient or the patient's physician (as a second opinion) wrote by post seeking advice. The letter would detail the patient's age, constitution, habits, and symptoms and a reply would be sent by post without ever having examined the patient. An exceptional record of these *consulti* from 1680 to 1693 was kept by Malpighi in which he detailed over 217 *consulti* sent from all over Europe.

Sydenham's pupil was Englishman Walter Harris (1647-1732) who, in 1689, wrote a Latin text entitled *De morbis acutis Infantum* in which he articulated for the first time in modern medical literature the challenge to physicians that pediatric care requires an enormity of skills to glean from the *infans* ("the voiceless") all of the signs and symptoms necessary for diagnosis and treatment. The book contained no original descriptions of disease, although in the absence of any concept of microbes, Harris was the first to note the predictable seasonal nature of seasonal diarrhea: "From the Middle of July to about the Middle of September, the Epidemical Gripes of Children are so rife every Year that more of them usually die in one Month, than in three or four at any other Time...." Harris credits Sydenham for encouraging him to write the book that made him famous. The great Sydenham begrudgingly acknowledged Harris' celebrity, writing: "I never flatter anyone, and I say it without any compliment, you are the first I ever envied. It is my sincere opinion that this little book may be of greater service to mankind than all I ever wrote."

By the end of the 17th century surgery attained greater legitimacy in medicine and barbers were relegated to wound drainage and dressings. A few surgeons stand out in this epoch. Surgeon Marco Severino (1580-1656) of Calabria authored the first illustrated textbook on surgical pathology in 1632. During an epidemic of diphtheria in Naples he performed tracheotomies that saved many lives, and during the 1656 Naples epidemic of plague he bravely remained in the city caring for the sick and consequently succumbed to the pestilence himself.

Richard Wiseman (1625-1686), an army surgeon and surgeon to James I, was the first to advocate amputation as the primary treatment of gunshot wounds of the limbs. In general he favored non-surgical intervention when possible, such as compression for the treatment of aneurisms. Wiseman rendered a classic account of the "King's evil" (scrofula) and was the first to describe *tumor albus*, the white swellings of joint tuberculosis. Richard Morton (1637-1689) gave a very detailed description of tubercular pathology in his *Phthisologia* (1689), but his studies and writings were little recognized.

Johan Jacob Wepfer (1620-1695) worked on the vascular system of the brain and the pathology of cerebrovascular disease. His observations led him to hypothesize that the symptoms of a stroke or cerebral apoplexy were caused by bleeding in the brain and that the same symptoms could be elicited by a blockage of the arteries that supply the brain. His autopsies focused on the carotid and vertebral arteries, and in 1658 he published a treatise on strokes entitled *Historiae-apoplecticorum*.

Frenchman Jean-Louis Petit (1674-1750) was a child prodigy who at the age of eight began to assist Alexis Littre (1658-1726) in the teaching of anatomy. By eighteen he was on the army surgical staff. Petit is credited with inventing the tourniquet. His case reports on hemorrhaging and on bone diseases earned him great praise. He wrote about the metastasis of cancer and advocated aggressive surgery despite the known and certain morbidity and mortality.

John Floyer (1649-1734) is chiefly remembered for his invention of the pulse-watch which facilitated a more accurate measurement of cardiac rhythm, and in 1698 he published the first treatise in English on asthma. "[I] have assign'd the immediate Cause of Asthma to the Straitness, Compression or Constriction of the Bronchia ... properly the Periodic-Asthma."

Francois Mauriceau (1637-1709) was an *accoucheur* (a male midwife – a profession that came into its own with the new medical discipline of obstetrics) who wrote an authoritative work, *Des maladies des femmes grosses et de celles qui sont accouchées* (1668) that was translated into English by Hugh Chamberlen (1630-1720) (see ahead). It contained richly illustrated and accurate images of fetal positions and presentations. Although they lacked the artistic finesse and richness that characterized the obstetrical plates of William Hunter (see ahead), they were very original for the times. He popularized delivery in bed rather than a birthing chair. Mauriceau studied pelvic confirmations, unusual fetal positions, devised bimanual extraction of the head, described cord strangulation and developed a strategy for placenta praevia. He was the first to refer to tubal pregnancy, to correct the prevailing wisdom that the pelvis separated during labor and that amniotic fluid was a mixture of menses and milk. The latter was based on a belief that a nonexistent kiveris or "milk" vein travelled from the uterus to the breast and which was depicted by Da Vinci in *Human Coition* (Fig 11).

Paracelsus, as noted, described ailments related to work and occupations, but the first extensive and systematic treatise on occupational diseases was written by Bernadino Ramazzini (1632-1717) in *De morbis artificum* (1700). He recognized metal intoxications from mercury, lead and antimony by closely studying those engaged in forty-two occupations, including miners, gilders, midwives, painters and bakers. He presciently warned against polypharmacy and excessive bleeding.

> In unsuitable combinations the quality of drugs changes and one should not combine different remedies where one does not exactly know their compatibility.

> ...it seems as if the phlebotomist grasped the Delphic sword in his hand to exterminate the innocent victims rather than to destroy the disease.

In 1663 John Graunt (1620-1674), a London haberdasher, had produced an important epidemiologic and demographic study using the *Bills of Mortality*, the publication that recorded the week's deaths, causes of death and the number of burials. Charles II (1630-1685) and his officials had presided over the inception of the *Bills* in 1603 as a system to alert the populace of impending epidemics, especially that of the plague. The publication, however, was circulated and merely gossiped about by a public fascinated by the lists of the numbers of deaths and their causes. Nevertheless, John Graunt perceptively appreciated its epidemiological potential, and in 1663 published *Natural and political observations mentioned in a following index and made upon the Bills of Mortality*.

One more seventeenth century work deserves mention, one that focused on the mind and depression. Robert Burton (1577-1640) was a scholar at Oxford and although a not a physician wrote an influential book on the study of melancholia. Burton suffered depression all his life which informed his famous *The Anatomy of Melancholy* (1621) in which he redacted the opinions of many writers and addressed many human emotions. He said of himself, "I write of melancholy by being busy to avoid melancholy." Burton included grief in the sphere of melancholia believed by writers of the 16th and 17th centuries to be deleterious to health. Wrote a student of Linacre, Thomas Elyot (1490-1546), "There is nothing more enemy to life than sorrow." Sorrow, sadness or grief was thought to produce an excess of melancholia – a humor believed to sap vital spirit. Continued Elyot in *The Castle of Health* (1543) grief and sorrow "exhaust both natural heat and moisture of the body and doth extenuate or make the body lean." Even the London *Bills of Mortality* listed "grief" as a cause of death. Certainly Shakespeare informs us of the same sentiment when he has the guilt-ridden Enobarbus die in *Anthony and Cleopatra* declaring: "Throw my heart against the flint and hardness of my fault / which being dried with grief will break to powder / and finish all foul thought."

Seventeenth century Summary
An emerging medical sophistication at the advent of the Age of Reason – the Enlightenment – produced the unique individuals named above who established spheres of medicine with new intensity and passion, introducing yet to be fully defined new disciplines, such as epidemiology and occupational medicine. The 17th century in general marked advances in microscopy, anatomy and physiology. Universities for the first time set core curricula and the experimental process became institutionalized. The reexamination of natural science was conjoined with medicine, but innovative advances were slow to be incorporated into the *practice* of medicine which lagged far behind its scientific counterparts. Galen continued to be discredited, but his tenets, long etched in stone, were difficult to expunge from general clinical medicine. Paracelsus prescribed the study of nature to encourage natural remedies. For a short period of time the iatro-schools controlled theory and methodology. Descartes conceived of the body as machine, and Jan von Helmont (1580-1644) said it was "all chemistry," but no one described how to make diagnosis or offer treatments until Sydenham, who studied medicine from a classic approach and steered medicine back to the bedside of Hippocrates' *Prognostics*. In his time Sydenham influenced the most insightful of his peers, but confounded lesser minds still in search of a "System."

VI: Eighteenth Century Medicine

Timeline:

1702 Queen Anne ascends throne
1704 Isaac Newton's *Optics*
1707 Free clinics for the poor in French schools
1714 Fahrenheit's 212° thermometer
1715 First Jacobite uprising
1721 Defoe's *Journal of the Plague Year*
1733 Flying shuttle invented by Kay
1735 Linnaeus' *Systema Naturae*
1740 Frederick the Great is crowned
1742 Celsius' 100° thermometer
1749 Goethe is born
1752 Ben Franklin's lightning rod
1762 Rousseau's *Social Contract*
1767 Mason-Dixon line
1769 James Watt steam engine
1771 Karl Scheele discovers oxygen
1775 Lavoisier isolates oxygen
1776 American Independence
1778 Voltaire dies
1780 Franklin invents bifocals
1783 Montgolfier balloon
1789 Storming of the Bastille
1791 Guillotine appears publicly
1796 Jenner's vaccination
1799 Rosetta stone found

If, by the term *elements*, we mean to express the simple and indivisible molecules that compose bodies, it is probable that we know nothing about them; but if on the contrary, we express by the term *elements* or *principles of bodies* the idea of the last point reached by analysis, all substances that we have not yet been able to decompose by any means are elements to us.
                Lavoisier: *Traité Elémentaire de Chimie* (1789)

In the Year of Christ • MDCCLV• George the Second Happily Reigning • Philadelphia Flourishing • This Building • By the Bounty of the Government • And of many Private Persons • Was Piously Founded • For the Relief of the • Sick and Miserable; • May the God of Mercies • Bless the Undertaking
                Cornerstone of the Pennsylvania Hospital:
                Author – Benjamin Franklin

Men who are occupied in the restoration of health to other men, by the joint exertion of skill and humanity, are above all the great of the earth. They even partake of divinity, since to preserve and renew is almost as noble as to create.
                Voltaire (1694-1778): *Philosophical Dictionary*

These are the books your son will learn under my direction, the others are fit for very little.
                John Hunter: Pointing out cadavers to the
                father of Philip Syng Physick (c. 1790).

The fate of these people [chimney sweeps] seems singularly hard: in their early infancy, they are most frequently treated brutally, and almost starved with cold and hunger; they are thrust up narrow and sometimes hot chimneys, where they are bruised, burned, and almost suffocated; and when they get to puberty, become peculiarly liable to a most noisome, painful, and fatal disease.
                Pott: *Chirugical Observations* (1775)

EighteenthCentury
The Enlightenment was marked by two major and uniquely human qualities: intellectual fervor and a thirst for good and just governance. Neither the cerebral pursuits nor the political activism were original to the times. They had thrived in the seats of power and among the intelligencia in the golden age of Greece and the humanism of the Renaissance. Emmanuel Kant (1724-1804) invoked Horace's (65-8 BCE) *First Epistle* in challenging the human spirit to seek knowledge – *sapere aude* (dare to know). To this end Denis Diderot's (1713-1784) *Encyclopédie* (1751) was inspired by Pliny's *Natural History* and Samuel Johnson (1708-1784) catalogued the English language in his dictionary (1755). Linnaeus (1707-1778) accomplished the same for wonders of the natural world. All manner of writing blossomed, from poetry and prose to pedagogy and political polemics to science. It was the Age of Revolution, marked by the American Revolution, the French Revolution and the Industrial Revolution, successive phenomena that had the cataclysmic magnitude and power to irrevocably alter societal structures throughout the Western world. The mechanical innovations of what we call the Industrial Revolution produced machinery and factories that effected a metamorphosis of the world's rural and urban landscapes and the lives of the people who dwelled within them. The impact of the political revolutions in North America and in France continues to reverberate throughout the world, in concert with the social and economic impact of industrialization.

The progressive intellectuals of the age thought all problems could be solved by reason. In France, philosophers such as Baron de Montesquieu (1689-1755) and Jean Jacques Rousseau (1712-1778) had enormous impact on social and political reforms. The emphasis on "reason" invited conflict between philosophers who wanted to construct systems to explain natural phenomena and scientists who insisted on scientific experiments that showed how nature explained systems. Isaac Newton (1643-1727) was a philosopher, naturalist, mathematician and theologian. His *Philosophiae Naturalis Principia Mathematica* (1687) laid the foundations of modern physic mechanics and universal gravity, but also posed provocative questions on natural philosophy that led some investigators to question mechanistic views of the body and to ask broader questions about the nature of life.

There were philosophers who searched for genuine medical systems. They were mostly transitional figures in medical history whose perspectives were regrettably flawed. Their medical theories were doomed to obsolescence as new findings in pathology, physiology and physiological chemistry transformed medical knowledge and the nature of disease and made possible informed perceptions about the human body.

For example, Georg Ernst Stahl (1660-1734) from Halle devised the system of *Animism*, explained in his *Theoria medica vera* (1707). He believed disease was the result of disturbed *anima* – the energy of life or the agent of consciousness and physiological control over disease. This in fact was an ancient doctrine that the soul heals and attempts to correct incipient deterioration. According to this theory, anima permeated circulation and was detectable through pulse and temperature and spontaneous hemorrhage that released the vascular stasis of humors.

Friedrich Hoffmann (1660-1742), also from Halle, published *Medicina rationalis systemica* (1718-1740) in nine volumes that detailed his doctrine of *Tonus*: All living organisms are composed of fibers with tonus that contract and expand, an activity modulated and controlled by a central nervous system – "ether." Health comes from a normal tonus, and disease from tonus disequilibrium by plethora (excess), originating from the gastrointestinal tract (the ancient *whdw*). He introduced drugs to alter tonus from which we get the term "tonics."

William Cullen (1712-1790) was famed as a Professor of Chemistry and Medicine and served as master to apprentice William Hunter. He was the King's physician in Scotland and left behind an archive of thousands of consultation letters. Cullen revised the pedagogy of clinical teaching in Edinburgh and founded the medical school in Glasgow. His belief in the flawed tonus hypothesis, however, detracted from these achievements, as did his theory that the nervous system regulated all organs and that fluxes of the central nervous system produced disease. He introduced the term "neurosis" to classify these diseases.

His pupil John Brown (1735-1785) in Edinburgh modified and simplified the tonus doctrine with the formulation of his own view that disease was either *sthenic* (severe) or *asthenic* (mild) and that there were two treatments, stimulant or sedative, as found in cold water, emetics, moderate bleeding and alcohol or the use of the sedative opium. He subsequently modified this system by proposing that life was a state of constant energy stimuli and the balance of these stimuli constituted health (Brunonism).

Théophile de Bordeu's (1722-1776) *Vitalism* posited that *vita propia* resided in every organ almost *sui generis* and that nature regulated health through its own secretions that pooled in blood in a balanced concentration. In his *Recherches sur les maladies chroniques* (1775) he wrote, "...the living body is a collection of several organs which live in their own way and...general life is the sum of all the particular lives." He referred to the heart, brain and stomach as the "Tripod of Life."

Franz Anton Mesmer (1734-1815) experimented with magnets and theorized that energy emanated from the body through electrical currents, magnetism and hypnotic states and that positive and healing energy could be transmitted by placing hands on a diseased body. His technique involved sitting in front of a patient with knees touching and pressing the patient's thumbs in his own hands while steadily gazing into the patient's eyes. Then, to stimulate the patient's magnetism, he employed a series of movements, passing his hands from the patient's shoulders down along the arms. He sometimes pressed his fingers on the patient's hypochondrium for hours. Patients reported peculiar sensations such as paraesthesias or fluxes of fluid through their bodies, a sign Mesmer claimed, presaged a cure. He concluded his treatments by playing music on a glass armonica.

In Leipzig Samuel Hahnemann (1755-1843) proposed the theory of homeopathy (*hómoios*-similar/*pathos*-disease) – "like disease" – or *similia similibus*, which theorized treatment should mimic the symptoms of the disease as opposed to allopathy which sought to eliminate the symptoms – *contraria contrariis*. For example, he experimented with cinchona to produce fever, chills, and weakness that mimicked malaria and spent the rest of his life experimenting with other substances in efforts to mimic illnesses. Of the various theory sects, homeopathy is the only one still in use and is considered a form of alternative medicine that employs serial dilutions of substances which homeopaths contend excoriate toxicity. Interestingly there is a biological phenomenon that supports this concept. Called hormesis, it posits that a minute amount of a poison induces a contrary effect to what is observed at a larger dosage. In other words, a known toxin in tiny doses induces beneficial effects opposite to expected effects.

Franz Joseph Gall (1758-1828) believed the surface of the cranium disclosed intellectual and moral elements of the person and that by palpation of the skull it was possible to diagnose mental characteristics and emotions. He called this theory phrenology, and mapped out the topology of the head wherein these elements resided. Those who opposed his theory called it "bumpology," claiming there was no relationship between the cranium and the brain (Fig. 19).

As these various theories were discredited and fell into disfavor, genuine pioneers, whose groundbreaking experiments ultimately altered the course of medical theory and clinical science, were at work. Scottish physician Joseph Black (1728-1799) experimented with thermochemistry and discovered carbon dioxide (1757). He also observed that after oxygen had been consumed and carbon dioxide absorbed, some air remained that would neither support life nor ignite fire. It was a conundrum he submitted to his student, fellow Scot Daniel Rutherford (1749-1819), who in 1772 confirmed Black's findings and called the remaining air "phlogiston." Now known as nitrogen, it was believed to be a fire-like element that was part of combustible bodies liberated during combustion that resulted in oxidation and rust.

In 1766 "inflammable air" was described by Henry Cavendish (1731-1810), who noted that on combustion it produced water. These men amplified the work of Robert Boyle, Richard Lower, John Mayow and

Robert Hooke, fortifying their bedrock work on the physiology of respiration.

In Italy physician and physicist Luigi Galvani (1737-1798) experimented with electrical stimulation, noting that muscles of dead frogs responded to electrical stimulation. Alessandro Volta (1745-1827) developed the first electric cell. Collectively their experiments led to the field of bioelectricity and ultimately to a clearer understanding of nerve conduction and sequential cardiac contractility (and the eventual development of the EKG).

Swedish polymath cum physician Carl von Linné – Linnaeus (1707-1778) – established the foundation of modern taxonomy with his system of binomial nomenclature, *Systema Naturae*, printed in the Netherlands in 1735. In his medical writings he produced a system of nosology – *Genera Morborum* (1763).

Anatomy
During the 18th century the study of anatomy evolved to a new pinnacle. Leiden became a rival center of anatomy to Padua, and Edinburgh was the anatomy center in Great Britain. Scottish physicians prospered as leaders in surgery and obstetrics.

Three generations of the Monro family in Scotland flourished as a "dynasty" in anatomy. All named Alexander Monro, to distinguish among them they are referred to as "primus," "secundus" and "tertius." Alexander Monro primus (1697-1767) was the founder of the Edinburgh School of Medicine which evolved into the most famous in the British Isles. Monro primus published his lectures as *The Anatomy of Humane Bones*, an unillustrated text. He was elected a Fellow of the Royal Society in 1723. Monro primus held the chair in anatomy and was succeeded by his son, secundus (1733-1817) and grandson, tertius (1773-1859).

The influence of the school at Edinburgh began to suffer when local politics intruded on its domain. At the turn of the nineteenth century, the Tory City Council began the practice of appointing professors on the basis of their party affiliation rather than their abilities, and some viewed university chairs as hereditary entitlements. In the example of Monro tertius, he embodied the mediocrity this practice can produce. Charles Darwin attended Edinburgh University in 1825. He described Alexander Monro tertius as displaying "unimpassioned indifference" whose lectures were known to degenerate into riots. Darwin attended them and was repulsed by Monro's appearance. He would enter the lecture hall wearing bloody garments from the dissecting room. Darwin wrote, "I dislike him & his lectures so much that I cannot speak with decency about them. He is so dirty in person & actions." The school's decline was gradual as it lost its reputation as the premier institution of the day. It would only reestablish itself in the following century.

Parenthetically, one of the first European medical connections with America was established by William Shippen (1736-1808), who studied with both Monro secundus and the Hunter brothers (see ahead) before returning to Philadelphia in 1763. Shippen became a medical leviathan who taught anatomy and midwifery and served as Director General of Hospitals of the Continental Army – the precursor to Surgeon General. He was one of the originators of the College of Physicians.

There was another "dynastic trio" in Berlin and Bern: three consecutive generations of Meckels – Johann Friedrich (1714-1774), Philipp (1756-1803) and Johann (1781-1833) – who in turn headed the chair in anatomy. Johann Friedrich Meckel is referred to as the Elder to distinguish him from his grandson. Meckel the Elder concurred with the evolutionary and original beliefs of naturalist Jean Baptiste Lamarck (1744-1829), and he became a pioneer in the science of teratology. He is most popularly remembered for describing the remnant portion of the omphalomesenteric duct of the ileum present in only two percent of the population, now commonly known as Meckel's diverticulum. Son Philipp wrote an important dissertation on the middle ear *De labyrinthi auriscontentis* and was the favored obstetrician of the Russian Court. Johann became an eminent pathologist and comparative anatomist.

Surgery
In England, the Act of 1511 had regulated physicians in greater London, but throughout the British Isles the business of medicine continued to be conducted as a troika of physic, apothecary and surgeon/barber, and with a great deal of discord among the competing groups. Under the Pharmacy Wares Drug and Stuffs Act of 1540, apothecaries could diagnose and treat but charge only for the medication used. The act proscribed them to act as physicians but they were tolerated and often called "doctor." In 1745 disharmony and jealousies resulted in the dissociation from disaffected barbers and the formation of the Company of Surgeons. But the physic or traditional physician remained as the medical kingpin that carried the gold-handled cane. This hodgepodge of ersatz medicine would persist until the introduction of the 19th century hospitalist.

The most prominent English surgeon in the first half of the 18th century was William Cheselden (1688-1752). Cheselden insisted that anatomy be taught to all surgeons, and gradually dissociated all of them from the barbers guild. Among his students were Pott, Cooper and the Hunter brothers. There were twelve editions of Cheselden's text, *The Anatomy of the Human Body* (1713) that was complemented by splendid plates. It remained the preeminent English anatomy text for over one hundred years.

In the second half of the century, Percivall Pott (1714-1788) dominated English surgery. Potts was a popular lecturer at London's St. Bartholomew Hospital. He is best remembered for his description of what is called Pott's fracture (supra-condular tibial-fibular) and Pott's disease (tubercular carious vertebra). He was the first to describe "chimney sweep" cancer about which he wrote with a commendable social conscience. Among his many works are *That Kind of Palsy of the Lower Limbs which is Frequently Found to Accompany a Curvature of the Spine* (1779) – related to scrofula – and dissertations on hernia (1756), head injuries (1760), hydrocele (1762), fistula in ano (1765), fractures and dislocations (1768), cataracts, nose polyps, chimney sweep's cancer (1775) and spinal deformity (1779). In 1765 he was elected Master of the Company of Surgeons. Pott's overall philosophy of medicine merits quoting:

> It is to be presumed, that every practitioner wishes to cure his patients as soon as he can, by the least painful means, and in such manner as shall be productive of the least possible deformity or defect; taking care at the same time, not be inattentive to any evil which may arise, nor to omit or neglect doing whatever may be necessary during such cure.

William Hunter (1718-1783) lectured in his celebrated surgical theater in London's Soho district with his famous brother John Hunter (1728-1793). The Hunters taught anatomy, surgery, obstetrics and diseases of women and children. William wrote on all aspects of anatomy and made obstetrics a discipline of medicine. His most important book was *The Anatomy of the Human Gravid Uterus* (1774), illustrated with splendid obstetrical plates by Jan van Rymsdyck (1750-1784) (Fig. 20). Keenly aware of the tortuous suffering the unanesthetized patient suffered, he wrote: "Anatomy is the Basis of Surgery, it informs the Head, guides the hand and familiarizes the heart to the kind of necessary inhumanity."

John Hunter wrote *The Natural History of Human Teeth* (1771), *On Venereal Disease* (1786), *Animal Oeconomy* (1786) and *Blood Inflammation and Gunshot Wounds* (1794). His studies on the human jaw, its muscular structure, movement and teeth elevated the study of dentistry. He introduced novel dental terminology (incisor, bicuspid, molar, etc.) and the concept of calculous prophylaxis for preventing tooth and gum disease. A renaissance man, he focused on dissection, surgery and embryology. His anatomical studies were made possible by hundreds of cadavers pilfered by grave robbers. He discredited bleeding, purging and mercury as useless one hundred years before anyone else which put him at odds with his contemporaries. With respect to cancer, John Hunter understood a fixed tumor was a death knell, but in *Principles of Surgery* he emphasized "...to know if a cancer is proper for operation...if the tumour is moveable... then there is no impropriety in removing it...." The lasting influence of John Hunter's work derives from the scientific legitimacy he gave surgery, the authority of his teaching and experimental methods, and his philosophy of minimal surgical intervention. Hunter taught his students to be intellectually honest, autonomous and curious; to rely on what was seen, not what was read. His eminence and the heightened level of respect he earned for surgery as a profession are reflected in his election as a Fellow to the prestigious Royal College in 1767 and the acquisition by that body of his unique anatomical and odontological collections. Hunter also left his mark because of his many renowned students, among whom were Edward Jenner, Astley Cooper and through Cooper, John Keats (1795-1821).

Pierre-Joseph Desault (1744-1795), founder of the first surgical journal (1791) followed in anatomist Petit's path and became France's leading surgeon during the second half of the 18th century. Desault placed great emphasis on the teaching of anatomy to surgeons and had begun to reconstruct surgical pedagogy when the Revolution completely disrupted France and its institutions. When the ten year old imprisoned *Dauphin* was sick, Desault attended him and consequently he himself became ill with fever and toxemia and died at the age of fifty-one.

Antonio Scarpa (1752-1832) of Modena wrote multiple works on anatomy and several anatomic entities bear his name: Scarpa's nerve (naso-palatine), Scarpa's triangle (thigh), Scarpa's fascia (cremasteric) and Scarpa's tympanum (membrane). Abraham Vater (1684-1751) of Wittenburg wrote *Dissertatio Anatomica* (1720). One of his many discoveries is the ampulla of the common bile duct.

Pathology would not fully flourish until the 19th century, but the fundaments of the discipline began with Florentine pioneer Antonio Benivieni (1443-1502) who used the autopsy as a method for both anatomical study and to understand the causes of death. His one hundred and eleven autopsies led to *De Abditis Morborum Causis* published postmortem in 1507 and he has been called "the father of pathological anatomy."

However, autopsy methodology and fundaments truly were established in 1761 with Giovanni Morgagni (1682-1775) of Padua, the first of the great pathologists. Morgagni published *De sedibus et causis morborum per anatomen indagatis* (the sites and causes of disease studied through anatomy) based on seven hundred autopsies that correlated clinical diseases and pathology (some of the cases belonged to Malpighi and some to his teacher, Valsalva). This work gave impetus to the mechanisms of disease – the fountainhead of modern medicine – and it systematized clinical medicine. Morgagni emphasized disease was not defined by symptoms, but rather by the diseased organ (the ontology of the disease).

For example, he observed the correlation of pulmonic stenosis and cyanosis, the destroyed infarct of cardiac apoplexy, and the hardening of the coronary arteries (atherosclerosis). His observations were the vectors on the course to understanding pathophysiology. His book proved so popular it was translated in nearly all European languages. In the words of Sherwin Nuland (1930-2014) "[w]ith the publication of *De Sedibus,* the first distinct sounds of the humoral theory's death knell were heard."

Morgagni in turn gave tribute to Théophile Bonet's (1620-1689) *Sepulchretum* (1679) as a work that greatly influenced his own understanding of the pathologic processes since Bonet's book discussed a compendium of some 3000 autopsies classified by disease and symptoms. In Morgagni's words, "[Bonet] form'd them into one compact body; and thereby caus'd those observations ... to become extremely useful, when collected together and methodically dispos'd." In Britain nascent pathology was commonly referred to as morbid anatomy, and the first text on the subject was written by Scottish physician Matthew Baillie (1761-1823), who studied under his uncle John Hunter. In *The Morbid Anatomy of Some of the Most Important Parts of the Human Body* (1793) Baillie described transposition of the great vessels and *situs inversus* – the right-sided heart, emphysema and alcoholic cirrhosis.

The complement to gross pathology is histopathology. Marie François Bichat (1771-1802), a student of Desault, is credited with developing the discipline of histology. Bichat was a gifted man who, in his short thirty-one years, wrote *Traite des membrane* (1800), *Sur la vie et la mort* (1800) and *Anatomie generale* (1801). He devised a system of pathology based on twenty-one tissues studied by microscopy, among them nervous, muscular, vascular, mucous and connective. While working at the Charité in Paris he wrote about the membranous peritoneum, a seminal observation his student Laennec would expand into his classic study of peritonitis.

Physiology
One of the great leaders of 18th century physiology was Albrecht von Haller (1708-1777) of Bern. Haller was a naturalist, botanist and physician. Among his many works his most famous is the eight volume *Elementa physiologiae corporis humani* (1757-1766). Arguably, his most important contribution was the Doctrine of Irritability (muscle response to nerve stimuli) and the fundamental division of fibers according to their reactions. Contraction, he argued, was as inherent to muscles as receptivity was to nerve fibers.

Lazzaro Spallanzani (1729-1799) put to rest the fallacy of spontaneous generation with his study of ova and fertilization in many species, thus establishing the principle of *omne vivum ex ovo.* He also demonstrated that systole sustains circulation down to the capillary level and that respiratory death is not cardiac but anoxic.

In 1778, chemist and mathematician Antoine Laurent Lavoisier (1743-1794), demonstrated that oxygen* was the "vital substance" extracted from the air by the lungs. It was a landmark event. Following up on the work of Cavendish, in 1783 Lavoisier reproduced and confirmed his own experiment, but expunged Cavendish's reference to "inflammable air" and renamed the element "hydrogen" ("water-maker"). Lavoisier was instrumental in developing the metric system of measurement and he organized the first compendium of known elements. With the first version of the Law of Conservation of Mass, Lavoisier noted that when matter changed in form or shape its mass always remained the same. He has often been called the Father of Modern Chemistry and his work in energy and combustion contributed in no small measure to the concepts and understanding of modern nutrition (see ahead).

Lavoisier, a prominent aristocrat, political liberal and social reformer was involved in several administrative posts before the French Revolution and was, during the Revolution, denounced by physician and radical journalist Jean-Paul Marat (1743-1793). For supposed crimes against the people, he was wrongfully guillotined.**

English physiologist and veterinarian the Reverend Stephen Hales (1677-1761) wrote *Statical Essays* in 1731 in which he described his studies in plant hydrostatics. This led him to his most important experimental work in 1733, the calibration of blood pressure in animals. His techniques, however, were invasive and did not lend themselves to clinical application. The practical measurement of blood pressure would not be possible until the work of Riva-Rocci (see ahead).

---

*Isaac Asimov (1920-1992) referred to Swede chemist Karl Wilhelm Scheele (1742-1786) as "hard-luck Scheele" because he made several discoveries for which others received credit: oxygen before Joseph Priestly (1733-1804) and Lavoisier, and, molybdenum and chlorine before Humphrey Davy (1778-1829). Parenthetically, around 1805 Davy described the carbon-arc light but did not pursue its practical application. However, fifty years later Desormeaux would employ the intense gas arc light for an early optic endoscope (see ahead).

**In 1789, "a machine that beheads painlessly" was proposed by English-born French physician Joseph-Ignace Guillotin (1738-1814). Although he did not design the device, his name, to his family's everlasting ignominy, became associated with decapitation and the infamous instrument that created the "Terror" of the French Revolution.

Clinical medicine

William Withering (1741-1799) in his *Account of the Fox-Glove* (1785) introduced *Digitalis purpurea* for the treatment of cardiac dropsy or congestive heart failure. He had heard about a folk herbalist in Shropshire, a Mrs. Hutton, who used foxglove in a polyherbal formula of her concoction to treat dropsy. Overtime and with extensive experimentation, Withering deduced that the active substance of the polyherbal was the foxglove. For a decade he tested different preparations of various parts and proportions of the plant and described the effects and the most salubrious method of administration.

Herman Boerhaave (1668-1738) of Leiden was an advocate of Hippocratic medicine who focused on the patient's condition. He (1) examined the patient, (2) formulated a diagnostic theory and (3) treated accordingly to his findings instead of what had become 2-1-3 during the epoch of search for a medical system. He influenced all of European medicine for generations because of the students he attracted from many countries and the multiple editions of his works *Institutiones medicae, Aphorisms* and *Opera medica omnia.* Such was his fame that he was once sent a letter from China addressed to "the illustrious Boerhaave, physician in Europe" and in due course it reached him. Personages such as Peter the Great (1672-1725), Voltaire and Linnaeus traveled to Leiden specifically to meet him.

Leopold Auenbrugger (1722-1809) of Vienna came from a family of oenologists. Inspired by the process of wine cask percussion, he described chest percussion employing the same methodology. He conducted experiments on cadavers into which he injected water into the pleural cavities and demonstrated it was possible to detect the limits and levels of a pleural effusion and, moreover, determine when and where to drain it. He described his process in *De inventu novo* (1761), but it went largely unnoticed until Napoleon's physician, Jean Nicolas Corvisart, popularized it.

William Heberden (1710-1801) is known for his description of angina pectoris and rheumatic nodules. In 1745 he published *Essay on Mithridatum and Theriaca*, effectively dismissing them from the pharmacopoeia. However, to the interest of pediatricians and public health officials, in 1767 he was the first to detail varicella – chickenpox – as a disease *sui generis* in *Commentaries* (1802). His accurate assessment of the disease made more facile the differentiation of severe varicella from the invidious, virulent, variola or smallpox.

Smallpox

The recurring smallpox epidemics that ravaged populations, recorded from as early as 200 BCE, remained a feared worldwide scourge in search of a cure. In the 18th century it is estimated that four hundred thousand people a year died in Europe from the disease. A third of survivors lost their sight. Hundreds of thousands were disfigured.* Headway was made when in 1715 Ottoman Greek physician Emmanuel Timonius (1670-1718) observed that Circassian women who pricked the body with detritus from small pox pus induced a benign form of the pox. In Constantinople, Lady Mary Worthy Montagu (1689-1762) – herself disfigured by smallpox – reported how Turkish women gathered in their homes to inoculate each other and their families. Writes Montagu, "[She] immediately rips open that [vein] you offer to her, with a large needle (which gives you no more pain than a common scratch) and puts into the vein as much matter [pox detritus of a recovering patient] as can lie upon the head of her needle, and after that, binds up the little wound with a hollow bit of shell...." Montagu had her son inoculated presumably *a la Turca*. When she returned to England in 1721, determined to popularize the procedure, she had her daughter inoculated with prominent physicians looking on. Variolation in short order became an accepted practice. Despite known risks of fever and infection, it greatly reduced the number of cases of smallpox and it remained in vogue until Jenner and vaccination (see ahead).

In America the pox also plagued the population. Word of "inoculation" had reached the ears of Cotton Mather (1663-1728), and he encouraged Boston physician, Zabdiel Boylston (1679-1766) to experiment with the method. During the sixth epidemic of small pox in Boston, Boylston inoculated his six year old son by lancing the skin and applying nine to fourteen days old pustule detritus from a small pox patient. The experiment worked and he inoculated an additional two hundred and eighty individuals, of whom sixty-five were children under fifteen years of age. Six patients, none of them children, died. The results of two hundred and seventy-five successfully inoculated were ignored in the highly charged atmosphere of suspicion and fear and inoculation failed to gain acceptance until, in 1771, John Cochran (1730-1807) opened a smallpox hospital in Bound Brook, New Jersey, where he inoculated successfully with little morbidity and few side effects.

Inoculation became an acceptable practice in 1777 when General George Washington (1732-1799) appointed Cochran surgeon general to his troops and ordered that they be inoculated.**

---

*Victims disfigured by smallpox used ceruse – white lead powder in wax to hide the pox marks and shaped mouse skins for new eyebrows.

**This was in part a response to reports that the British were using the pox as a biological weapon, first in 1763 at Fort Pitt where blankets contaminated with small pox detritus were sent to disaffected tribes, the Ottawa, Mingoes and Delawares. Again in 1775 four British soldiers admitted to spreading the pox around Boston and in Quebec. The last account comes from Virginia during the period of 1775 to 1781 when Cornwallis was conducting his doomed campaign and had to deal with deliberately infected manumitted slaves that were sent to his camp.

In England it had long been rumored that dairy maids did not get smallpox, an observation physician Benjamin Jesty (1737-1816), among others, made. During an epidemic in 1774, he vaccinated his wife and two sons with cowpox from a nearby herd. They did not contract the disease.

Country doctor Edward Jenner (1749-1823) successfully vaccinated eight year old James Phipps in 1796 with detritus from milkmaid Sarah Nelmes, and, like Jesty, was mocked and ridiculed despite the successful experiment (Fig. 21). He thereafter conducted carefully documented trials on many patients before publishing *An Inquiry into the Causes and Effects of the Variolae Vaccine* (1798) that had data of the overwhelming and irrefutable success of the clinical trials and vaccination soon became the standard preventive procedure. It replaced inoculation, which was outlawed in England in 1840. Cowpox serum was shipped to America where Benjamin Waterhouse (1754-1846) introduced it clinically. America would become a major proponent of the modality with establishment of a Federal Vaccine Agency in 1813 under President James Madison (1751-1836) and in 1855 Massachusetts passed the first state law requiring vaccination of all school children. New and different vaccines were made by the end of the 19th century but an antivaccination movement arose abetted by antivivisectionists who considered the development of vaccines a threat to the well-being of animals. However, in 1905, the Supreme Court ruled in *Jacobson vs. Massachusetts* the government's right to mandate vaccination as a public health measure.

Obstetrics
The "*accoucheur*," a male-midwife trained in anatomy, joined the female counterparts that attended French birth deliveries in the 18th century and edged forwards obstetrics as a distinct medical discipline. Forceps had been introduced in the last half of the 17th century by French Huguenot Peter Chamberlen (1560-1631). For three generations the forceps had been a well guarded secret by the Chamberlen family. In 1670, Hugh Chamberlen tried to sell the invention to the French government but failed. He divulged the design and function to Amsterdam based surgeon Roger van Roonhuysen (c. 1660) on condition it be kept secret, as it was for another 60 years, by which time the instrument and its function became generally known (around 1750). By the end of the 18th century forceps made of leather covered metal were in common use.

Scot William Smellie (1697-1763) trained in obstetrics in Paris in the 1740s then he devoted his care to the poor of London's Eastend. He taught obstetrics from his home, devised teaching models made of leather (see ahead: Leboursier-Decoudray) and was teacher to William Hunter at the University of Glasgow. His *Treatise on Midwifery* (1752) was based on over 1100 deliveries and contained the first systematic discussion on the use of forceps. Smellie designed forceps with two significant innovations: a lock and a pelvic curve. He established the clinical criteria when forceps should be used and designed maneuvers for the delivery of a breech presentation.

Pediatrics
Celsus in antiquity, as may be recalled, grasped that children should be treated differently than were adults – *"Ex toto non sic pueri ut viri curari debent."* Yet, with few exceptions like Phaer and Ferrari, only in the 18th century did the concept of children's unique and special needs as patients begin to be acknowledged and understood.

In 1741 Nicholas Andry (1658-1742) resurrected Celsus' dictum in his best known work – *L'orthopédie, ou l'art de prevenir et de corriger dans les enfans les difformités du corps, etc....* Illustrated and didactic, it was written in plain prose with practical suggestions for parents to implement at home. Andry focused on ailments he believed altered symmetry and mechanical function of the body. He associated the development of some deformities with faulty daily routines that ignored children's unique physiology and small stature. He coined the word *orthopedics* (*orthós* and *paidéia*) a discipline intended to correct malformations in children. The term thereafter was applied to all bone deformities in all ages. In 1789 Jean Andre Venel (1740-1791) converted an old building – l'Abbaye – into the first institute for deformed children.

Following Andry's work, by 1799 forty-three additional books dedicated specifically to the care of children were published. The major works were Anonymous: *A Full View of all the Diseases Incident to Children*....(1742), Jean Astruc (1684-1766): *A...Treatise on the Diseases Incident to Children*....(1746), Leyden graduate William Cadogan (1711-1797): *An Essay upon Nursing*.... (1748), William Buchan (1729-1805): *De Infantum Vita Conser-vande* (1761), Neils von Rosenstein (1706-1773): *Underrattelser om barn sjukdomar*....(1764), George Armstrong (1719-1789): *An Account of the Diseases Most Incident to Children*....(1777) and Michael Underwood (1737-1820): *A Treatise on the Disorders of Childhood with general directions*....(1784).*

---

*The titles of many of these works on the treatment of children are so long that the authors have taken the liberty of abbreviating them.

Despite the number of books published about childhood diseases, the medical achievements of the 18th century that contributed to the evolution of the discipline of pediatrics were relatively slight. Collectively, however, their impact was significant.

Cadogan's essay on nursing contributed greatly to the elimination of the deplorable custom known as baby farming. The practice was responsible for more than a fifteen percent mortality rate among newborns that were sent by their wealthy mothers to wet-nurses in rural areas – over and beyond the London infant fatality rate of fifty percent. Jenner's success in developing the smallpox vaccination significantly reduced morbidity and mortality rates in children.

Scotsman Robert Whytt's (1714-1766) clinical elucidation in 1768 of tubercular meningitis and that of tetanus in 1789 by Joseph Clark (1758-1834) had great influence on the care of children. Neither Whytt nor Clark identified the causes of these diseases, but their faultless descriptions of the progress and prognosis would have clear application after the germ theory was presented and accepted.

Among children's major benefactors was George Armstrong, who founded the London Dispensary for the Infant Poor in 1769. Two other institutions founded in the 18th century reflect the interest in and commitment to social issues regarding children that would dominate the nineteenth century. In1785 Valentin Havy (1745-1822) founded a school for blind children, and in 1784 theologian and lawyer Charles-Micel de l'Epée (1712-1789) founded a deaf-mute school. Jacob Rodrigues Pereira (1715-1780) fled Portugal to escape the Inquisition and settled in Bordeaux where he formulated a system of signs for numbers, punctuation and handshapes to help the deaf communicate. His handshapes corresponded to a vocalized sound so his deaf students actually spoke. For this accomplishment he was honored and invited into the Royal Society of London in 1759.

The new world colonies – Spain, France, England, and America
French and Spanish settlements preceded those of the British in the colonies and their medical facilities were far more sophisticated. The Spanish had established and staffed permanent hospitals throughout their new territories early on. By 1525 there were over 125 in Mexico alone; by 1551 the University of Peru was granting medical degrees, and, by 1570, the university medical printing press had published the *Opera Medicinalis* of Francisco Bravo. In 1595, Alphonso Lopez de Hinajoso published *Summa y Recopilación de Cirugia* in Mexico City. Francisco Hernandez (1517-1587)

translated from the Latin 3000 botanicals used by the Aztecs in *Codex barberini*. In Canada by 1640 French Quebec had two hospitals.

When the *Mayflower* landed at Plymouth Rock in 1620 there was one physician, Samuel Fuller (1580-1633), among the one hundred and two passengers. He practiced the traditional European modalities of phlebotomy, purgatives and plasters. Within six months 44 of the settlers had died and he himself died in the smallpox epidemic of 1633.

Both the philosophic principles of the Age of Reason and the new science traveled slowly across the Atlantic, and even in the 18th century British colonial America remained shackled to puritanical values and, in medicine, the inexact science of pulse diagnosis. John Floyer's (see above) *The Physicians Pulse Watch* was the text of choice. The revolutionary thought of Laennec and Auenbrugger had not yet reached the distant American physician (see ahead).

There were as yet few physicians in North America. American families with no access to doctors relied on Benjamin Franklin's (1706-1790) *Poor Richard's Almanack* (1763) and *Hutchin's Almanack* (1778) that contained guidelines for diagnosis and treatment of adults and children. Medical encyclopedias for the home were popular reference sources, especially *Domestic Medicine* by William Buchan (1729-1805) and the *Primitive Physick* (1747) by John Wesley (1703-1791). Wesley was the founder of Methodism which extolled a healthy holistic life of unseasoned diet, drinking only water, daily exercise, light supper and early to bed. Bathing was always in cold water. Benjamin Franklin* printed *Every Man His Own Doctor or the Poor Planter's Physician* written in 1734 by Virginia born John Tennent (c.1700-1760). It focused on botanicals and therapeutics endogenous and available in the Americas.

Families often relied on home remedies, concoctions and plasters from botanicals grown and gathered in their gardens or purchased at the nearby apothecary. For those who could afford them, complete medical chests, such as Dr. Crawley's Family Medical Chest (c. 1790), were available for purchase. The concept of health insurance as we know it today of course did not exist, but the American anlagen appeared towards the end of this century borrowed from a concept borne in the English motherland. (See appendix-F).

---

*Benjamin Franklin is credited with inventing bifocal eyeglasses in 1784.

Harvard, Yale and William and Mary had colleges very early on devoted to the education of clergy, but there were no American schools of medicine until the latter half of the 18th century. The School of the College of Philadelphia (University of Pennsylvania) was founded in 1755. It was followed in 1767 by King's College (Columbia's Physicians & Surgeons) and Harvard College in 1782. Dartmouth followed in 1797 and Transylvania University (Kentucky) in 1799. As the century ended education predominantly was based on an apprentice system in which students trained with medical practitioners and there were only three general hospitals in the country: New York's Bellevue Hospital (1736), Pennsylvania Hospital (1751), founded by Ben Franklin and Thomas Bond (1712-1784), and New York Hospital (1771). Only Pennsylvania Hospital and New York Hospital had libraries. These hospitals housed books almost exclusively, since medical journals and periodicals were in a fledgling state of being published.

18th century Summary

Progress in the 18th century was marked by discovery and the development of medical specialties. Anatomy evolved as a respected science essential to the study of medicine and anatomical/surgical theaters increased in number, as did the number of dissections thrusting forward the understanding of pathophysiology. Obstetrics became a distinct discipline and was linked with pediatric care as "diseases of women and children." Surgery became accepted as co-equal with medicine and modern pathology took root. The small pox vaccine vanquished a dreaded disease and population statistics began to validate clinical results. Medical schools and hospitals were founded in America, modeled after European counterparts, and contributed to the advance of science and medical knowledge. The more rapid diffusion of scientific discovery, the reorganization of disciplines and new research in universities, with equal dignity, accorded to all of medicine's new branches characterized the new medicine. After all the political upheavals of the century settled and debate about philosophical conundrums ebbed, the recognition that *anatomy, physiology and pathology constituted the underpinnings* of medical study enabled a pedagogical structure for medicine of the 19th century to emerge.

VII: Nineteenth Century Medicine

Timeline:

1800 Volta invents the battery
1804 Lewis and Clark expedition
1807 English slave trade abolished
1815 Battle of Waterloo
1821 Mexican independence
1822 Brazil gains independence
1823 Thomas Wakley's *Lancet*
1827 Beethoven dies
1829 Daguerre's photographic plate
1833 English child labor act
1837 Victoria assumes English throne
1840 Morse's code
1854 Florence Nightingale active
1859 Darwin: *On the Origin of Species*
1862 Emancipation proclamation
1865 Billings' Medical Library
　　　End of American Civil War
1867 Lister and antiseptic surgery
　　　Atlantic cable laid
1869 Suez canal opens
1876 Koch's germ theory formulated
　　　Telephone invented by Bell
1880 First *Index Medicus* catalogue
1885 Pasteur's rabies vaccine
1891 Quincke: lumbar puncture
1893 Henry Ford's first car
1895 Roentgen describes x-rays
1898 Curie describes radium

[Sir Francis Bacon] blames physicians for not making the euthanasia a part of their studies: and surely though the recovery of the patient be the grand aim of their profession, yet where that cannot be attained, they should try to disarm death of some of its terrors, and if they cannot make him quit his prey, and the life must be lost, they may still prevail to have it taken away in the most merciful manner.
                       Heberden: *Commentaries on the History and Cure of Disease.* 51 (1802).

...A boy of 12 should not work in a coal mine at 4 cents an hour and the 4 cents withheld from him and his starving family on account of a debt incurred by his father who was killed in the same coal mine. Perhaps you can convince the commonwealth more if you doctors would go into politics.
                       Jacobi: (1830-1919): cited in *The Doctors Jacobi* by Rhoda Truax

It is a most gratifying sign of the rapid progress of our time that our best textbooks become antiquated so quickly.
                       Billroth: *The Medical Sciences in the German University* Pt.II

I have steadily endeavoured to keep my mind free so to as to give up any hypothesis, however much beloved (and I cannot resist forming one on every subject) as soon as facts are shown to be opposed to it.
                       Darwin: quoted by Francis Darwin (1848-1925) in *Charles Darwin* 2.

This hypothesis [natural selection] may or may not be sustainable hereafter; it may give way to something else, and higher science may reverse what science has here built up with so much skill and patience, but its sufficiency must be tried by the tests of science *alone*, if we are to maintain our position as the heirs of Bacon and the acquitters of Galileo.
                       Thomas Huxley (1825-1895):
                       Letter to the *Times* 26 December 1859

NineteenthCentury

A shift in focus in the 19th century began at its onset with a transition to hospital centered learning that facilitated scientific exploration in many disciplines. France's traditional institutions, casualties of the 1789 Revolution's excesses, had been suppressed or closed. Medical instruction continued modestly enough in hospitals and over time these grew in number and scope until they became the centers of medical education where bedside teaching, postmortem theaters and the laboratory became the benchmarks of medical education. At first the forced radical change in medical education appeared a modest shift, but in fact had a profound effect as original clinical innovations steadily deployed to all other countries in Europe. Large numbers of patients could be studied in the hospital and coordinated patient history, signs and symptoms, gross pathology observed at autopsy and microscopic analysis of postmortem tissues became the optimal learning tools. In France, by the end of the century, a seismic transformation had occurred that in essence advanced medicine in a mere hundred years beyond all of the accomplishments that had been achieved in the prior two millennia.

Another important factor in the century's progress in medicine was inspiration and influence drawn from new knowledge, culled from the work of discoveries made by prominent trailblazers in other scientific disciplines: Georges Cuvier (1769-1832) importantly established vertebrate paleontology and comparative anatomy and organismal biology; Julius Robert Mayer (1814-1878) made an impact with his theory of Conservation of Energy; Charles Darwin's (1809-1882) and Alfred Russell Wallace's (1823-1913) revolutionary and controversial theory of the Law of Natural Selection caused an uproar of protest in many quarters and animated creative energies in all sciences; Gregor Mendel (1822-1884), an Augustinian friar isolated from the academic world of science, elucidated the mechanisms of particulate inheritance. His treatise was printed in 1865 but escaped attention until 1902 when William Bateson (1861-1926) wrote *Mendel's Principles of Heredity.* These and other progressive scientific ideas invigorated medical research with original and unconventional perspectives and in particular ensnared medicine in a sense of new optimism and hope that all disease was conquerable.

In France new paradigms of the physician appeared such as Corvisart and his pupils Bayle, Laennec, Bretonneau, Dupuytren and Trousseau. New specialists emerged at the so-called Paris school: psychiatrist Philippe Pinel, pediatrist and pathologist Charles Billard, pathologist Jean Cruveilhier, otologists Jean Marc Gaspard Itard and Prosper Meniere and neurologist Francois Magendie (see ahead). The work of Pinel, Itard, Meniere and even Magendie laid the foundation for accurate neurological studies and descriptions that for the most part were an achievement dominated by French physicians.

Philippe Pinel (1745-1826) wrote *Traite medicophilo-sophique sur l'alienation mentale* (1801) that asserted mental disease was brain pathology. In 1793 the Revolutionary Council in Paris had appointed Pinel director of the Bicêtre Insane Asylum. The inmates had always been kept in dark chambers and chained to walls. Pinel recognized that traditional methods of purgatives and bloodletting to treat their affliction were useless. He advocated sunlight, discussion of personal problems between doctor and patient, exercise, cleanliness and meaningful work, and he was granted permission to unchain his patients. There was immediate improvement when these compassionate and innovative measures were implemented. The humane and noninvasive treatment Pinel pioneered ameliorated mental symptoms and saved lives. Over half the patients admitted to Bicêtre died in their first year of confinement until Pinel became director, after which mortality fell to thirteen percent. After his program was well established at Bicêtre, Pinel applied his treatment model while director of Paris' Salpêtrière asylum for women. His initiatives quickly became known throughout Europe, and were widely adopted by other mental institutions.

A student of Pinel and Laennec, otologist Jean Marc Gaspard Itard (1775-1838) published the first book on diseases of the ear in 1821. He became a champion for the education of deaf students. Following Itard as physician-in-chief at the Institute for Deaf-Mutes, otologist Prosper Ménière (1799-1862) conducted studies on an ailment marked by unexpected attacks of vertigo, nausea and tinnitus with unilateral deafness. He reported his observations in an 1861 essay "On a particular kind of hearing loss resulting from lesions of the inner ear." Aural vertigo continues to be referred to as Ménière's disease.

Jean Nicolas Corvisart (1755-1821), physician to Napoleon Bonaparte (1769-1821), wrote a well received treatise on heart disease: *Essai sur les maladies et les lesions organiques du Coeur et des gros vaisseaux* (1806), but, most importantly, Corvisart revived and popularized Auenbrugger's work on percussion that had been largely ignored. After using percussion for some twenty years, he published a new translation and revision of Auenbrugger's book. He was a renowned educator who trained a generation of progressive physicians, including Gaspard Laurent Bayle (1774-1816). In 1801 Laennec came to study with Corvisart.

Bayle's extensive work in pathology – he conducted more than nine hundred autopsies – culminated in the classification of the lesions of tuberculosis (phthisis) and pulmonary cancer, which he documented in *Recherches sur la phthisie pulmonaire* (1810). A colleague of Laennec, his original pathological descriptions of tubercular lesions provided the basis for some of Laennec's clinical auscultatory observations.

In 1802 René Théophile Hyacinthe Laennec (1781-1826) published his thorough and novel treatise on peritonitis and described the cirrhosis associated with alcoholism, but his most influential work was *De* *l'auscultation mediate* (1819 and 1823). In 1819 he formulated the concept of the stethoscope, at first using a rolled-up piece of paper. He then invented a functional wood model (Fig. 23). Importantly, and for the first time, he differentiated bronchiectasis, pneumothorax, hemorrhagic pleurisy, infarct and emphysema from pulmonary tuberculosis. A talented flutist, he used musical terminology in his annotations of the characteristics of auscultatory sounds – "brassy horn" "bassoon reed" or "diminutive 3rd murmur." Some sounds he described as rales, fremitus, egophony and he introduced a whole aural dialogue to report on auscultation (a word he himself coined) findings. Many of these terms continue in use. Like Louis (see ahead), he confirmed his clinical observations through the autopsy. Ironically, he died of tuberculosis at the age of 45, having his diagnosis confirmed through auscultation by his colleagues. Examination of patients employing Laennec's auscultation* and Auenbrugger's percussion facilitated physical diagnosis in a way that would not be equaled until the invention of x-ray.

The first clinician to understand the significance of Laennec's methods and consistently apply them was Viennese physician Josef Skoda (1805-1881). With its emphasis that auscultation and percussion must be a routine part of the physical examination, his book, *Abhandlung über perkussion und auskultation* (1839), shaped the scientific basis of modern physical examination.

Pierre Bretonneau (1778-1862) wrote an early monograph on typhoid fever (1819), but is best remembered for his work with diphtheria. He importantly recognized that a single disease had been studied and discussed at cross purposes as several separate entities, making treatment random and diverse. He gave the currently used name diphtheria (1826) to the malady and thereby discarded the litany of other terms (canker, throat-distemper, cyanche trachealis, aphthaemalignae, phlegmone anginosa, garrotillo, morbus stangulatorius, angina puerorum, angina membranacea, cyanche stridula and soffacatio stidula) that in their usage had impeded both research into the cause of the disease and the most efficacious treatment. Bretonneau also introduced tracheotomy (1825) in the treatment of croup and diphtheria.

François Magendie (1783-1855) in 1822 wrote a thorough description of the motor and sensory characteristics of the anterior and posterior spinal roots. In 1804 Englishman Charles Bell (1774-1842), who had described the V and VII cranial nerves, published *An Idea of a New*

---

*In 1852, George Cammann (1804-1863) produced the first binaural (2-earpiece) stethoscope. Laennec's pupil, Jean Alexandre LeJumeau (1787-1877) first described auscultation of the fetal heart using a wood fetoscope in 1821.

Anatomy of the Brain in 1811 on essentially the same topic. An intense rivalry ensued between Bell and Magendie, as the experiments they both had conducted on the nervous system affirmed the differentiation between sensory and motor nerves in the spinal cord. The British claim that Bell published his observations first is indisputable, but Magendie's work* was undeniably more comprehensive. The discord was resolved when their work was recognized as the Bell-Magendie Law, that is, the anterior branch of spinal nerve roots contains only motor fibers and the posterior roots contain only sensory fibers. Bell was accorded a renowned eponymous reference – Bell's palsy – for his description of the unilateral idiopathic paralysis of facial muscles.

Jean Cruveilhier (1791-1874) in 1836 was appointed as the first chair of pathology at the University of Paris. He wrote a two volume *Anatomia Pathologique du corps humain* (c. 1841) and used case histories to describe the pathology of the lesions seen in multiple sclerosis. The work was complemented with beautiful illustrations by physician/water-colorist Robert Carswell (1793-1857). Cruveilhier correlated the symptoms of weakness of extremities, spasms, dysphagia and visual intrusions with the neurologic plaques on the upper portion of the spinal cord. His concept of pathology unfortunately was flawed by his assertion that "phlebitis dominates all pathology" (a theory that would be dismantled by Virchow) and distorted his original and objective observations.

Armand Trousseau (1801-1887), one of the great masters of French medicine, wrote outstanding descriptions of hypocalcemic infant tetany and the carpopedal spasm now referred to as "Trousseau's sign." He additionally conceived of new methods for treating pleurisy, croup and emphysema. Trousseau broke new ground with the practice of intubation and thoracentesis to remove pleural fluid. A professor of the French faculty and a highly regarded teacher and physician at the Hôtel-Dieu, he wrote on

---

*Magendie was, among others, a notorious vivisectionist. He was singled out by Irish MP Richard Martin (1754-1834), who called him a "disgrace to society" and introduced a famous bill that banned animal cruelty in the British Isles. Martin made particular reference to Magendie's public dissection of a greyhound, in which the dog was nailed down ear and paw, half the nerves of its face dissected, and then abandoned overnight for further dissection the following day. Other British medical luminaries such as William Harvey, John Hunter and Astley Cooper were active vivisectionists and equally indifferent to animal suffering, but their discretion saved all of them from notoriety. Harvey's classis *De motu cordis* relied almost entirely on direct vivisection observations of animal hearts. Harvey later expressed remorse regarding his vivisection experiments.

Parkinson's, aphasia, chorea and asthma (which he himself had) in *Clinique médicale de l'Hôtel-Dieu* (1861). With a nod to Bretonneau's tutelage, he routinely performed tracheotomy for diphtheria. It became the standard treatment until New York's Joseph O'Dwyer (1821-1898), after repeated success with intubation for gravid diphtheria in the late 1800s, published his findings in 1885 and tracheotomy as a primary treatment virtually disappeared.

Clinician Pierre C. A. Louis (1787-1872) taught that the signs uncovered by the physician in the course of examination were more objective than the symptoms reported by the patient and therefore more conducive to diagnosis. Louis was an ardent advocate of numerical analysis that prompted him to devise a methodology for clinical statistics. He demonstrated the useless and detrimental nature of bleeding by employing statistical data and conducted over 5000 autopsies to confirm his statistical observations. In 1825 he analyzed 2000 cases of tuberculosis correlating mortality with age, sex and symptoms. Louis' work is considered by some to be a precursor of modern clinical epidemiology. Louis taught a number of Americans, the most prominent of whom were O. W. Holmes, W.W. Gerhard, H.I. Bowditch and John Warren (1753-1815). These physicians, inspired by the methodology they learned, were instrumental in restructuring American hospitals into teaching institutions along the French model.

In America William Wood Gerhard (1809-1872) differentiated typhus and typhoid. His greatest contribution was the description of tubercular meningitis in children. Henry Ingersoll Bowditch (1808-1892) also studied tuberculosis and was the first to perform pleural effusion taps with a pump. Oliver Wendell Holmes (1809-1894) contributed to the recognition of puerperal fever transmission from unwashed hands of doctors – a judgment violently opposed by Charles Meigs (1792-1869) among others (see ahead).

A physiologist at the Collège de France Marie Jean Pierre Flourens (1794-1867) demonstrated the respiratory center in the medulla and the function of the cerebellum in muscular coordination. Experiments conducted in 1825 confirmed that specific parts of the brain were responsible for specific functions. Hereafter, a careful physical examination could pinpoint where in the nervous system a lesion existed.

Jean Baptiste Bouillard (1796-1881), professor at La Charité, was a student of Franz Joseph Gall and a founding member of the Société Phrénologique organized in Paris three years after Gall's death. In 1825 Bouillard published a paper that presented clinical evidence indicating that speech corresponds to a specific center of the anterior lobes of the brain, a confirmation of Gall's opinion regarding that particular part of the brain as responsible for articulate language. Sorbonne professor Paul Broca (1824-1880) described a patient with long-standing language deficit who had recently died and at autopsy revealed widespread disease of the frontal lobe. Over the next several months he presented similar cases and concluded the speech center resided at the third convolution of the left frontal lobe. Broca is regarded as the Father of Modern Neurosurgery.

The leading French exponent of medical care specific to children was Charles-Michel Billard (1800-1832). In 1826 Billard was an intern in the Paris *Hôpital des Enfants Trouvés* – the Hospital for Foundlings. There was a shockingly staggering mortality rate in the large patient population. Billard, inspired by the work of Morgagni, began to keep meticulous clinical records on his observations of dying infants and postmortem findings, following Morgagni's dictum to pursue the study of the pathology of childhood disease. He compiled them as case records that provided the basis for a six hundred and sixty-eight page volume published in 1828 entitled *Traité des Maladies des Enfans Nouveauxnés et à la Mamelle* (A Treatise on Diseases of Newborn and Suckling Infants). Arranged by pathology rather than by signs and symptoms, the book contained a separate folio atlas of plates of his water-colors and drawings. Billard's *Traité* was the original model for the modern methodical study of pediatrics. The book almost instantly was translated into multiple languages and widely distributed.

French influence crossed the channel to inspire Dublin's prominent hospitalists Robert Graves, William Stokes and Dominic Corrigan and, in London, at Guy's Hospital, where Richard Bright, Thomas Addison and Thomas Hodgkin conducted clinical research (see ahead). The French model reached Vienna and Germany, countries that dominated medical research and progress in the second half-century.

Anatomy

With autopsy as the optimal learning tool, focus on the study of anatomy became even more intense. Scotsman John Bell (1763-1820) wrote several monumental works, *Discourses on the Nature and Cure of Wounds* (1795) and *Principles of Surgery* (1801-07) with original engravings of ligatures of the great vessels, fractures, and tumors. With his younger brother Charles Bell (above referenced with Magendie for work on the nervous system) he wrote and illustrated the *Anatomy of the Human Body*. The book enjoyed several editions and was translated into German, but it never attained the legendary status of what surely is the most famous and classic text of anatomy published in English, Henry Gray's (1827-1861) *Anatomy Descriptive and Surgical* (1858), a book still in press popularly known as "Gray's Anatomy" and at this date in its fortieth edition. It is a work known even to the general public. The illustrator was Henry Vandyke Carter (1831-1897), a Demonstrator of Anatomy at St. George's Hospital. Gray recognized the exquisite nature of Carter's engravings, but apparently was not willing to fully credit his considerable contribution to the text. In the original proofs Gray reduced the font size of Carter's name and deleted his job title.

Gray was a promising investigator who wrote prize-winning essays on the optic nerve and the spleen. He maintained the post of Lecturer of Anatomy at St. George's Hospital, London, and was a candidate in 1861 for the post of Assistant Surgeon, but contracted smallpox and died at the early age of thirty-four at the height of his career. Carter rose to the rank of Deputy Surgeon-General in the Indian Medical Service and served in India in varying capacities until his retirement in 1888.

Throughout Europe and the United States the image of the anatomist was somewhat tarnished by grave robbing scandals that undermined an understanding of the indispensible role the cadaver played in medical education. In America the demand for cadavers began in 1745 when the University of Pennsylvania offered a course in anatomy. The only bodies available were those of executed criminals. Other bodies were obtained by robbing graves. Episodes of missing bodies were recorded in Ohio, New York and New England. The public was scandalized. In 1846 the family of nine year old Ruth Sprague in New York was only one of scores who were outraged. The Sprague outcry on their daughter's tombstone bears testimony to the additional burden of grief imposed by the violation of graves:

> Her body stolen by fiendish men,
> Her bones anatomized,
> Her soul, we trust, has risen to God,
> Where few physicians rise

Massachusetts led the reformation. In 1784 the court declared judges could sentence the body of a duel victim and the murderer to dissection, and again in 1805, the law was expanded to include all murderers. These laws were passed primarily to deter the crimes and secondarily to provide cadavers for dissection, but they also intensified the abhorrence of dissection by associating it with criminality. Finally, the Anatomy Act of 1831 authorized local officials to deliver any unclaimed bodies to schools of dissection. Similar laws soon followed in other states, and by 1913 almost every state had an anatomy act allowing unclaimed bodies for study.

In 1788 the New York doctor's riot occurred on April 13-15. Outside the anatomy laboratory of New York Hospital children were playing when one dissection student, a John Hicks, mischievously waved a cadaver arm out the window at the children. As a result of the incident citizens became suspicious and coffins were unearthed, inspected and many were found empty. The hospital was raided, anatomical specimens were destroyed and many townspeople and students were injured. Freed black New Yorkers also found it necessary to petition the City Council to stop the bodysnatching of their African burial grounds.

In England, stealing a body from its burial site or "unlawful disinterment," was a misdemeanor punishable by fine or a few months in jail, since a dead body belonged to no one and was not considered property; to remove even a single object from the grave, however, was a crime punishable by hanging. Grave robbers (also called body-snatchers, sack-em-up men, shusy-lifters, Burkers and noddies) were careful to leave behind every item in the coffin – even the shroud – and make away only with the crumpled cadaver in a sack or basket. Watch houses or towers were built in graveyards where guards observed for nocturnal activity – the "graveyard shift." Sometimes "mortsafes" – iron cages with heavy stones – were placed over graves for a week, after which the body was not fit for dissection.

Anatomists of great fame admitted to dealing with these nefarious snatchers, among them John Hunter, Charles Bell and Astley Cooper. Not only surgeons but dentists relied on the guile and gall of snatchers for wares. Young, strong, noncarious teeth were used for making dentures and a good tooth fetched one shilling, while an entire matching set could fetch one to two guineas. In 1831 a fresh adult corpse averaged eight to twelve guineas, while children and fetuses were sold by the inch. Almost all creatures were anatomized, and a dog or cat cost up to half a crown.

The most notorious episode of "resurrection men," evolved in Scotland. Robert Knox (1791-1862) of Edinburgh was a famous teacher of anatomy. In contrast to the monotonous pedantry of teachers like Monro tertius, Knox's teaching style was lively, engaging and included demonstrations of expert and complete dissections with student "hands on" participation. His immense popularity resulted in swollen class sizes that necessitated increased numbers of cadavers for study. The need was met with resourceful and then nefarious grave robbing. The most disreputable of the felons were William Burke (1792-1829) and William Hare (d. c. 1858). In Hare's lodging house an old Highlander died in bed, and Hare delivered the body to No.10 Surgeon's Square and was paid seven pounds, ten shillings. The easy money aroused criminal instincts. Another old lodger lay ill and dying and Burke and Hare sped his demise by suffocation. Knox unwittingly bought this murdered body for ten pounds. The pair began an iniquitous murdering spree of vagrants, peddlers, beggars, prostitutes and the destitute, people whose deaths were most likely to go unnoticed. Eventually they were caught, and in their defense claimed they bought fresh bodies from families wanting to save funeral costs. Hare received immunity for testimony. Burke was convicted and executed, but not before the pair had murdered sixteen people.* This episode was the catalyst for the Warburton Anatomy Act of 1836 that provided unclaimed bodies to anatomists, effectively ending grave robbing in the British Isles.

Knox did not know about the murders and was never charged as an accessory to any crime, but his reputation was tainted and public feelings were well expressed in a rhyme:

> Doon the close and up the stair
> Butt and ben wi Burke and Hare
> Burke's the butcher, Hare's the thief
> And Knox the boy that buys the beef!

But medical schools persisted with an insatiable appetite for cadavers and they found places to hide bodies when the authorities appeared in search of missing loved one. The cupola of many a school often served as an architectural conceit as well as a hiding place.

Basic sciences most flourished in the Germanic states, especially in Austria during the 19th century. Unfettered by the anti-dissection attitudes among the public that grave robbing had engendered, advances in dissection and microscopy dramatically enhanced the discipline of anatomy and the evolving disciplines of histology, embryology and physiology.

Building on the work of Bichat, Albert von Kölliker (1817-1907) wrote the first complete text on histology. He introduced new tissue preparation techniques such as hardening, sectioning and staining that improved the study of microscopic anatomy. Johannes Purkinje (1787-1869) was the first to use the microtome and introduced the term"protoplasm" which still evokes the substance of biology. The work of Kölliker and Purkinje made histology central to the understanding of microscopic pathology, a discipline the Father of Cellular Pathology – Virchow – institutionalized (see ahead).

---

*In 1831, in London, three years after the Edinburgh scandal, John Bishop, Thomas Williams and James May were arrested on suspicion of murder after they attempted to sell the still-warm body of a young Italian boy. Bishop had had a long history of grave robbing. During his trial he admitted to having sold over 500 bodies to surgeons working in the three London schools of Medicine: Guy's, St.Thomas' and the private school of Grainger's on Webb Street. May admitted only to extracting the boy's teeth and was sentenced to transport, but Bishop and Williams were found guilty of murder and executed. After their very public trial and executions grave robbing declined. But, the "Asiatic cholera" of 1832 killed over 5000, while a typhus epidemic in 1837 and again cholera in 1848 filled more graves, and the fear of an infectious miasma thought to linger in grave yards was a deterrent of the sordid and heinous crime far greater than fear of the Anatomy Act of 1832.

Medical polymath Johannes Muller (1801-1858) of Bonn defined the Law of Specific Nerve Energy that stated every sensory organ responds to a stimulus by its own specific sensation. He extensively experimented with phonation and vocal cord motions. Muller wrote the *Handbuch der Physiologie des Mensches* in 1830. This remarkable physiologist also was an anatomist par excellence and was editor of *Archiv für Anatomie und Physiologie*. He mastered microscopic anatomy and trained Hermann von Helmholtz and histologists Virchow, Schwann and Henle.

Jakob Henle (1809-1885) was an outstanding histologist who cofounded the journal *Zietschrift fur rationalle medizin*. He described the renal tubules, vascular endothelium and smooth muscle. While predominantly remembered for the "loop of Henle" – that portion of the nephron in the kidney medulla that provides a concentration gradient – epidemiologists commemorate his original work, *Von den Miasman und Kontagien*, which provided an early foundation for the germ theory. During his lifetime, Henle's thinking on germs and contagion was universally opposed and ridiculed, but he lived long enough to be vindicated by the findings of his student Robert Koch (see ahead).

Karl Rokitansky (1804-1878) of Vienna was a renowned gross pathologist who worked at the 2000 bed Vienna General Hospital. Every patient that died was transported to his postmortem table and over his lifetime performed 56,786 autopsies. He was twenty-three years old when he performed his first, on Beethoven (1770-1827), revealing pathology that suggested Paget's disease of the bones. (Massive lead intoxication is still in debate as the cause of Beethoven's death). His *Handbuch der pathologischen anatomie* made new contributions about goiter, arteries, congenital cardiac anomalies, acute yellow atrophy, gastric ulcer and many other conditions. He both established and standardized proper autopsy method and was at the forefront as the pedagogical torch of medical education passed from France to Germany.

In 1838 Theodor Schwann (1810-1882) theorized that all living structures consist of cells. That same year, lawyer and botanist Matthias Schleiden (1804-1881) recognized that growth was due to cellular hypertrophy and hyperplasia, but Robert Remak (1815-1865) was among the first to show that cell proliferation and tissue growth were both through cell division and cell growth (1852). These simple concepts of cellular growth revolutionized the disciplines of histology, physiology and biochemistry to the degree that it is inconceivable that further progress and understanding in these sciences would have been possible without Schleiden's insights. Moreover, his work established a biological reductionism to the cellular level that fundamentally influenced the progress thereafter of all scientific understanding.

Cellular pathology became the definitive modality to study the mechanisms of disease. It became a movement led by the peerless Rudolf Virchow (1821-1902), a great cell pathologist whose elemental microscopy observations discovered and named, among other findings, leukemia, amyloid and myelin. He distinguished thrombic pathology from embolic – a concept that was completely novel. A pupil of Johannes Muller, Virchow demonstrated that the seat of all disease stems from the cell, and that cells reproduce by nuclear division. His *Cellular Pathology*, published in 1853, facilitated the modern concept of mechanisms of disease. His pupils Daniel von Rechlinghausen (1833-1910) and Julius Cohnheim (1839-1884) demonstrated a fundamental cellular mechanism of inflammation with their study of the migration of white blood cells (diapedesis) through vessel walls.

In 1884 a Russian zoologist, Elie Metchnikoff (1845-1916), described amoeba-like cells that engulfed bacteria. He called the phenomenon *phagocytosis*, which, together with diapedesis, helped shape a comprehensive understanding of cellular defense against microbes. He shared the 1908 Noble Prize in medicine and physiology with Paul Ehrlich (1854-1915), who using new dyes for staining cells described the white cell neutrophil, eosinophil and basophil. (Fig. 22). It had taken nearly one thousand years to explain how pus formed and refute what had long been regarded as "laudable" pus.

Embryologist Kaspar Wolff (1733-1794) in *Theoria Gernerationis* (1759) described the process of germ layers whereby specialized organs develop from unspecified tissue – refuting the prevalent theory of preformation and set the pathway for developmental biology. Karl Ernst von Baer (1792-1876) conducted comparative biology studies and described the ovum in 1827. In his two-volume textbook *Überdie Entwicklungge-schichte der Thiere* (On the Development of Animals) (1837) he also proposed the germ-layer theory of development and advanced the concept that all embryos begin as similar structures that evolve into complex heterogeneous forms.

Eminent biologist Ernst Heinrich Haeckel (1834-1919) mapped the genealogical tree of the phylogenetic system. His pupil Wilhelm Roux (1850-1924) introduced experimental embryology and studied the relationship of embryology to evolution. Still another embryologist, Wilhelm His (1831-1904) invented the microtome, an instrument capable of cutting very thin sections, measured in microns, that allowed the study of reconstructed embryos by means of microscopic serial sections. In 1893 his son Wilhelm His Jr. (1863-1934) described the specialized tissue in the heart – the bundle of His – that transmits the electrical impulses that synchronize contraction of the cardiac muscles. The work of Sydney Ringer (1835-1910), who devised solutions to keep myocardium viable for physiologic study, proved invaluable for *in vivo* observations.

A survey of other notable 19th century anatomists and physiologists would have to include Ivar Sandstrom (1852-1889) who identified the parathyroids, Paul Langerhans (1847-1888) who isolated the pancreatic insulin groups, Franz von Leydig (1821-1908) who investigated testicular interstitial cells, Wilhelm von Waldeyer (1836-1921) who studied tonsillar lymphoid cells and Willy Kühne (1837-1900) student of Bernard, who isolated trypsin and founded the Doctrine of Enzymes. Ivan Petrovich Pavlov (1849-1910) studied gastric and pancreatic secretion and is remembered for his work on conditioned reflexes commonly referred to as "Pavlovian conditioning."

Herman von Helmholtz (1821-1894) experimented with the physiology of sight and sound and in 1857 invented the ophthalmoscope and thereby demonstrated that the macula is sensitive to light. He measured the velocity of nerve signal propagation in frogs and in 1847 he formulated the Law of Conservation of Energy, stating that energy can be transformed but not destroyed.

Ernst Weber (1795-1878) established the notion of "threshold" in studies on how human subjects react to physical stimuli and experiments, with two point discrimination of tactile response. He published his results as *De Tactu* in 1834. Together with his brother Eduard Weber (1806-1871), he measured pulse velocity and conducted experiments that stopped the heart by vagal stimulation – vagal inhibition. Their work promoted further study of the heart and the field of neurophysiology.

Physiological chemistry as a field of study began with the work of Justus von Leibig (1803-1873). He classified foods into proteins, carbohydrates and fats (see ahead). He also described urea excretion and measured protein metabolism by measuring urinary nitrogen. Working and teaching at the German University of Giessen, his genius produced a generation of great biochemists that included Carl von Voit (1831-1908). Von Voit, together with Max von Pettenkofer (1818-1901), established that metabolism initiates in the cell, not the blood, and therefore oxygen requirements are the result of metabolism, not the cause. Studying thin slices of fresh organs in gasometric vessels allowed Otto Warburg (1883-1970) to begin analysis of metabolic pathways, a methodology refined by Hans Krebs (1900-1981) to elucidate the citric acid cycle and the urea cycle. The new and original understanding of the chemistry of the body gradually eroded whatever remained of the theories of animism, tonus and mesmerism. The work of these men made possible a new venue of medical care: disease prevention through good nutrition.

By the end of the 18th century, the collective work of Boyle, Hooke, Lavoisier, Lower, Mayow and Priestly revealed that the "vital substance" of respiration was indeed oxygen. But how was it transported via blood from the lungs? In 1851 Otto Funke (1828-1879) crystallized and identified a red pigment in red cells called hemoglobin, which his colleague Felix Hoppe-Seyler (1825-1895) proved carried oxygen forming oxyhemoglobin. But the physical chemistry of how oxygen was transported and released by the molecule was not elucidated until 50 years later by Dane Christian Bohr (1855-1911) who in 1903 described the complex interaction of hydrogen, carbon dioxide and oxygen in the hemoglobin binding affinity – now referred to as the Bohr Effect. Having defined oxygen delivery the next phase of concentration during the 20th century would center on oxygen utilization.

As noted, in the latter half of the 19th century, German dominance in the basic sciences was exceptional, but there were, additionally, extraordinary French researchers. Most illustrious among the physiologists was Claude Bernard (1813-1878), pupil of François Magendie, who began as a playwright and wrote *La Rose du Rhone* and *Arthur de Bretagne*. Critics in Paris were not impressed with his plays and a friend suggested he try medicine, to which Bernard acquiesced. After completing his medical studies, Bernard concentrated on physiology. He clarified the role of pancreas in digestion, studied glycogen and vasomotor nerves. His concept of the "internal milieu" (the underlying principle of cellular homeostasis) revolutionized physiology. Using fistulas, he separated the role of the pancreas in fat and carbohydrate digestion, and in 1857 he defined hepatic glycogen metabolism. His *Introduction to Experimental Medicine* (1865) established modern physiology.

Charles E. Brown-Sequard (1817-1894) adopted Bernard's premise of the doctrine of internal secretions. He conceived of "organotherapy" and in 1856 demonstrated that extirpation of the adrenals resulted in death. In his later years he was ridiculed for his experiments of the injection of testicular extracts as an elixir to prolong life.

Paul Bert (1830-1886), student of Bernard, studied the effects of barometric pressure and the clinical aspects of hypotension and hypertension. His *La pression barometrique* (1878) was the beginning of balloon (aviation) medicine and the discussion of blood gases, caisson disease and oxygen at high pressure.

The success of the new physiology, chemical extraction and analysis, along with methodology in quantification, made possible the discipline of modern pharmacology. The isolation of pure substances is the hallmark of this new science which facilitated animal experimentation and assessment of physiological effects. Morphine was first to be purified by Friedrich Sertürner (1783-1841) in 1806, and Pierre-Joseph Pelletier (1788-1842) extracted strychnine from *nux vomica* in 1818 and quinine from Peruvian bark in 1820. Caffeine from coffee was purified by Friedrich Runge (1795-1867). Oswald Schmiedeberg (1839-1921) worked with digitalis and histamine. Thomas L. Brunton (1844-1916) analyzed heart drugs and introduced the use of amyl nitrite. Karl Binz (1832-1912) studied the pharmacology of anesthetics, and Thomas Fraser (1841-1920) pioneered work on physostigmine. Robert Cushny (1866-1926), Professor of Pharmacology at both University College London and Edinburgh University, wrote the textbook *Pharmacology* in 1899. It was well received but did not achieve the popularity of the fourteen editions of *Therapeutics* written by American H. C. Wood (1841-1920). Wood's *Therapeutics* would remain the authorative English language text in pharmacology for decades. He used many animal models for his studies on the effects of amyl nitrate, hyoscyamine, atropine and several other drugs.

Germ-Theory

The Contagion theory had been set forth by Fracastoro in the 16th century and defended by Kircher in the 17th century. In the 18th century Reverend Cotton Mather wrote about infectious fomites:

> Every Part of Matter is Peopled. Every Green Leaf swarms with inhabitants. The Surfaces of Animals are covered with other Animals. Yea, the most Solid Bodies, even Marble itself, have innumerable Cells, which are crouded with imperceptible Inmates. As there are Infinite Numbers of these, which the Microscopes bring to our View, so there may be inconceivable Myriads yett Smaller than these, which no glasses have yet reach'd unto. The Animals that are much more than Thousands of times Less than the finest Grain of Sand...may insinuate themselves by the Air, and with our Ailments, yea, thro' the Pores of our skin; and soon gett into the Juices of our Bodies.
> *The Angel of Bethesda* Cap. VII (1724)

Scientific investigation into the germ theory can be said to have begun in earnest with Agostino Bassi's (1773-1857) investigations of the blight that all but destroyed the thriving Northern Italian silk production industry (1825-1835). Bassi's experiments led to the conclusion that silkworm *mal de segno* was caused by the fungus *Botrytis paradoxa* and he made an insightful generalization: "While many, if not almost all scientists…believed and still believe that contagious materials are of a special kind, they are actually living substances – that is to say – animal or vegetable parasites."

Concepts of microorganisms (germ theory) versus miasma (noxious vapors) were to that time ill-defined theories of the cause of disease. It was recognized that epidemics tended to occur in polluted densely populated urban or coastal areas and both concepts could in part account for transmission of disease. The fallacious belief in miasma therefore was not yet discounted as a possible trigger of transmissible diseases.

Epidemic typhus is caused by louse-borne pleomorphic bacteria called *Rickettsia prowazekii* and presents with fever, rash, muscle and joint pains, confusion, cough and pneumonia. Epidemics have been recorded over centuries, particularly during wars, in prison camps, and during poverty crowding conditions. During the Spanish siege of Granada in 1489, 17,000 died of typhus as did ten percent of the English population from 1577 to 1579. An English inquiry in 1759 determined that one quarter of the jailed population died of "gaol fever." During Napoleon's retreat from Moscow in 1812 more soldiers died from typhus than war wounds. In the years 1816-1819, 700,000 cases occurred in Ireland and during the 1840s 9000 refugees crossing the Atlantic to escape the potato famine died in the holds of the "coffin ships" from typhus. In America several epidemics occurred in major eastern cities during 1865 to 1873. WWI saw over 3 million die of typhus and only major efforts of DDT-delousing contained epidemics during WWII. Howard Taylor Ricketts (1871-1910) lent his name to Rickettsia after studying Rocky Mountain spotted fever and ironically, he died of typhus while studying an outbreak of the disease in Mexico City.

Cholera, endemic to the Indian subcontinent, in 1829 entered an epidemic phase that spread across Russia, China, North Africa and Europe. Patients presented with violent emesis and "rice-water" stools, marked by a hollow face, cyanotic lips and marked dehydration. Deaths were swift. The London cholera epidemic of 1848 killed fifty-three thousand people. Physician John Snow (1813-1858) correctly suspected a contagious agent as a cause of cholera long before Koch (see ahead) isolated the organism. Snow conjectured water as the infective source, but was unable to prove his theory until cholera broke out in Soho in 1854. Using city maps of Soho that showed the sites of city water pumps, he determined that the majority of cases of cholera clustered near one specific pump on Broad Street. When the city cut off the pump's water supply, incidences of cholera ceased. Snow also compared the number of cholera victims in two neighborhoods and reported there were many more cases of the disease where there was contaminated water and far fewer where people had clean water. His thoughtful, careful studies are early examples of epidemiological investigation that would evolve into the branches of public health and preventative medicine.

In America epidemics occurred in 1832, 1849, 1854 and 1866 striking primarily in St. Louis, New Orleans, New York and Chicago and believed to have stemmed from Irish immigrants. Little or no cholera was recorded during the twentieth century.

An extraordinary infectious disease investigator was Karl Friedrich Meyer (1884-1974) who made multiple contributions to the field and to the understanding of brucellosis and botulism and the canning industry. He produced an effective yellow fever vaccine, studied the vectors of psittacosis (parrot fever) and the transmission of *Chlamydia psittaci*, the coccidiomycosis of Valley fever and leptospirosis as a zoonosis. A great achievement was to uncover the hidden reservoirs of the plague – the ground squirrel and sylvatic plague – and to develop a vaccine which was used to protect troops during the Vietnam war. He was a remarkable intuitive investigative epidemiologist.

In the 17th century Antony van Leeuwenhoek (1632-1723) had described microscopic animalcules with little understanding of their significance. He did not name these organisms he had observed. The term "bacteria," based on the Greek *bakterion* (a small rod), was first used in 1853 by the German botanist Ferdinand Cohn (1828-1898), who categorized three types of bacterial microorganisms – bacteria (short rods), bacilli (long rods) and spirilla (spiral rods).

In 1850 Casimir Davaine (1812-1882) and Pierre Rayer (1793-1867) had discovered anthrax in the blood of dying animals. They proved the organism was the vector of the disease by transmitting it to healthy animals (one of Koch's postulates). The feverish and hemorrhaging animals succumbed to *Bacillus anthracis*.

Louis Pasteur (1822-1895), a chemist and one of the most important figures in microbiology, in his experiments proved in 1857 that fermentation and souring of wine were due to microorganisms. His seminal research resulted in the differentiation of bacteria from yeast. He invented a method to control the growth of organisms in wine and beer with heat (pasteurization). The German chemist Franz von Soxhlet (1848-1926) successfully proposed Pasteur's process for milk in 1886, rendering it disease free without destroying nutrition.

Pasteur, who had left industry by 1876 in favor of laboratory research of disease, focused on cholera transmission and, importantly, on anthrax infectivity. By 1881 he developed a vaccine for anthrax and by 1885 a vaccine for rabies, a significant achievement since knowledge of viruses was unknown at the time.

Pasteur's extraordinary contributions to the entire field of microbiology were monumental and generated an unprecedented era of investigative focus on infection that had been a baneful adversary since the beginning of time.

Physician Robert Koch (1843-1910), abetted by his assistant Julius Richard Petri (1852-1921), like Pasteur, did research on anthrax and developed new bacteriologic media, fixation and staining. His four postulates revolutionized the study of infectious diseases, providing consistency and reproducibility to experiments. Although polymerase chain reaction (PCR) technology (see ahead) has made his postulates somewhat obsolete, Koch's work was in its time critical to the evolution of microbiology and fundamental to the philosophy of science for over one hundred years:

> In order to establish the specificity of a pathogenic microorganism, (1) the germ must be identified in all cases of the disease, (2) inoculation of the germ must produce disease in the host, (3) from the host it must again be obtained and (4) able to be propagated as a pure culture. (1890).

The following cascade of discoveries in infectious diseases reflect important achievements worthy of mention that simply are too numerous to detail in this condensed history of medicine. In 1882 Koch and Paul von Baumgartner (1848-1928) discovered the tubercular bacillus and in 1883 the organism responsible for cholera. In 1875 the protozoa causing amoebic dysentery was described by Fedor Loesch (1840-1903). Gonorrhea was identified in 1879 by Albert Neisser (1855-1916) and in 1880 typhoid fever by Karl Eberth (1835-1926) and Georg Gaffky (1850-1910). Armauer Hansen (1841-1912) in 1873 discovered the leprosy bacillus, and Charles Laveran (1845-1922) in 1880 detected the malaria parasite. The organism responsible for horse glanders was recognized by Friedrich Loeffler (1852-1915) in 1882, and Friedrich Fehleisen (1854-1924) in 1883 cultured the erysipelas bacteria. The diphtheria bacteria was characterized in 1884 by Edwin Klebs (1854-1913) and Loeffler. Shibasaburo Kitasato (1856-1931) isolated the tetanus organism, and streptococcus pneumoniae was cultured by Albert Fraenkel (1864-1938). In 1887 the meningococcus bacteria was found by Anton Weichselbaum (1845-1920), and Malta fever Brucella was defined by David Bruce (1855-1931). The gas gangrene bacterium was identified by William Welch (1850-1934) in 1892.

In 1894 the plague bacteria was monumentally cultured by Alexandre Yersin (1863-1943) and Kitasato. In that same year the bacterium causing botulism was isolated by Emile van Ermengem (1851-1932). In 1898 Kiyoshi Shiga (1871-1957) worked with the bacillary dysentery germ, and in 1901 David Bruce and Joseph Dutton (1874-1905) visualized the parasite that causes sleeping sickness. Fritz Schaudinn (1871-1906) discovered the agent of syphilis, and in 1906 Jules Bordet (1870-1961) found the cause of whooping cough.

Around 1884 Friedrich Loeffler and Emile Roux (1853-1933) observed that a number of diseases were caused by organisms or substances that escaped the Charles Chamberland (1851-1908) porcelain filter. It led to a breakthrough in microbiology that ultimately recognized these causative agents to be toxins or viruses. Alexandre Yersin (1862-1943 and Roux demonstrated that the essential pathology of diphtheria was toxin driven and Knud Helge Faber (1862-1956) made the same conclusion with regard to tetanus. By 1890 Emile von Behring (1854-1917) and Shibasaburo Kitasato (1856-1931) had developed antitoxin for both tetanus and diphtheria.

Serum diagnosis began in 1896 with Fernand Widal's (1862-1929) agglutination test for typhoid. This was followed in 1906 by August Wassermann's (1866-1925) syphilis agglutination test.

Until the roles of the healthy human carrier and insect and animal vectors were defined, the dilemma remained of how epidemics began. Germ theory and evolving concepts in disease transmission advanced research and treatment in the field of tropical medicine, a burgeoning specialty as a consequence of imperial and colonial expansionism. The high mortality of tropical infections such as malaria, yellow fever, trypanosomiasis, filariasis and other organisms checked the pace of expansionism of the colonial powers and their trade and economic visions. It can be said that a self-interested economic factor spurred the motivation to eliminate or effectively treat tropical diseases.

That was not the case with regards to Scottish customs medical officer, Patrick Manson (1842-1922), a dedicated scientist who while serving in south-east China pioneered the new discipline of tropical medicine. In 1877 he determined that the mosquito carried *Filiaria bancrofti* that caused the horrendously disfiguring disease elephantiasis. It was the first demonstration of an insect vector responsible for disease, a transmission model that would catapult the study of infectious diseases into an entirely new arena.

Manson then suggested to his colleague Ronald Ross (1857-1932) that the mosquito might be the vector of malaria. The malaria parasite had first been noticed in 1880 by French army surgeon Charles Laveran (1845-1922) while he was serving in Algeria, but he proposed no mechanism of disease. In 1897 Ross worked out the life cycle of the parasite and described how the plasmodia parasite was carried by mosquitoes and transmitted from bird to bird. Furthermore, he discovered that only a female mosquito of the genus *Anopheles* was the vector. Independently, Italian Giovanni Grassi (1854-1925) also related malaria to the anopheles mosquito, and in 1899 demonstrated mosquito transmission to the human. For malarial research Ross was awarded the Nobel Prize in 1901, and Laveran, the 1906 prize. For reasons known only to the Nobel committee, Grassi was not recognized.

During the 18th century yellow fever plagued the Eastern coast of America striking the big cities as far north as Boston. In the 1793 outbreak Philadelphia lost 10% of its population, prompting Noah Webster (1758-1843) to ask, "Why should cities be erected if they are only to be the tombs of men?" Yellow fever remained endemic in the Caribbean basin and it took enormous tolls, both during the Spanish-American War and during the construction of the Panama Canal. Cuban Carlos Finlay (1833-1915) demonstrated that yellow fever was transmitted by the mosquito in 1881. Finlay's discovery enabled Americans Walter Reed (1851-1902) and James Carroll (1854-1907) to do extensive research that uncovered the specie, *Aedes aegypticus*, which was also determined to be the vector of dengue. A successful mosquito eradication program was conducted in Havana by William Crawford Gorgas (1854-1920) and then repeated in the Panama Canal Zone, eliminating yellow fever. Gorgas then brought malaria under control with a program of drainage, kerosene spray over water and prophylactic quinine. In effect he eliminated both diseases in that area, enabling laborers to complete the Canal by 1914. In that same year, Gorgas was named Surgeon General.

During the 1930s, Max Theiler (1899-1972) developed a yellow fever vaccine by propagating the virus in chick embryos until it reached the safe attenuation to provoke a safe immune response.

Still, novel agents of infection were being discovered. In 1885, Romanian physician Victor Babes (1854-1926) found the intraerythrocyte babesia as the cause of febrile hemoglobinuria in cattle. Theobold Smith (1859-1934) and Frederick L. Kilborne found the tick *Ixodes dammini* as the vector and established for the first time an arthropod could transmit an infectious agent. Human babesiosis was not described until 1969 and is now a major zoonosis. Similarly, Lyme disease caused by bacteria species of the genus *Borrelia,* discovered by Willy Burgdorfer (1925-2014), is transmitted by tick species of *Ixodes* and was named after the towns of Lyme and Old Lyme in Connecticut, where cases were described in 1975. The zoonosis is marked by fever, headache, fatigue, rash and late onset arthritis, carditis and neuropathy However, observations of the disease date back to the 17th century and even "Ötzi the Iceman" has revealed DNA evidence of *Borrelia.*

Asepsis
As stated, in 1843 American Oliver Wendell Holmes, after significant clinical observations, concluded puerperal fever was caused by infective agents transmitted to women from the unwashed hands of doctors. Holmes' theory was strongly opposed, most notably by Charles Meigs who haughtily pronounced that "a doctor is a gentleman and gentlemen's hands are clean." Not long after, however, the defining experiments regarding puerperal fever were conducted by Ignaz Semmelweis (1818-1865), an assistant obstetrical lecturer at the prestigious Allgemeines Krankenhaus in Vienna (1844). Studying hospital records, he noted in 1847 that one hospital ward with the most mortality from puerperal fever was used by students and professors who rotated from a cadaver dissection class to the obstetric service, while another obstetric unit that was the province of midwives had a lower incidence of death. Semmelweis surmised that hands coated with postmortem detritus from the dissection lab were contaminating the parturition scene. That same year he introduced chlorine solution for the

washing of hands at his institution and there was a dramatic reduction of deaths from fifteen percent to three percent. When he further stipulated the washing of instruments and isolation of feverish patients, the mortality fell to one percent. At first, Semmelweis did not report his findings. Instead colleagues von Hebra, Rokitansky and Skoda publicized his work. His extraordinary research conducted between 1847 to 1849 was not published by him until 1861 as *Die Aetiologie des Begriff und die Prophylaxis des Kind-bettfiebers*. But like those of Holmes, his findings were ignored by his contemporaries and remained a subject of vituperative debate which took a toll on Semmelweis' health. He died a broken man of what is now believed to have been Alois Alzheimer's (1864-1915) presenile dementia and beatings at the hands of "asylum caretakers." Acceptance of the cause of puerperal fever would not be validated until the work of Pasteur.

In 1879 during a meeting of the Academy of Medicine in Paris, a physician at the podium expressed skepticism that puerperal fever was spread by unwashed hands. Louis Pasteur, having in that same year reported finding streptococcus in the blood of afflicted women, thereby validating with laboratory findings the cause of the disease, rose to his feet, irate and exasperated, and protested: "The thing that kills women with [puerperal fever]...is you doctors that carry deadly microbes from sick women to healthy ones."

Joseph Lister (1827-1912), Professor of Surgery at Glasgow, noted the differences in mortality between open and closed fractures. Cognizant of Pasteur's theory that bacteria were airborne, in 1865 he devised and used a carbolic acid antiseptic spray over the operative field that greatly reduced the incidence of intraoperative infections (Fig. 24). Lister credited both Pasteur and Semmelweis and in a paper entitled "On the Effects of the Antiseptic System of Treatment upon the Salubrity of a Surgical Hospital," published in 1870, Lister presented compiled statistics of the mortality rate over a two year period in which he used his carbolic spray. Despite figures that showed deaths dropped from nearly fifty percent to fifteen percent, his method was met with indifference in Great Britain, but warmly embraced in mainland Europe where studies and application confirmed Lister's results. One of the pioneers in adopting Lister's methodology was Ritter von Nussbaum (1829-1890) who in 1880 published *Einfluss der Antiseptik auf die gerichtliche Medicin aus dem Schluss-vortage der Winter-klinik* describing his success using antisepsis. Latvian Ernst von Bergman (1836-1907) further augmented the asepsis concept by promoting the steam sterilization of instruments and sterile catgut by iodine treatment was available by 1906.

American William Stewart Halsted (1852-1922) studied several years in Europe where he observed the work of accomplished masters of surgery, Theodor Billroth (1829-1894), Anton Wölker (1850-1917), and Theodor Kocher (1841-1917). On his return to America, he became the first Professor of Surgery at Johns Hopkins University in Baltimore, Maryland, in 1889. Halsted's European experience had made him a staunch proponent of Lister's asepsis techniques. He introduced rubber gloves, silk sutures and cocaine skin infiltration into the operating theater and greatly reduced infections and mortality. He was the first in America (1882) to propose and perform the radical mastectomy, a most profound cancer surgery.

Anesthesia
In a letter to William Morton in 1846, Oliver Wendell Holmes had suggested a term appropriate for modern soporification: "anesthesia" (Greek: *an* – "without" and *esthesia* – "sensibility"), which was adopted into the medical lexicon.

The first gas recognized for sleep induction was nitrous oxide, isolated by Joseph Priestley (1733-1804) in 1772. Bristol scientists Thomas Beddoes (1760-1808) and Humphrey Davy (1778-1829) in 1795 reported that it produced relaxation of muscles and apparent pain insensitivity, and it was suggested as an anesthetic. Davy in *Researches Chemical and Philosophical Chiefly Concerning Nitrous Oxide* (1799) wrote, "As nitrous oxide in its extensive operation appears capable of destroying physical pain, it may probably be used with advantage during surgical operations in which no great effusion of blood takes place."

Physicist and chemist Michael Faraday (1791-1867) in 1810 had noted nitrous oxide was used recreationally at social occasions to induce inebriating effects. He referred to it as nothing more than "philosophical bandy." In 1818 he perceived ether's similar effects, but fell short of recommending either nitrous oxide or ether as anesthesia agents. This concept was not put into use until thirty years later when in 1842 William Clark (1819-1898) and in 1844 Horace Wells (1815-1847), both dentists, used nitrous oxide for extractions.

Ether was described as far back as 1275 by Raymundus Lullius (1232-1315) from Catalonia. He called it "sweet vitriol." Valerus Cordus had described its synthesis, and Paracelsus had noted its tendency to induce sleep. More than six hundred years later, in 1842, Crawford Long (1815-1878) became the first to use sulfuric ether as an anesthetic. A humble country doctor in Georgia, Long did not think to report his use of ether for eight years.

Dentist William Thomas Morton (1819-1868) and physician Charles Jackson (1805-1880) used ether in Massachusetts, and tangled throughout their careers over the issue of who discovered anesthesia. In 1846 they approached Boston surgeon John Collin Warren (1778-1856) to sponsor their anesthesia experiment, and Warren agreed to use the ether in an operation. Morton and Jackson successfully anesthetized a twenty year-old, and Warren removed a congenital vascular malformation from the neck without pain sensation for the patient. Warren's purported reaction to the phenomenon was "Gentlemen, this is no humbug" in what may be the understatement of the ages.

In 1847 James Simpson (1811-1870), Professor of Obstetrics in Edinburgh, pioneered the use of chloroform for painless delivery. He scandalized the Calvinist Scots who rejected anesthesia during labor, citing *Genesis 3:16:* "Unto the woman" he said, "I will greatly multiply thy sorrow and thy conception; in sorrow thou shalt bring forth children."

In addition to his notable achievements regarding the cause of cholera, John Snow became a prominent anesthesiologist who devised a method to regulate chloroform delivery. He was the first to appreciate that anesthesia required the proper and precise mix of anesthetic with air and that the process was temperature dependent. He developed a clinical scale to determine the depth of anesthesia and emphasized that it was crucial that someone other than the surgeon administer and monitor the anesthesia. After Queen Victoria (1819-1901) requested Snow use chloroform anesthesia for an impending delivery (Snow elected to use the innovative drip method), obstetric anesthesia became widely accepted.

In America Charles Meigs also opposed anesthesia for women in labor. In 1856 he spoke against what he termed the "doubtful nature of any process that the physicians set up to contravene the operations of those natural and physiological forces that the Divinity has ordained us to enjoy or to suffer." This opinion was widely held until, the subsequent year, Fanny Longfellow (1821-1891), the wife of the popular poet John Wadsworth Longfellow (1807-1882), was given ether during labor. Thereafter public acceptance of obstetric anesthesia was inevitable.

Through the ages topical or local anesthesia had been achieved with counter-irritants, such as ice or a good smack. Carl Koller (1857-1944) in 1884 used cocaine topically, a far more effective measure. General anesthesia was administered via inhalation until August Bier (1861-1949) introduced spinal injection in 1898. Thereafter several injectable nerve blocking agents were introduced that facilitated local and regional anesthesia.

Surgery

Until the evolution of streamlined 19th century hospitals, surgeries were typically performed by barber-surgeons, specialized itinerant dentists, oculists, lithotomists and hernia-masters and under the most unsanitary conditions – on kitchen tables, in teaching theaters, below decks of ships and on the battlefield. As scientifically trained and technically skilled surgeons achieved equal status with clinicians and pathological anatomy, anesthesia and asepsis insured rapid and exceptional progress in the discipline, and surgical outcomes improved dramatically.

In France Guillaume Dupuytren (1777-1835) conducted teaching clinics at the Hôtel Dieu. Former physician to Napoleon, he wrote on the surgery of aneurysms and fractures, and in 1831 described palmer fascia contractures. His successor at the Hôtel Dieu was P.J. Roux (1780-1854) who was a swift and skilled amputator as well as an accomplished plastic surgeon, particularly of staphylorrhaphy (repair of the cleft palate).

In England Astley Paston Cooper (1768-1841), pupil of John Hunter, was a proficient surgeon who ligated aneurysms, deftly amputated hip joints and identified many ligaments. He was an avid dissector and paid huge sums to body snatchers. He practiced vivisection and among his many experiments, he tied off one testicular artery of a dog and the vas deferens of the other testicle. Six years later he sacrificed the dog, and demonstrated the testis with the tied artery had atrophied. The other testis was normal. It was probably the first experimental vasectomy. In 1817 he ligated an abdominal aorta. Cooper wrote a scholarly treatise *On the Anatomy of the Breast* (1840) which detailed the lymphatic drainage and lactating glands and ducts. He was a masterful teacher who attracted students in numbers that overcrowded the lecture hall, and such was his reputation that the *Lancet* serialized his lectures.* As observed by writer Druin Burch, Cooper believed a surgeon required "an eagle's eye, a lady's hand, and a lion's heart, and a thorough grounding in anatomy."

English surgeon and pathologist James Paget (1814-1899) is considered by some to share with Virchow honors for founding modern pathology. Paget is a star example of a surgeon who was an astute medical observer. In his early microscopy studies (1834) he demonstrated the cause of trichinosis. He is best remembered for several eponymous diseases, among them Paget's disease of the bone and Paget's nipple (intraductal carcinoma affecting the breast nipple). He authored *Lectures on Tumours* (1851), *Surgical Pathology* (1863) and *Clinical Lectures and Essays* (1875). His son, Stephen Paget (1855-1926) is credited with proposing the "seed and soil" theory of metastasis.

Scottish surgeon Robert Liston (1794-1847) was best known for his skill in rapid amputation – a leg in 2.5 minutes. He performed the first operation in Europe employing ether to which he said, "This Yankee dodge beats mesmerism hollow." His student James Syme (1799-1870) became

---

*With the encouragement of journalist William Cobbett (1763-1835), Guy's surgeon Thomas Wakley (1795-1862) founded *The Lancet* (1823). To sell his journal he serialized Cooper's lectures, unauthorized, with the editorial statement: "As the lectures of Astley Cooper, on the theory and practice of surgery, are probably the best of the kind delivered in Europe, we have commenced our undertaking with the introductory address of that distinguished professor given in the theatre at St Thomas's Hospital on Wednesday evening last. The course will be rendered complete in subsequent numbers." *The Lancet* succeeded beyond expectation and today remains one of the most eminent, respected medical journals. Wakley also served as a member of Parliament (1835-56) and as coroner (1839-62).

the first European surgeon to universally adopted ether and welcomed the antiseptic theory. Yet, contrary to his mentor, he eschewed amputation whenever possible preferring excision as he expounded in *Excision of Diseased Joints* (1831).

Active during the American Revolutionary war, American John Warren (1753-1815) worked as hospital surgeon during the siege of Boston and in the New York-New Jersey campaign. He was in charge of the Continental Army Hospital in Boston and served on the original faculty of Harvard Medical School as Professor of Anatomy and Surgery. Warren gave public lectures on anatomy and demonstrated his surgical acumen by successfully amputating at the shoulder joint (1781), executing an abdominal resection (1785) and removing a cancerous parotid gland (1804).

American Philip Syng Physick (1768-1837) studied with John Hunter in London. Appointed in 1805, he occupied the first American chair of surgery that was separate from the chair of anatomy at the University of Pennsylvania. He became a most admired surgeon who pioneered absorbable sutures. (In 1868, Lister would make them even safer by sterilizing catgut in carbolic acid and extending their duration from one week to two by permeating them with chromic acid). In 1813 his observations and ideas were published posthumously in *Elements of Surgery*.

In 1815 John Collins Warren (1778-1856) succeeded his father as Harvard's Professor of Surgery. He was a student of Cooper and Dupuytren, and would later become the first American to operate using ether anesthesia. In 1811, he was a founder of the august periodical, the *New England Journal of Medicine and Surgery*.

The great Western American migration produced pioneer surgeons like Ephraim McDowell (1771-1830) and William Beaumont (1785-1853). McDowell trained in medicine as an apprentice, and traveled to Edinburgh to study with surgeon John Bell. On his return to America he settled in rural Kentucky. It is notable that he performed the first successful ovariotomy in 1809 and in his lifetime performed an additional twelve such operations.

Beaumont was an army surgeon stationed in the wilderness of Fort Mackinac, Michigan when he attended trapper Alexis St. Martin's shotgun injury to the upper abdomen. Expected to die, St. Martin survived but was left with a gastrocutaneous fistula (an abnormal connection between stomach and skin) that never healed, and he agreed to participate in Beaumont's experiments on gastric juices. (By 1823, English physician William Prout (1785-1850), had proved gastric secretions contained hydrochloric acid). Between 1825 and 1834 Beaumont conducted a series of digestive experiments employing bits of food tied to a string. He published his findings in *Experiments and Observations on the Gastric Juice and the Physiology of Digestion* (1833).

In America at the turn of the 19th century, those physicians who sought surgical skill from the masters travelled to Europe. Those who did not go abroad to study, who were predominantly self-taught, learned surgical procedures from books. Successful surgeons in private practice had no practical or financial incentives to share or teach techniques. It was not until 1899 that William Halsted at Johns Hopkins, a teaching institution with salaried teachers, recognized the value of structuring a formal course of study in surgery and established a surgical residency program, regarded as a momentous evolutionary development in the history of surgery.

Samuel David Gross (1805-1884) wrote *Elements of Pathological Anatomy* in 1839 and a two-volume *System of Surgery* in 1859. In 1856 he was named Professor of Surgery at the Thomas Jefferson Medical College in Philadelphia, Pennsylvania, where he garnered fame for his innovative treatment of trauma and his many writings on the genito-urinary system. However, throughout his lifetime, he remained a steadfast opponent of antisepsis – disparaging referred to as Listerism. Gross was immortalized by Thomas Eakins (1844-1916) in an acclaimed monumental (8 ft by 6 ft, 6 in) painting, *The Gross Clinic*, which now hangs in the Philadelphia Museum of Art. A reproduction is at Jefferson University.

Two other important surgical innovations appeared in the latter half of the 19th century. One was the artery clamp (1862) designed by French surgeons Eugene Koeberlé (1828-1915) and Jules Péan (1830-1898) that permitted stemming the flow of blood without damaging the fragile artery. The other involved pathologists Johann Veit (1852–1917) and Carl Ruge (1846-1926). In 1878 they demonstrated that a large number of unnecessary surgeries were being performed for presumed cervical cancer. They acknowledged that a simple visual and tactile examination was insufficient for accurate diagnosis, and devised the frozen biopsy of the cervix that more accurately determined whether the patient presented with cervical cancer or a more benign condition treatable without resection. Thereafter the frozen section became the standard for questionable cancer resection of all tissues. In Germany, with animal experimentation Gustav Simon (1824-1876) showed that excretion remains functional with one healthy kidney. In 1869 he performed the first successful planned nephrectomy on a human patient. Together with Bernhad von Langenbeck (1810-1887) and Richard von Volkmann (1830-1889) he founded the journal *Deutsche Gesellschaft für Chirurgie* in 1872.

Orthopedics also witnessed innovations, now in common use. In 1852 Dutch Army surgeon, Antonius Mathijsen (1805-1878) first used plaster of paris to immobilize fractures, then Carl Hansmann (1852-1917), in 1886 first applied screws and plates for fixing broken bones. Geghard Küntsher (1900-1972) introduced the intramedullary nail for long bone fractures in 1939.

With greater understanding of pathology, anesthesia that allowed prolonged procedures, new instruments and aseptic measures, surgeons, endowed with newfound confidence, were able to operate on the peritoneal cavity – an area of the body that had been previously too risky to attempt electively. Among the pioneers of abdominal surgery was the aforementioned Theodor Billroth from Bergen, Prussia, who resected in the esophagus in 1872, the larynx in 1873 and the bowel in 1878. In 1881 he removed the pylorus with partial gastrectomy for carcinoma, a procedure Péan had unsuccessfully attempted. Billroth effectively sutured the remnant stomach pouch to the duodenum, a method that is now called the "Billroth II" procedure. His *Allgemeine chirurgische pathologie und therapie* (1863) was translated into ten languages.

French surgeon Mathieu Taboulay (1860-1913) introduced side-to-side gastroduodenostomy and in 1894 performed the first hemipelvectomy. Taboulay experimented with vascular anastomosis and among his students was Alexis Carrel.

American, Charles McBurney (1845-1913) also specialized in abdominal surgery and as chief surgeon at Roosevelt hospital in 1888 began novel studies in appendicitis. He described progression, presenting symptoms and signs and defined the point of greatest tenderness – now called McBurney's point. He described operative incisions and surgical techniques of various abdominal operations.

One of the most common and seemingly uncomplicated ailments – the inguinal hernia – remained problematic for surgeons of the period. Although the anatomy of the inguinal region was well known, as were the types of hernia and their complications, surgical repair was faulty, and recurrences and complications were common. Even with asepsis and anesthesia, repairs at best resulted in temporary relief, with nearly a one hundred percent recurrence within four years. An innovative surgical approach by Edoardo Bassini (1844-1924) from Pavia reversed the statistics, and other surgeons adopted Bassini's technique (described in the *Archiv fur Klinische Chururgie*, 1890), referring to it as the "triple layer" repair.

American J. Marion Sims (1813-1883) successfully corrected congenital malformations such as club feet and harelips. In 1855 he opened the New York Women's Hospital that catered specifically to "female troubles." In 1878 he performed a cholecystectomy. His observations regarding the case were original and insightful at the time. Sims mainly left his mark in the field of gynecology. He devised a vaginal speculum, introduced the knee-chest "Sims position" for pelvic exams and pioneered the repair of vesico-vaginal fistulas.

Gynecology and obstetrics became recognized surgical subspecialties. Englishman Thomas Wells (1818-1897) performed his first ovariotomy in 1857 and by 1881 reported on one thousand cases of ovariotomy to the Royal Medical and Surgical Society, boasting that in the last one hundred cases mortality was just eleven percent. Wells was one of the earliest surgeons to make common use of anesthesia.

Robert Tait (1845-1899) performed a hysterectomy in 1871 and then risked treating a hitherto catastrophic clinical condition – ruptured ectopic pregnancy – which was almost always a death knell. By 1888 he had reported thirty-nine cases, with only two mortalities.

Karl S. Crede (1819-1892) developed original obstetric techniques such as placental expression (1861) and introduced silver nitrate for the treatment of newborn ophthalmia neonatorum. Early in the century that followed, the diagnosis of a great gynecological scourge – cervical cancer – was greatly facilitated by the cytodiagnostic vaginal smear designed by George Nicholas Papanicolaou (1883-1962).

Except for the trephine employed to relieve pressure without penetrating the dura, the skull was rarely entered without fatal consequences. Asepsis facilitated cutting into the skull with a reasonable chance of success. It was the beginning of the field of neurosurgery. In 1879 William Macewen (1848-1924) of Glasgow reported successfully removing a meningioma. Ten years later another innovator, Victor Horsley (1857-1916), expanded the scope of neurological surgery by removing a spinal tumor employing laminectomy. Thereafter he became skilled in the treatment of injuries to the spine and the skull. He was the first to use intra-operative electro-stimulation to localize epileptic foci. In 1908, together with Robert Clarke (1860-1926), he devised a stereotactic guide and technique used in animal experiments to localize lesions with exactitude.

Another pioneer was Norwegian Wilhelm Magnus (1871-1929), who in 1908 removed an epileptogenic tumor from a patient. Over the next twenty years he performed over one hundred and eighty-nine brain surgeries, removing supratentorial tumors (cerebral region) with a mortality rate of 7.7 percent and infratentorial tumors (cerebellar region) with a mortality of 17.8 percent.*

Progress in neurosurgery in America was chiefly due to the work of Harvey Cushing (1869-1939), considered the greatest neurosurgeon of the twentieth century and called the Father of American Neurosurgery. He learned his surgical techniques from Halsted at Johns Hopkins and neurosurgery in England and Germany. Upon a review of Hopkins' hospital

---

*The treatment of epilepsy took a curious and provocative turn in 1866 when Isaac Baker Brown (1811-1873) suggested clitoridectomy for a cure. Great controversy arose and Brown's career ended when he was accused of performing the procedure without patient consent. At their meeting in 1887, the Obstetrical Society expelled him from membership.

records, Cushing realized the diagnosis of brain tumor was rarely made antemortem and that when intervention was attempted, the surgery was almost universally fatal. Cushing began his career in neurosurgery using Halsted's asepsis methodology and moved to Peter Bent Brigham Hospital in Boston. He became Professor of Surgery at Harvard and, from 1933 on, Professor at Yale University. Cushing operated on the friable tissue of the brain with success, employing critical hemostasis with cotton pledgets and tiny silver clips, using layered interrupted fine silk sutures, and he scrupulously avoided shock by constant monitoring of blood pressure. With each surgical procedure his skill improved, so that by the end of his career he had removed over two thousand tumors with an overall mortality of 8.7 percent. He wrote extensively on brain tumors (and a Pulitzer Prize winning biography of Sir William Osler). He was renowned as a teacher who trained an entire next generation of neurosurgeons who themselves became eminent worldwide.

The monitoring of blood pressure, so crucial to Cushing's operative cautions, was the result of an international effort that had spanned more than two centuries after Englishman Hales had experimented with animal blood pressure. In 1847 German Karl Ludwig (1816-1895) used his kymograph to record human blood pressure obtained through a catheter inserted into an artery. Fifty years of study to devise a noninvasive method to measure blood pressure yielded unsatisfactory results. Samuel Siegfried von Basch (1837-1905) in 1881 had designed a kymographic unit that recorded radial artery pressure at the wrist uninvasively, but the unit was large and unwieldy. Then, Italian Scipione Riva-Rocci (1863-1937) constructed the now familiar mercury sphygmomanometer in 1896. Cushing traveled to Italy specifically to meet Riva-Rocci and brought back a sphygmomanometer to America for use in his operating room. The use of the instrument was furthered by the description in 1905 of the pulsating tones by Russian Nicolai Korotkov(1874-1920).

Medicine
In the 19th century English clinicians assimilated the concepts of Laennec and Bichat and melded them into the clinical matrix developed by Sydenham. Richard Bright (1789-1858) was one of the impressive numbers of great physicians at Guy's Hospital in London who differentiated renal dropsy from the cardiac form. He correlated urinary signs with physical signs and with autopsy findings to define chronic renal disease. His description of acute glomerulonephritis was for generations known as Bright's disease.

Bright, Addison and Hodgkin inaugurated an era of clinicopathological study, a bedrock of modern medical practice. Together with Addison, Bright published the first volume of a textbook of medicine:

Elements of the Practice of Medicine. Surprisingly, the book had little success and the proposed second volume was never published.

Thomas Addison (1793-1860) is recognized for his characterization of chronic adrenal insufficiency and pernicious anemia, but he made other important contributions. He published a thorough account of appendiceal abscess in "Inflammation of the caecum and appendix vermiformis," and described biliary cirrhosis, originally discussed by dermatologist Pierre-François-Olive Rayer (1793-1867) in *Traité théorique et pratique des maladies de la peau* (1835). Addison developed an interest in dermatology and founded a department at Guy's Hospital devoted to the discipline. His wax model collection of skin diseases is extant. "On a certain affection of the skin, vitilogoidea plana tuberose," he described the xanthomata of hypercholesterolemia, and, with William Gull (1816-1890), he described xanthoma diabeticorum and circumscribed scleroderma (morphoea).

In 1832, in an essay entitled "On Some Morbid Appearances of the Absorbent Glands and Spleen," Thomas Hodgkin (1798-1866), pathologist at Guy's hospital, described the disease we now know as Hodgkin's lymphoma, a malignancy that affects the spleen, liver, lymphoid tissue and other tissues. His *Morbid Anantomy of Serous and Mucous Membranes* (1829) became a respected text in modern pathology. Hodgkin left another significant mark in the field of preventive medicine in 1841 with his publication *On the Means of Promoting and Preserving Health.*

About this time the status that Edinburgh enjoyed as a center of medical training began to decline and Irish schools began to ascend in prestige. Dublin drew students from all over the world, due in no small measure to the lectures of Robert Graves (1796-1853) and William Stokes (1804-1878). Peripatetic Graves spent several years studying in the capitals of Europe where he became impressed with the manner of bedside clinical instruction. Upon his return to Ireland he inspired Stokes to join him in changing the pedagogy. They developed and taught methodologies for most effectively interviewing patients to obtain a complete medical history, taught the techniques of Auenbrugger and Laennec and the proper and succinct method to record clinical notes. In 1843 Graves published *Clinical Lectures on the Practice of Medicine* which was well received all over Europe. Trousseau wrote the introduction to the French edition, and suggested that exophthalmic goiter – the syndrome of hyperthyroidism – be called Graves' disease. Graves broke the universal rule of "starve a fever" by demonstrating that fasting in no way diminished fever but only served to weaken the patient. He playfully suggested his epitaph be "He fed fever."

Stokes evolved a special interest in the heart and lungs and wrote two significant works, *A Treatise on the Diagnosis and Treatment of Diseases of the Chest* (1837) and *The Diseases of the Heart and Aorta*

(1854). The references to Cheyne-Stokes breathing (agonal breathing) and Stokes-Adams disease (transient syncope) endure.

John Cheyne (1777-1836) was a Scotsman who joined the Dublin school in County Meath. With Stokes, he is credited with perceptive description of agonal breathing. As a pediatrist, Cheyne wrote *Essays of Diseases of Children* in 1801 and in 1809 *Pathology of the Membrane of the Larynx and Bronchia*.

In 1832 Dominic Corrigan (1802-1880) published *On Permanent Patency of the Mouth of the Aorta*, which incisively described aortic regurgitation. He described the accompanying *bruit de soufflé* and *fremissement* felt at the carotid and chest. Memorably, during the Irish famine, Corrigan endeavored to persuade the English government to provide wholesome food to the starving populace: "The generation that has suffered cannot again be what it has been...and the offspring will inherit for generations to come the weakness of body and apathy of mind which famine and fever have engendered." All the same, Corrigan accepted the position of physician-in-ordinary to Queen Victoria and the title of Baronet of the Empire – honors rarely bestowed on Catholics.

James McKenzie (1853-1925) of Edinburgh devised the polygraph that allowed cardiac studies to simultaneously record the jugular and apex pulses, a modality that helped to classify cardiac arrhythmias. While Cushing introduced the sphygmomanometer into the operating room, P.C. Potain (1825-1901), who was the first to classify gallops in *Theorie du bruit de gallop* (1885), recognized its value at the hospital bedside.

The dawn of the stethoscope in 1819 and the evolving understanding of cardiac anatomy and pathology gave a new impetus to auscultation of the chest for both pulmonary and cardiac disease. All heart sounds were scrutinized and an eponymous list of heart murmurs entered the medical vocabulary. Beginning alphabetically, the Austin Flint (1812-1886) murmur, a mid-diastolic rumble, was associated with aortic regurgitation. Barlow's syndrome murmur named after John Barlow (1924-2008) is heard secondary to mitral valve prolapsed. Described in 1968 it can be asymptomatic or cause palpitations and syncope. Robert Cabot (1868-1939) and Frank Locke (1871-1949) in 1905 described the diastolic murmur of severe anemia which disappears with treatment. Carey Coombs' (1879-1932) book *Rheumatic Heart Disease* (1924) was based on over 600 cases in which he described a mid-systolic murmur of an inflamed mitral valve. William Dock (1898-1990) in 1967 reported a diastolic murmur due to a stenotic left coronary artery and in 1906 George Gibson (1854-1913) described the continuous murmur of persistent ductus arteriosus. The Graham Steell (1851-1942) of pulmonary insufficiency was also found by George Balfour (1823-1903), but Steell published several in depth papers on the murmur and thus carries his name. Charles Aston Key (1793-1849) worked with Thomas Hodgkin and the two together described the murmur of syphilitic aortitis – a raspy diastolic sound now eponymously referred to as the Key-Hodgkin murmur. Henri-Louis Roger (1809-1891) named the holosystolic murmur of ventricular septal defect. Finally, Still's murmur is named after the Father of British Pediatrics, George Frederick Still (1868-1941). It is a long systolic ejection musical murmur which is benign and believed to arise in the chordate tendineae or from an aortic gush.

The thermometer, an experimental device since the 1600s, finally became widely used in hospitals about the 1870s and, in the process, revolutionized the understanding of the body's physiologic response to infection. For centuries fever had been considered a disease entity and texts entirely dedicated to the different kinds of temperature elevation had been written. Books described fevers that were ephemeral, putrid, hectic, continuous, tertian, quartan, and quotidian, fevers that were simple childhood conceits and fevers that came with the heat of adult passions. Experiments with primitive oral thermometer had led Santorio Santorius in 1614 to attribute the cause of fever to abnormal metabolism.

In 1714, Gabriel Fahrenheit (1686-1736) improved the reliability of the alcohol thermometer by substituting mercury that allowed more accurate calibration. The improved device permitted a narrower range of temperature measurement between ninety-five to one hundred and eight degrees. Nevertheless, the clinical significance of body temperature did not become apparent until 1868 when Carl Reinhold Wunderlich (1815-1877) wrote *Das Verhalten der Eigenwarme in Krankheiten* (*Medical Thermometry*). This seminal work explained the importance of temperature as a harbinger of disease and, most importantly, identified a measurable unit – the degree – as a correlate of disease gravity. Medical historian Fielding Garrison (1870-1935) commented that Wunderlich "found fever a disease and left it a symptom." Only when Thomas Clifford Allbutt (1836-1925) invented the short clinical thermometer in 1867 in the now familiar form of a small glass capillary tube with a bulbous end, however, did the thermometer become a practical clinical aid that replaced the cumbersome foot-long contrivance that had required hand support and an interminable twenty minutes wait before registering a temperature.

In Baltimore, Maryland, William Osler (1849-1919) became the first Johns Hopkins University Professor of Medicine, and as such became a part of a formidable coalition of scientists at this institution: pathologist William Henry Welch (1850-1934), gynecologist Howard Kelly (1858-1943) and the surgeon William Stewart Halsted. Osler described multiple syndromes, but carved his name in medical history for his description of platelets, as a widely acclaimed teacher of basic medical principles and for his landmark book, *Principles and Practice of Medicine* (1892), which was medical study's core text until 1950, when Tinsley Harrison (1900-1978) published *Principles of Internal Medicine* (now in its seventeenth edition). In 1904, his legacy secure, Osler left Hopkins to assume the position of Regius Professor of Medicine at Oxford University, a position held until his death.

Abraham Flexner's (1866-1959) 1910 report on the condition of the American medical schools advocated the Johns Hopkins University model designed by Billings, Welch and Osler. He cited it as the pedagogical model that would make study of the basic sciences axial to the medical curriculum. This adopted model of medical education dismantled the extant apprentice-system.

America's evolution in medicine was an idiosyncratic gallimaufry. While most of the scientific advances reported from Europe were accepted favorably, in many quarters traditional American medical education and methodology were challenged. With medical giants emerging in pedagogy and clinical and academic progress on the gallop, nevertheless, America had a core of eccentric nonconformists who believed traditional medicine was at best ineffectual and at worst harmful and they spurned it and every new medical breakthrough, foreign and domestic, in almost every specialty.

Sylvester Graham (1794-1851), a Presbyterian minister from Connecticut, eschewed the commonly accepted medical practices and advocated a vegetarian diet, temperance and sexual restraint to sustain good health. He produced a tasty additive-free graham cracker that continues to be stocked on grocery shelves, albeit with modern chemical additives. His considerable numbers of disciples "Grahamites" followed *The New Hydropathic Cookbook* (1855).

Several mavericks with large followings and ideologies that deviated from mainstream medical thought and practice of the times have persisted, but only after significantly amending their theories to conform to sound prevailing clinical norms. Andrew Taylor Still (1828-1917) believed that the proper alignment of the musculoskeletal system was essential to good health, and he developed a system he called osteopathic manipulative medicine. His theory was a good one, but only when it was conjoined with the theories and practice of mainstream medicine did it evolve into a well respected field of medical practice that is current and flourishing. Still was a strong proponent of preventive medicine.

Daniel David Palmer (1845-1913) popularized the treatment of misaligned vertebrae and major joints. He focused on determining a unifying cause of all disease and concluded that a subluxed vertebra caused ninety-five percent of all maladies and the other five percent were due to other dislocated joints. In 1897 he founded a school of chiropractic medicine, and his method is widely practiced in our time as an alternative therapy outside the medical mainstream.

Mary Baker Eddy (1821-1910) decreed all illness originated in the spirit and the mind and that one could cure oneself of illness by divine inspiration, reading scripture and sustaining a strong will to be cured. She founded a religious sect called Church of Christ Scientist which shuns all medical intervention and remains extant although controversies regarding the care of children has seen Church members steadily dwindled for the last sixty years.

Dermatology

Englishman Robert Willan (1757-1812) advanced the discipline of dermatology and syphilology. He treated a plethora of skin pathology at the London Carey Street dispensary for 20 years. Willan differentiated lupus from eczema. He published *Cutaneous Diseases* in 1808 in which he established a classification system for dermatology, grouping lesions by appearance. About the same period Jean Louis-Marc Alibert (1768-1837) a student of Desault, Bichat and Pinel, administered to patients with syphilis, leprosy and skin ailments, and developed a classification system for skin diseases published in *Descriptions de maladies de la peau* (1806) and *Monographie des Dermatoses* (1835). Fellow Frenchman Philip Ricord (1799-1889) distinguished gonorrhea from syphilis in *Traité pratique des Maladies vénériennes* (1838) and described the three stages of Lues and the nature of the chancre. Ferdinand von Hebra (1816-1880) of Vienna devised a system of dermatology based on pathology. His *Atlas der Hautkrankeiten* (1860) was liberally illustrated with remarkably colored and detailed plates of many skin diseases. His coauthor was Moritz Kaposi (1837-1902) who described the sarcoma now know to be caused by a specific herpesvirus.

For most of the 19th and well into the 20th century dermatology was mostly a descriptive discipline in which lesions were classified and various emollients, lotions and astringents applied. Gradually excision, dermabrasion, cryosurgery and anti-inflammatory were introduced as major treatment modalities and, starting in the 1980s, the laser was used to remove pigmented lesions, tattoos, hair and for cosmetic resurfacing.

Neurology

In neurology the outstanding figure of the 19th century was Jean Martin Charcot (1825-1893), clinician and teacher at Salpêtrière, who became the Founder of Modern Neurology. Several conditions were named after him: Charcot's joint (diabetic arthropathy), Charcot's disease (amyotrophic lateral sclerosis) and Charcot-Marie-Tooth disease (peroneal muscular atrophy). The physicians he trained are part of his legacy to medicine. Among them are Sigmund Freud (see ahead), George Gilles de la Tourette (1857-1904), Alfred Binet (1857-1911), Pierre Marie (1853-1940), and Joseph Babinski (1857-1932).

Pierre Marie, professor at Paris, was Charcot's great pupil. He described many new entities, among them peroneal muscular dystrophy, congenital cerebellar ataxia and hypertrophic pulmonary arthropathy, or clubbing. Babinski is recognized today for his eponymous toe sign which he wrote about in 1896. His short 28 line report simply stated: "In certain cases of paralysis, the toes on the affected side, instead of flexing when the sole is stimulated, execute an extensor movement." As a student he challenged Charcot and openly disagreed with his professor's reliance on medical history and observation for diagnosis. Babinski insisted thorough physical and neurologic examinations were also essential components for a correct diagnosis, separating organic or somatic disease from the functional or psychological.

In 1884 Tourette described nine patients with multiple involuntary motor and vocal tics that were repetitive and rapid. He labeled the disorder "maladie des tics." Charcot, impressed by Tourette's insightful report, renamed the malady Tourette's illness, now universally referred to as Tourette syndrome.

Binet became famous as a psychologist and today his name is immediately recognized as the developer of the test that determines IQ scores (1905).

English surgeon, geologist and paleontologist James Parkinson (1755-1824) is best remembered for *An Essay on the Shaking Palsy* (1817) in which he rendered this description of neurodegenerative paralysis agitans: [the patient demonstrates] "Involuntary tremulous motion, with lessened muscular power, in parts not in action and even when supported; with a propensity to bend the trunk forward, and to pass from a walking to a running pace: the senses and intellects being uninjured." His most remarkable work, however, was in his other passion – paleontology – and was called *Organic Remains of a Former World* (1804).

Alois Alzheimer first saw patient "Auguste D," a 51 year old female in 1901. She had become forgetful, frequently got lost and had progressive memory loss. She died in 1906 and Alzheimer performed an autopsy noting general brain atrophy and in micropathology "peculiar changes of the neurofibrils …clustering together in thick bundles which emerged at the surface of the cell and miliary foci distinguishable by the deposit in the cerebral cortex of an peculiar substance which can be recognized without stain and is, in fact, very refractory to staining." Thereafter, sporadic cases were described by others, who along with Alzheimer believed they were atypical cases of senile dementia, but Emil Kraepelin recognized a difference and coined "Alzheimer disease" as a presenile dementia with rapid progression, young onset and distinct pathology.

In 1881, Italian physiologist Angelo Mosso (1846-1910) was attending to a patient with frontal cranial bone trauma when he noted cerebral artery pulsations increase as church bells were ringing in the distance. He checked the patient's peripheral pulse and blood pressure which remained unchanged then asked the patient what he was thinking about to which he replied, it was time for prayer. Thus Mosso correlated blood flow with mental activity, the basis of the modern cerebral PET neuroimaging.

German Adolph Kussmaul (1822-1902), a pupil of Virchow, was an extraordinary observer and innovative clinician who was the first to report a series of conditions: "word blindness" or dyslexia, polyarteritis nodosa, progressive bulbar paralysis and embolism to the mesentery. The Kussmaul sign is a paradoxical rise in the jugular-venous pressure on inhalation that often is associated with constrictive pericarditis and chronic obstructive pulmonary disease. Kussmaul breathing is seen with severe diabetic ketoacidosis. He pioneered gastric lavage and performed the first gastroscopy when in 1868 he inserted a gastroscope into a patient's throat. The man, as it happens, was a sword-swallower – a factor that may have facilitated the procedure.

Guillaume Duchenne (1806-1875) made several valuable observations on many new diseases such as progressive bulbar palsy and pseudohypertrophic muscular paralysis. He was, curiously enough, also an advocate of physiognomy and phrenology, and believed that the human face and features could be codified and classified to reveal a taxonomy of inner being. His thinking was a reference to a concept that not had been seriously considered in medicine after Franz Gall. He experimented on human subjects, applying electrodes and contorting facial muscles into grotesque expressions which he then meticulously photographed and classified, convinced the face revealed the soul.

John Hughlings Jackson (1835-1911) was a founding neurologist at the National Hospital for the Paralyzed and Epileptic. Rather than positing specific brain centers and/or autonomic reflexes as causal, he believed the disintegration of higher functions – cognitive thought, memory, speech, etc. as fundamental to clinical nervous ailments, his – "dissolution theory" – thus integrating neurology with psychiatry and evolution.

Histological staining methods for both fixed tissues and vital staining had advanced significantly, but analysis of the nervous system tissue was beyond the method's capabilities. Conventional staining techniques highlighted the cell nucleus, but the dendritic processes could not be seen. Camillo Golgi (1843-1926) from Pavia introduced the silver stain which made the dendrites and cytoplasmic inclusions highly visible. His work was expanded by Santiago Ramon y Cajal (1852-1934) who analyzed the network of cells and proposed a cytological structure for the central nervous system. In 1906 Cajal and Golgi shared the Nobel prize for the neurohistology work that facilitated further research into synaptic transmission. Wilhelm His (1831-1904), already recognized for his embryological research, and Charles Sherrington (1857-1952) formulated a theory that axon transmission is cellulifugal and dendrite cellulipetal, which led to the concept of synapse and reflex-arc function – synaptic transmission, the process whereby nerve impulses are conveyed.

Access into the spinal dural space for relief of increased cerebral pressure was first described by Walter Essex Wynter (1860-1945) who in 1891 in the *Lancet* reported on four tubercular cases with increased pressure. Wynter made a small incision down to the dura, then introduced a Reginald Southey (1835-1899) tube for drainage. Heinrich Quincke (1842-1922) acknowledged Wynter's work, but improved on the process by inserting a "very fine cannula 2 cm deep between the 3rd and 4th lumbar spinal arches." Once access to cerebral spinal space was simplified, analysis of the fluid aided in confirming diagnosis and culturing for microbes.

A new class of nervous system disease, degenerative neuropathy, would enter the medical vocabulary in the 20th century. An umbrella term for generally slow and progressive disintegration of neurons it included *inter alia* amyotrophic lateral sclerosis, Parkinson, Alzheimers, and Creutzfeldt-Jakob disease. Some are caused by abnormal deposition of protein within neurons and are called tauopathies, of which Alzheimers is a common example. Others may be caused by prions – misfolded transmissible proteins – as is the case for the spongiform encephalopathy named after Hans Creutzfeld (1885-1964) and Alfons Jakob (1884-1931). The prion was discovered and named by Stanley B. Prusiner (b. 1942) by combining "proteinaceous" and "infectious."

Endoscopy

In 1805 Philipp Bozzini (1773-1809) had described an apparatus he called a *lichtleiter* (light guider) that consisted of a candle, a reflecting mirror and a cannula for examining orifices, particularly the urethra and rectum. It was largely ignored at the time. Fifty years later Antoine Desormeaux (1815-1894) used the apparatus and improved it by employing a gas arc lamp that gave a more reliable, strong, light. With these crude beginnings endoscopy began to take form.

In 1877 Max Nitze (1848-1906) and Josef Leiter (1830-1892) invented the cystourethroscope which made possible a careful examination of the urethra and bladder. Other specialists took notice and by simply altering the design of the cannula or speculum, a thorough examination of the ear, nose, pharynx, stomach, rectum and vagina also became possible.

George Kelling (1866-1945) of Dresden in 1901 injected air into the abdomen of a dog that resulted in a pneumoperitoneum, and inserted a cystoscope to study the dog's viscera, a procedure that was referred to as "closed cavity" endoscopy. Ten years later Swede Han Christian Jacobaeus (1879-1937) published on his experiments with human laparoscopy, "The Possibilities for Performing Cystoscopy in Examination of Serous

Cavities," that introduced the revolutionary laparoscope as a diagnostic and operative tool. Arthroscopy closely followed. Severin Nordentoft (1866-1922), from Denmark, in 1912 presented a paper before a Berlin congress of surgeons entitled "Endoscopy of Closed Cavities by the Means of my Trokart-Endoscope" in which he described the internal structure of the knee.

Pediatrics

The most common chromosomal abnormality in children was named after John Langdon Down (1828-1896) who in 1862 rendered the best description of the syndrome. Jérôme Lejeune (1926-1994) and Marthe Gautier (b. 1925) discovered the cause as trisomy 21.

In the 19th century more than twenty-five textbooks on pediatrics were published. The pediatrist had come of age. Abraham Jacobi (1830-1919), considered the "Father of American Pediatrics," was instrumental in establishing hospitals for children throughout the nation:

> My plea is for the establishment of children's hospitals....Infants, who are so much more liable to be taken with acute and life-endangering maladies than the class we generally meet with in hospitals, are not admitted. Thus, those who require most aid receive none.

Jacobi received the first appointment in academic pediatrics in America at New York Medical College in 1860. In 1879, he successfully lobbied Congress to fund the publication of John Shaw Billings' (1838-1913) *Index Medicus*, and the following year he organized a pediatric section of the American Medical Association (AMA). A prolific writer, Jacobi published books on teething, intestinal diseases, the thymus gland and a three edition book on infant diet. Among his more important monographs were studies on diphtheria and intubation, intestinal obstructions and infant nutrition. In 1909 Jacobi's published works were compiled into eight volumes.

A common pediatric problem, the swallowed or aspirated foreign body, was studied by otolaryngologist Chevalier Jackson (1865-1958) who developed instruments for their extraction which he accomplished successfully without anesthesia nearly 5000 times.

Several physicians, beginning in 1860, contrived incubators to save premature infants. Their success was compelling and the equipment evolved from units that simply provided a warm and humid environment to sophisticated automated machines that sustained an infant's fragile life until incubation was no longer necessary. Karl Franz Crede (1819-1892) designed an immobile model in 1860, and Thomas Morgan Rotch (1849-

1914) designed a mobile unit in 1893 capable of being employed in different areas of a hospital. Stephan Tarnier (1828-1897) and Pierre Budin (1846-1907) made a very simple incubator in 1883 that could be duplicated with facility (Fig. 25). At that time most units were designed to hold more than one newborn. Pierre Auvard (1855-1941) designed a model for one infant.

Despite the long established awareness of the degree to which prematurity contributed to infant mortality, physicians, particularly proponents of social Darwinism, initially resisted the use of incubators. R.S. Ransom detailed their rationale in the Minnesota *Northwestern Lancet*, December 15, 1898:

> It is maintained by some that it is inconsistent with the best physical development of the men and women of our nation to rear these little creatures, it being assumed that they will have impaired physical vigor and transmit this to their offspring.

Popular acceptance of the incubator did not occur until the 20th century and only after public pressure. Awareness about the success of the incubators increased as a result of magazine and journal articles on mothering that described the innovation.*

Nutrition

The progenitor of the discipline of nutrition began with the work of Antoine Lavoisier, who as had been noted, was famous for his studies of oxygen and oxidation in the 18th century. His experiments with "biological combustion" were in effect the precursor to the calorimeter. Lavoisier placed a guinea pig into a bi-shelled chamber containing ice on the outside. The metabolic heat produced by the guinea pig melted the ice, and the collected water, when

---

*In 1896, Martin Couney (1860?-1950) had been asked by his old mentor, Pierre Budin, to arrange an exhibit of incubators for the Berlin World Exposition in the hope of enlisting public support for their use in hospitals. Couney obliged with six incubators, a group of nurses and six tiny babies from the Berlin Charité. The public display, called *Kinderbrutanstalt* was an instant sensation that drew huge crowds that paid to see what clearly was a human hatchery sideshow. Couney got whiff of a windfall. The exhibit moved on to London (1897), Omaha (1898), Paris (1900), Buffalo (1901) and St. Louis (1904) and finally, became an annual feature at Coney Island, New York. Thousands of dollars were generated by as many as three thousand patrons a day who wanted to see premature babies in incubators. Couney had exhibits in San Francisco in 1915, Chicago in 1933 and at the New York World Fair in 1939, all of them successful ventures.

measured, reflected calorimetric expenditure, so that 1 kg of melted ice equated to 80 kcal of heat. From this experiment Lavoisier construed that metabolism was "*une combustion.*" Lavoisier's idea of metabolic conversion inspired Justus von Liebig (1803-1873) as he studied food groups and their caloric values. Gradually the concept of proper nutrition and those foods that defined it emerged and with it the realization that some diseases were triggered by specific deficiencies. A case in point is scurvy, long a scourge of seafaring men. The nutritional cause of scurvy had been confirmed by John Woodall (1570-1643). As early as 1617 in *The Surgeon's Mate*, he accurately described scurvy, and posited that lemons were both preventive and curative of the disease. His recommendation that lemons be added to sailors' diet, however, was ignored by the Admiralty and scurvy persisted. It was not until 130 years later, in 1747, that British Navy physician James Lind (1716-1794), while serving aboard the *HMS Salisbury*, conducted an experiment on twelve scorbutic sailors whose symptoms included bleeding gums, skin hemorrhages and loose teeth. He divided them into six pairs with a shared basic diet. He supplemented one different food to each pair's dietary regime: cider, seawater, garlic, mustard/horseradish, vinegar and a citric fruit – an orange or a lemon. Those who had been given citrus developed no scurvy. Although his data was persuasive, it took the Admiralty ten years to add lemon juice to the diet of sailors at sea (1757). The essential ingredient in citrus – vitamin C – remained unidentified until, in 1928, Albert Szent-Gyorgyi (1893-1986) isolated it.

John Grant Malcolmson (d. 1844) in Madras, India, in 1835 chronicled the symptoms of beriberi; fifty-two years later, in 1887, Dutch physiologist Christiaan Eijkman (1858-1930) recognized it as a nutritional deficiency disease. Eijkman had been sent to Indonesia to study the puzzling condition that was marked by lethargy, weakness and congestive heart failure. He noticed from chance observation that chickens fed polished rice developed symptoms of peripheral neuropathy. When he fed the chickens unpolished rice, the fowls recovered, leading Eijkman to surmise that an "anti-beriberi factor" was unknowingly being removed from polished rice during decortication. Fifteen years later, in 1912, Casimir Funk (1884-1967) isolated the missing compound and called it thiamine. He noticed it was a "vital amine" and coined the word "vitamin" from it.

Laboratory studies, slow and methodical, had up to that time used large farm animals such as sheep in experiments. In 1912 Elmer Verner McCollum (1879-1967) began to use small animal models such as mice and rats, whose more rapid metabolism and shorter normal life spans were more suitable for laboratory research. Using the rat model, McCollum discovered vitamin A. McCollum also demonstrated that vitamin D prevented rickets.

Biochemist Frederick Gowland Hopkins (1861-1947) in 1901 had discovered the amino acid tryptophan, and in 1912 wrote a seminal article entitled "Feeding Experiments Illustrating the Importance of Accessory Food Factors in Normal Dietaries," published in *The Journal of Physiology*. His work, and that of Eijkman, was ground-breaking, and both were credited for their vital contributions to the elucidation of specific vitamin factors in foods. A surge of vitamin and specific nutrient discoveries flowed into the twentieth century (Appendix D).

Milk, a major source of nutrition – particularly for children – nevertheless by 1870 was noted by members of the international medical community to cause significant morbidity. As early as 1874, Otto von Bollinger (1843-1909) from Munich had demonstrated that milk could carry tuberculosis. Ignorance, poverty and poor hygiene exacerbated the illnesses caused by contaminated milk. The containers from which infants sucked were problematic. Nursing bottles, made from blown glass, pewter or pottery were not always properly cleaned, as was the case with nipples of chamois and pickled calf teat. Rubber nipples that had been introduced in 1840 were easier to clean.

It was only gradually recognized that these feeding devises also harbored bacteria, as did contaminated milk that commonly caused infectious diarrheas, dehydration and death in children. In 1886 German chemist Franz von Soxhlet (1848-1926) successfully applied Pasteur's process to milk, and in 1891 proposed a simple method to sterilize milk bottles in the home. Decades would pass before germ free milk was widely used. Henry Chapin (1857-1942), from the New York Infirmary, in 1893 presented a paper in which he described milk studied after being centrifuged: "the detritus was found by microscopic examination to contain pus and blood corpuscles, dirt and hair." To save money, some dairies fed their cows residuals from distillery mash that resulted in "swill milk," attributed at the time to some eight thousand infant deaths. Additionally, to increase the yield or to alter the appearance of milk, corrupt dealers added molasses, chalk, and even plaster of Paris. A New York Commission of Health reported in 1902 that fifty-three percent of more than two thousand samples of milk tested were adulterated.

An organized and resolute movement began to remove all contaminants from milk and certify, for the public's edification, that it was safe to drink. Nathan Straus (1848-1931), merchant and philanthropist, with his wife established a private milk pasteurization plant as early as 1892, and began to create certified milk distribution stations. Ultimately there were almost three hundred such stations. They published a book about milk contamination and its dangers. Henry Coit (1854-1917), founder of Babies Hospital in Newark, at the meeting of the pediatric society in 1901 presented a paper that convincingly associated summer epidemics of diarrhea with contaminated milk. Meaningful, effective change occurred, however, only when laws were passed requiring milk be pasteurized and, by 1925, the morbidity and mortality rates for infants and children had dramatically decreased.

Nineteenth century wars, among them the Crimean, Italian War of Independence, and American Civil War resulted in horrendous numbers of dead and wounded. Jean Henri Dunant (1828-1910) witnessed the aftermath of the Battle of Solferino in 1859. Over 5000 died and nearly 30,000 were wounded – bayoneted and shot – sprawled all over the battlefield and unattended. Dunant initiated the organization of the civil population to assist and evacuate the wounded and bury the dead. This experience deeply touched his Calvinistic upbringing and he returned to Geneva where he courted public figures and began talks and negotiations that led ultimately in 1863 to the founding of the International Committee of the Red Cross. The iconic Red Cross symbol is the reversed Swiss national emblem. In Muslim countries the cross was replaced by the crescent. One year later, the diplomatic conference ended in twelve nations signing the first Geneva Convention that guaranteed neutrality and care for wounded soldiers. Dunant received the Nobel Peace Prize in 1901.

19th century Summary

The most critical development of 19th century medicine was the redefinition of the physical examination by Laennec, Auenbrugger and Wunderlich. Physical examination and macro (gross) and microanatomy (histology) became the optimal learning tools, as medicine learned to coordinate patient history and signs and symptoms with pathology. Moreover, this innovative approach definitively ended any remaining schism between physicians and surgeons. Revitalized, the medical profession was once again united. Furthermore, other disciplines and theories were universally accepted. Physiology became the center of the experimental process. The germ theory and asepsis were universally recognized as valid concepts and, together with anesthesia, propelled the modern science of surgery into the 20th century. The study of tropical medicine contributed a vast amount of important assets, including the new concept of insects as disease and parasite vectors. All of the medical advances were recorded in proliferating numbers of specialized medical journals. The facile dissemination of medical news via journals meant that post graduate medical education could be achieved without the need for expensive and time consuming travel.

A scientific domino effect in medicine had become quantifiable in the 19th century. The axiom that discoveries lead to more questions and those to more investigation to more discoveries has particular relevance. A quantum surge in understanding and comprehension of all that went before resulted in clinical progress never equaled in history. The knowledge garnered in this century gained pendulous momentum and, like a medical meteor, slammed into the 20th century with an explosion of new and audacious ingenuity and invention.

VIII: Women in the History of Medicine

Women in the history of medicine stands alone as a chapter to highlight the barriers throughout millennia that prevented women from educational and vocational possibilities. From a 21st century viewpoint, one can only image the potential that was wasted and the frustration and suffering societal dictates caused talented women. A very few – and in disparate fields – broke the gender barricade, and what follows is a beadroll of illustrious persons who, beginning in antiquity, made immeasurable contributions to the care of women and children and to medical education, especially of women. In our more open and less discriminatory modern times, women have joined the ranks of their male counterparts as original and innovative scientists responsible for breakthrough discoveries as well as equal partners in the clinical practice and teaching of medicine.

Historiography of women in medicine begins with historian Gaius Hyginus' (c. 64 BCE-17 CE) *Fabulae* (274:25-35) and his references to Agnodice (fl. 340 BCE) of Alexandria. She was a midwife and gynecologist said to have studied anatomy with Herophilus. Agnodice dressed as a man in order to study and practice, and an anecdote has it that a patient in labor was unwilling to have a man attend her, so Agnodice exposed herself to the woman who only then accepted her administrations. Thereafter Agnodice attracted many female patients. A group of jealous physicians charged her and she was tried, convicted and sentenced to death for "seducing patients." Wives and daughters of the judges and senators and women in general were outraged, and successfully protested the trial and verdict. Consequently, the Ptolemy government changed the law, and women such as Phillista (318-272 BCE), reputed to have been a popular lecturer in medicine, were permitted to study, practice and teach medicine.

Other Greek women active in medicine were spouses of famous men: Theano (c. 546 BCE) was the wife of Pythagoras. She studied mathematics and physik and practiced and taught medicine in her husband's school. Pythias (c. 365-335 BCE), Aristotle's wife, was his assistant who coauthored many of his works in biology and embryology. Artemisia (d. 355 BCE) was queen of Caria. Pliny described her as a healer famous in her time for her great knowledge of botanicals and their effects.

Aspasia of Phoenicia (470-400 BCE), gynecologist and midwife, was mistress of Pericles. Aetius quoted her in his *Tetrabilion*. Her writings were considered among the obstetric standard until the works of Trotula appeared in the 12th century. Among her many accomplishments, Aspasia described fetal positions and recommended hot olive oil and mallow to promote cervical dilatation. She devised contraceptives made from lint wrapped around small pieces of wood soaked in astringents like oak gall, myrrh and wine to insert into the vagina. (Ancient Egyptians used similar disposable contraceptives made from softened papyrus).

The historiography of early Rome, as in Greece, indicates women were active in medicine. No specific names have been recorded but there remain many tomb inscriptions to *medicae* – i.e. woman physicians. Celsus described women in Rome who practiced urinoscopy and leeching and who used poppy juice as anesthesia prior to lancing procedures for boils, abscesses, or bleeding.

The establishment of houses of healing in early history appears to be primarily at the instigation of women. Roman noble woman Fabiola (?-400 CE) studied medicine and opened the first Christian *nosokomeion* in Ostia in the year 390 and another in Rome specifically for the poor. Fabiola had been profoundly influenced by St. Jerome's teachings during his stay in Rome in 382-384, after which she began a life dedicated to the poor and suffering. Of her Jerome said, "How often did she wash the putrid matter from wounds another could not bear to look upon." Eudocia (396-460), wife of Theodosius II (401-450), tetrarch of the Eastern empire, founded hospitals in Jerusalem. She also founded two schools of medicine – one in Syria and one in Edessa. The Merovingian queen, Radegonde (525-587), studied medicine and founded a convent hospital in Poitiers for lepers. She pressed her husband, King Clotaire (497-561) to allow her to take holy orders, and she became abbess to a nunnery that devoted itself to healing.

Women functioned as hospital healers until the Synod of Orleans in 533 that suppressed female deacons "by reason of the frailty of their sex." But within the confines and privileges of monasteries and nunneries, proscription often was not observed. Bridget of Ireland (453-525), Hilda of Whitby (614-680), Berthildis of Chelles (625-702), Mathilda of Quedlinburg (895-968) and Hroswitha of Gandersheim (935-1000) – all abbesses – all practiced healing. Hilda was a particularly gifted polymath who taught and practiced medicine as well as the *trivium* and *quadrivium*.

In the 12th century Age of *Universitas* the famous *mulieres Salernitanae* – the first women professors of medicine – made their appearance. Trotula of Salerno, whose fame in the early Renaissance, known even to Chaucer (1340-1400), has been discussed. In his *Canterbury Tales* Chaucer had the abbess in the Wife of Bath take a copy of Trotula's manuscript to Paris

> In which book eek ther was Tertulan,
> Crisippus, Trotula, and Helowys,
> That was abbesse nat fer fro Parys.
> (*WB* Prol 676-78).

Other professors of medicine, trained at Salerno, were Rebecca Guarna (13th century), Abella (14th century), and Constancza Calenda (c. 1415), who taught about the diseases and surgery of the eye. Guarna used the pseudonym Mercuriade for her papers *On Pestilent Fever, Cure of Wounds, Fevers, On Urine* and *On the Embryo*. Her reputation endured at least a century, and she is said to have been the inspiration for one of Giovanni Boccaccio's (1320?-1375) tales in the *Decameron* (1350-1353). Abella's works include *De atrabile* and *De natura seminis humani*. None of the works of these physicians survive; the Naples archives, however, attest to their existence and licensures. The preamble to their licenses reads:

> "Since, then, the law permits women to exercise the profession of physician, and since, besides, due regard being laid to purity of morals, women are better suited for the treatment of women's diseases, after having received the oath of fidelity, we permit the practice...."

Post Reformation and during the 16th century, the numbers of women as physicians were minimal. As noted, in London's 1651 publication *The Ladies Dispensatory*, English women were confined to service as herbalists, leechers or midwives. At least one woman, Elizabeth, Countess of Kent (1582-1651) circumvented these conventions. She was noted for her medical skills as well as for her midwifery. Posthumously, in 1670, her *Manual of Choice Remedies or Rare Secrets in Physic and Surgery* was published. Its nineteen editions attest to its remarkable success and influence.

In Germany Margarita Fuss (1555-1626) studied medicine in Cologne and Strasbourg. Her fame and talents were such that she was appointed court physician and midwife to the monarchs of *Heiliges Römisches Reich* – Holy Roman Empire.

Marie Colinet (c. 1560 - c. 1640), as mentioned, was the wife of German surgeon Fabry and a skilled midwife and surgeon who devised original modalities of treatment (see above). Louise Bourgeois (1563-1636) wrote *Several Observations on Sterility, Miscarriage, Fertility, Childbirth and the Illnesses of Women and Newborns* (1609). She was midwife to Marie d'Medici (1575-1642) and assistant to Ambroise Paré at the Hôtel Dieu. She recommended rest for hemorrhage, labor induction for placenta praevia and outlined interventions for twelve fetal presentations. She recognized poor nutrition as a factor in anemia and recommended iron for adolescents. Bourgeois appears to be the first to observe and comment on the effects of syphilis on the newborn.*

Early in the seventeenth century, Bologna became a leading center of anatomical studies and during the coldest month of the year, January, the "Ceremony of the Anatomy Lesson" was conducted. Following the public execution of a criminal, public dissection was held in the anatomical theater for the edification of students and the curious. Later during the *settecento* to further promote the city as a center of learning, leaders, among them Benedict XIV (1675-1758) decided to invite women into the University and one of the first was Laura Bassi (1711-1778), who earned her degree in 1732 and became professor of anatomy in 1734. Paradoxically, because of her sex, she could only lecture at the invitation of the Bolognese Senate. She was additionally an accomplished physicist who introduced Newtonian physics and was an early teacher of Alessandro Volta.

In the latter half of the 17th century, into the 18th century, all of Europe with the exception of England had resumed educating upper-class women in medicine. Among prominent practitioners was Eleonora Maria Rosalia, Duchess of Troppau from Silesia, who published six books on medicine. Only *Treuvillig aufgesprungener Granatapfel des Christlicher Samartians* has survived.

Italian Anna Morandi Manzolini (1714-1774) was a lecturer of anatomy and sculptor of anatomical models in wax. She was married to Giovanni Manzolini (1700-1755), a Professor of Anatomy at the University of Bologna. When her husband became ill with tuberculosis, she received special permission to lecture in his place, and became Professor of Anatomy in her own right upon his death in 1755. As she became renowned for molding anatomical models, Manzolini was invited to several royal courts throughout Europe.

Frenchwoman Angelique-Marie Leboursier Ducoudray (1712-1789) served as Professor of Obstetrics and Anatomy for twenty-two years, and was a midwife at the court of Louis XV (1710-1774). She developed anatomical models of leather to teach methods of parturition. There were five editions of her textbook on obstetrics.

---

*The conventional treatment for syphilis was toxic mercury and the problem of congenital syphilis was not systematically addressed until 1780 when experiments were conducted at Paris' Vaugirard Hospital. There, wet nurses were given oral mercury in hopes that a milder dose of mercury would pass into breast milk. There was no evidence it helped the newborn and in a perverse turn, healthy nurses often acquired syphilis from the newborn. Nevertheless the practice continued into 1900.

The woman's suffrage movement in the 19th century had early roots in America. Harriot Hunt (1805-1875), after an apprenticeship with a Dr. Mott, established a practice in Boston in 1835. She was ostracized from the medical community and denied hospital privileges. In 1847 she applied to Harvard, which refused her entry on grounds of her age. Hunt persisted with the practice of medicine, and in 1853, she was awarded an honorary doctor of medicine by the newly founded (1850) Female Medical College of Pennsylvania (FMCP) in Philadelphia. The College was the first in the world to exclusively educate women in the field of medicine.

Elizabeth Blackwell (1821-1910) was the first American female admitted to and to graduate from a medical school. She was first in her class in 1849 from the Geneva Medical College of NY and trained further in England. Upon returning to America in 1857 she started a dispensary for working women and their children on Bleeker Street. Her sister, Emily Blackwell (1826-1910), like Elizabeth had been denied admission to several medical schools. She finally was admitted to Western Reserve University in Cleveland. She graduated in 1854 and went to Europe for further training, after which she became her sister's assistant at the Bleeker Street Infirmary. It evolved into the renowned New York Infirmary (1857) which, in addition to the care of women, established a college for the training of women in medicine. Emily was its administrator, practiced surgery and taught. She eventually became Dean of the college. Elizabeth focused on public health, was a tireless lecturer and an activist for the medical education of women.

Born in Germany, Maria Zakrzewski (1829-1902) trained at La Charité, Berlin, in midwifery. She emigrated to the United States in 1853 and, with the help of Elizabeth Blackwell and funds from the Harriot Hunt education fund, studied medicine at the Cleveland Medical College. Once an MD, she returned to New York and raised funds for Blackwell's Infirmary. She practiced there for two years. In 1859 she accepted a position as Professor of Obstetrics at the Samuel Gregory Female Medical College in Boston. After a quarrel with its director, Zakrzewski left the college and founded the New England Hospital for Women and Children.

The Boston Lying-In Hospital enjoyed a great reputation and, by its 25th anniversary, was staffed entirely by women. However, repeated epidemics of puerperal fever forced the closing of the hospital three times. Gradually the New England Hospital became the premier facility for *accouchements*. Rebecca Lee Crumpler (1833-1895) was a graduate of Zakrzewski's training program in 1864 – the first African-American physician.

Cordelia Green (1831-1905) graduated in 1853 from the FMCP and pursued postgraduate work at the Cleveland Medical College. In New York she lectured on preventive medicine, chaired the education committee of the Woman's Medical Society and became a member of the AMA.

Mary Edward Walker (1832-1919) was the first woman U.S. Army surgeon. A graduate of the Syracuse Central Medical College (1855), she served in the Union Army, and on multiple occasions entered Confederate territory to treat the wounded and retrieve Union soldiers. She was once captured by Confederacy forces, imprisoned for four months and released during a prisoner exchange. In 1865 she was awarded the Medal of Honor for her heroic service in the Civil War.

Ann Preston (1813-1872) was a member of the first graduating class of FMCP, and by 1853 Professor of Hygiene and Physiology. She became Dean of the college and championed the medical education of African-American, Native American and missionary women. Recognizing the students' need for clinical experience (they were barred from all of Philadelphia's hospitals and public clinics), in 1862 Preston founded the Woman's Hospital of Philadelphia. She persistently petitioned Philadelphia institutions to grant her students access in order to gain more clinical experience. By 1869 students were allowed to attend lectures at two teaching clinics, including that of the Pennsylvania Hospital. The women were subjected to vicious conduct from male students. At one clinical session, students spat tobacco juice along with vile invective. The women elected a dignified exit, dodging rocks being hurled at them. Ironically the publicity generated by the outrageous behavior influenced public opinion in favor of educating women as doctors.

Emeline Cleveland (1829-1878) studied medicine at FMCP (MD 1855) and obstetrics at the Maternité in Paris, and returned to FMCP as Professor of Anatomy and Histology. She established a training program for nurses and was named Dean of the college in 1872. Cleveland was one of the first women to perform gynecological and abdominal surgery. Surgeon Mary Harris Thompson (1829-1895) was a student of Elizabeth Blackwell. In 1865 she founded the Hospital for Women and Children in Chicago, and there began in 1871 the medical education of women.

Mary Putnam Jacobi (1842-1906) was awarded an MD from the FMCP in 1864 and interned at the New England Hospital for Woman and Children. She pursued further medical studies in Paris at the *École de Médecine*, from which she earned another MD, the second woman at that institution to do so. Upon her return to New York in 1871, she was appointed professor at the Woman's Medical College of the New York infirmary, where she founded a children's ward. In addition to being in the forefront of pediatric medicine, both she and her husband, Abraham Jacobi, were central forces in the struggle for improved health and social conditions in the community. Putnam Jacobi became a member of the AMA and was the first female member of the Academy of Medicine. She founded the Association for the Advancement of the Medical Education of Woman (1872) and wrote 120 scientific articles and 9 books.

The above account regarding some of the pioneering American women in medicine* eludes the enormous obstacles and derision they experienced. Resistance to women in medicine was virtually universal and many, including the most prestigious professors of medicine, based their objections on prevailing concepts of gender inferiority. Philadelphia gynecologist Charles Meigs, referring to "woman's nature," taught his students that a woman had a poor mind with a "…head almost too small for intellect but just big enough for love." His views were published in 1848 in *Females and Their Diseases*. Others claimed women's physiology and menses affected the central nervous system controlled by the uterus and ovaries, and that brainwork interfered with women's primary reproductive role. Harvard professor Edward H. Clarke's (182-1877) dogged opposition to education for women promulgated this thinking. In 1874 he published *Sex in Education: or a fair chance for the Girls* in which he opined, "Nature has reserved the catamenial week for the…perfection of the reproductive system." He contended educated women were fated to be sickly, and predicted they would be sterile or have difficult pregnancies because of smaller pelvises and large brained fetuses. He also asserted they would have inadequate breasts for nursing.

Julia Ward Howe (1819-1910) challenged Clark in a collection of essays entitled *A Reply to Dr. E. H. Clarke's "Sex in Education,"* and Mary Putnam Jacobi effectively refuted Clark with a scientific rebuttal in her book, *The Question of Rest for Women during Menstruation.* Her essay merited Harvard University's prestigious Boylston Prize. The rising power in the late 19th century of the woman's suffrage movement encouraged them to pressure universities to admit women. The exceptional women of the past who had fought individual, lonely, battles now acted collectively.

In England the suffrage movement was exceptionally stalwart, and several women insisted on being evaluated on merit. Elizabeth Garrett Anderson (1836-1917) attended a London lecture given by Elizabeth Blackwell. Inspired, she applied to several medical schools and was refused admittance to all of them. Undeterred, she studied privately with physicians, and succeeded in being certified by the Society of Apothecaries. Anderson worked the Marlebone Dispensary (later called the New Hospital for Women). Determined to become a physician, she was able to study medicine at the University of Paris and was granted an MD in 1870. She founded a medical school for women at the New Hospital and was the first

---

*Georgia Arbuckle Fix (1852-1918), a graduate of Omaha's College of Medicine, is representative of rural self-reliance and ingenuity common to the century's general practitioner. She attended a Nebraska farmer who had fractured his skull, exposing brain matter. With thoughtful equanimity she took a silver dollar from her purse, cleaned it with oxbile, anvil hammered it into a thin metal plate then skillfully sewed it to the skull.

woman awarded a medical post at the East London Hospital for Children. The New Hospital in 1918 changed its name to the Elizabeth Garrett Anderson Hospital in her honor.

Sophia Jex-Blake (1840-1912) exemplifies the determined resolve of women of the period who experienced rejection and abuse but implacably persisted in pursuing a career in medicine. Trained in mathematics, she applied to the University of London, School of Medicine after having studied in America with Elizabeth Blackwell. Rejected, she applied to the University of Edinburgh, which admitted her and a small group of women, including Edith Pechey (1845-1908).* Experiencing ridicule and riot, they completed the degree requirements with distinction, surpassing their male counterparts in academic achievement, but the university refused to award them the MD degree and the British Medical Association refused to certify them. Resolute, indomitable and combative, Jex-Blake appealed to Parliament. Through the efforts of Member of Parliament Russell Gurney (1804-1878), a bill was passed (1876) that mandated all medical schools provide education for women on the same terms as men. Jex-Blake's MD degree, however, was obtained at the University of Bern and, at the behest of the King's and Queen's College of Physicians in Dublin, was granted a license to practice medicine. The University of Edinburgh, having denied Jex-Blake her degree, now claims her as an alumna and has honored her distinguished place in the annals of medical education with a plaque that notes, "Physician, pioneer of medical education for women in Britain, and alumna of the university."

James (Miranda Stuart) Barry (1795-1865) masqueraded as a man to gain admittance to Edinburgh University's School of Medicine. Maintaining the subterfuge enabled her to serve as an army physician and surgeon in South Africa, India, the Caribbean and Canada, where she gained recognition as an exceptional surgeon. She rose to the rank of Inspector General, and promoted campaigns for better nutrition for soldiers and for improved sanitary conditions in hospitals. Ill, she returned to England in 1859 and died in 1865. Undertakers who prepared her body for burial discovered the life long held secret of her gender.

The field of nursing was more open to women and, in Kaiserwerth, Germany, Theodor Fliedner (1800-1864) established the Deaconess Institute (1836) to train nurses. Elizabeth Fry (1780-1845) studied at the institute, and in London applied the pedagogical methodology she learned. Fry founded the nursing order the Protestant Sisters of Charity in 1840.

---

*Edith Pechey-Phipson was one of a group of five women who with Sophia Jex-Blake fought from 1869 to 1877 to gain admittance to a British medical school. Queen Victoria sent Pechey to India where she spent 20 years attending English women serving there. Upon her return, she was admitted to the Irish College of Physicians.

In 1851 Florence Nightingale (1823-1910) also studied the nursing methods taught at the Kaiserwerth. In 1853 she travelled to Paris to study the institutional care provided by the Sisters of Mercy. These experiences formed the basis for her own principles of nursing which she famously implemented in the Crimean War of 1854 with a nursing team she assembled to attend the wounded. She and her staff became renowned for their nursing skills and dedicated service. To this day Nightingale is called the "Lady of the Lamp" in tribute to her tireless care of the wounded day and night. The standards for hospital cleanliness that she originated at the Scutari Hospital in Istanbul were responsible for a decrease in dysentery mortality rates from forty-two percent to two percent. Upon her return to England, she established the first secular nursing school at St. Thomas' Hospital, with a formal curriculum and rigorous standards of nursing care. Nightingale knew nothing of the germ theory – in fact she rejected it – but intuitively understood sanitation standards, and potable water prevented infection and disease. Her nursing philosophy was extensively influential. *Notes on Nursing* and *Notes on Hospitals* consolidated reforms throughout Europe and the United States that rendered order and system to the modern hospital model of today.

Jamaican nurse Mary Jane Seacole (1805-1881) also served during the Crimean War caring for the sick and wounded. She was not among the thirty-eight nurses selected by Nightingale, so she sponsored her own travel to the battlefield, where it was noted she distinguished herself attending to those on both sides of the conflict even under fire.

Revisionism has recently taken to excoriating Nightingale and promoting Seacole as the "real heroine" of the Crimean, but there is no historiography to support this claim and in fact Seacole's own book, *Wonderful Adventures of Mrs. Seacole in Many Lands* (1857), describes her role as a major hotelier and cook for officers.

Nightingale's American counterparts were Dorothea Dix and Clara Barton. Dorothea Dix (1802-1887) dedicated her life to reforming conditions in jails and almshouses in America and throughout Europe. She founded thirty-two institutions for the mentally retarded, insisting on humane treatment and sanitary conditions. Although not a nurse, Dix was named Superintendent of the Army Nursing Corps during the Civil War, and in her lifetime established several training facilities for nurses.

Clara Barton's (1821-1912) work nursing the wounded during the American Civil War and searching for the missing after the war merited her enduring reputation. She successfully lobbied for medical supplies to be stored and ready for distribution to the battle field. She had to petition for consent to ride in ambulances and administer care to the wounded being transported to hospital facilities. Inspired by the International Committee of the Red Cross, Barton was instrumental in founding the American Red Cross, and became its first president.

Social activists focused attention after the Civil War on the appalling infant mortality rates in large cities. American crusaders Josephine Baker (1873-1945) and Lillian Wald (1867-1940) played important roles in reducing infant mortality. Baker earned her medical degree in 1898, and in 1908 became director of the division of Child Hygiene in New York City. She instituted programs instructing mothers on how to prevent and deal with summer diarrheas, enforced licensing of midwives and organized the Little Mothers' League, an educational program for the older sisters of beleaguered families who cared for younger siblings. She actively influenced laws mandating the licensing of midwives. By 1923 the city had the lowest infant mortality rate of any city in America.

In 1893 Lillian Wald directed the Visiting Public Health Nursing Association located at New York's Henry Street Settlement. The organization had a staff of nurses who made home visits to new mothers and their babies to give them infant supplies and child care instruction as well as general medical attention.

Despite the many achievements of female physicians, women continued to confront discrimination. Emily Dunning Barringer (1876–1961) received her medical degree from Cornell in 1901, scoring the second highest grade in the qualifying exam for an internship at Governor Hospital in New York City. It took a year before she was accepted to the program, and then only because prominent political and religious figures intervened on her behalf. Barringer was the first American woman accepted in a post-graduate surgical training program and was the first female ambulance surgeon.

American pathologist Alice Hamilton (1869-1970) in 1919 was the first woman appointed to the Harvard medical school faculty. (Ironically and inexplicably Harvard did not admit women students until 1945). Hamilton became a social reformer who lived and served in Hull House community center (founded by activist Jane Addams (1860-1935), the second woman to receive the Nobel Peace Prize) where she delivered medical care to young mothers and their babies. She pioneered research in lead and phosphorus intoxication and became an authority in occupational medicine, which earned her the Lasker Award in 1947. Throughout her lifetime she returned yearly to Hull House to participate in the care of the residents.

Maude Abbott (1869-1940) was the only woman in her class at Bishop's College Medical School in Quebec. She was awarded an MD with honors in 1894 and studied three additional years in Europe. Ironically, having been rejected by McGill Medical School because she was a woman, McGill appointed her curator of its medical museum. She organized its collection of specimens into a world class medical museum and did research on congenital heart disease. The celebrated William Osler invited her to contribute a chapter on the subject for his *System of Modern medicine*

(1904). Abbott reclassified newborn cardiac anomalies along pathophysiological lines, and in 1936 wrote the *Atlas of Congenital Cardiac Diseases*. Recognized worldwide in her field, Abbott is among those listed in the Canadian Medical Hall of Fame.

At the inception of the 20th century a number of female "firsts" – women who distinguished themselves and the profession – underscores to some extent the diminution of bias that had to that point so hindered women from training for a career in science.

Physicist and chemist Marie Curie (1867-1934) was the first woman to earn a doctorate in science. She was the first woman Professor of Physics at the Sorbonne. She remains world renowned for her discovery of radium in 1898, and, in 1903, she became the first woman to win a Nobel Prize in Physics, shared with her husband, Pierre Curie (1859-1906). She was again honored with a Nobel in 1911 for Chemistry. In 1914 the University of Paris founded the Radium Institute to facilitate Curie's research and appointed her as Director of the Curie Center, where she and her team of research scientists worked to find practical clinical applications for the properties of radium.* In 1995 Curie and her husband were reinterred in the Pantheon in Paris, a singular honor.

In 1907 Roman physician Maria Montessori (1870-1952) opened her *Casa di Bambini* that focused on the nurturing and development of children employing sensorineural modalities. Montessori schools, based on her understanding of child development and how children learn, continue to flourish worldwide.

Margaret Sanger (1879-1966) trained and practiced as a nurse in New York, but devoted her life's work to the legalization of birth control and its availability to all. After visiting a Dutch clinic in 1915 she returned to New York to advocate the use of the diaphragm as the most efficacious contraceptive available. In 1916 and 1917 she wrote her famous *What Every Girl Should Know*, followed by *What Every Woman Should Know*. That same year she opened the first birth control clinic in Brooklyn, which was raided and closed by the police nine days later. Under the Comstock Act of 1873 she was repeatedly arrested for distributing contraceptives until an appeals court ultimately vindicated her work by amending the law to allow physicians to distribute contraception information. In 1921 she founded the American Birth Control League (Planned Parenthood). By 1950 Sanger realized that the diaphragm and condom were not the ideal forms of contraception and that a cheaper effective method was essential. In 1951 she met Gregory Pincus (1903-1967) and, together with John Rock (1890-1984), embarked on a course of funding, research and clinical trials that in 1960 resulted in the first oral contraceptive – Enovid. In 1965 the

---

*Like many of the doomed radium clock dial painters, Curie died of aplastic anemia.

Supreme Court decision (*Griswold vs. Connecticut*) recognized birth control as a right protected under the constitution of the United States. Sanger's British counterpart was Marie Stopes (1880-1958), a scholarly paleobotanist, who by 1910 started to turn her attention to suffrage. She met Sanger in 1915 and thereafter began her quest for providing contraceptive information. She authored *Contraception, Its Theory, History and Practice* in 1923.

Cicely Williams (1893-1992) received her degree in medicine from Oxford University in 1923. She worked in Ghana (then the Gold Coast), where she defined the syndrome of kwashiorkor, the still used African term for protein-calorie malnutrition. Williams continued her work with malnutrition and maladies affecting children in tropical environments. In Jamaica she studied ackee apple intoxication. In 2003 the Jamaican government posthumously awarded her the National Medal for Science for elucidating the cause of "vomiting sickness" and ackee apple (*Blighia Sapida*) poisoning.

American histologist Florence Rena Sabin (1871-1953) conducted innovative research on the origins of the lymphatic system, immune system cell and the pathology of tuberculosis. She was the first woman to graduate from Johns Hopkins University School of Medicine, and in 1917 was named its first female full professor. She was awarded the Lasker prize for her work in public health and in 2005 Johns Hopkins named Sabin Hall in her honor.

Dorothy Andersen (1901-1963) earned an MD from Johns Hopkins in 1916, interned in surgery at Strong Memorial Hospital and taught anatomy at the Rochester School of Medicine. Despite her training and experience, Strong Memorial refused to grant her a residency in surgery, and Andersen shifted her energies to research in pathology and endocrinology. By 1952 she was chief of pathology at Columbia-Presbyterian Medical Center in New York City. Andersen was the first to describe cystic fibrosis as a separate disease entity in 1935, and helped to develop a diagnostic test for the disease.

French physician Anne Spoerry (1918-1970) trained at Saltpêtrière and was active with the resistance movement in WW II. She was imprisoned in a Nazi concentration camp for two years and then travelled to Africa, where in the model of Alsatian Albert Schweitzer (1875-1965) who devoted his life to medical missionary work in Gabon, spent the remainder of her life serving the natives of Kenya. She became an airplane pilot to serve the medical needs of people in a wide-spread area.

Helen Brooke Taussig (1898-1986), another medical graduate of Johns Hopkins, in 1930 was appointed Director of Hopkins' Pediatric Cardiac Clinic. Considered the Founder of Pediatric Cardiology, her research in congenital heart disease focused on "the blue baby syndrome." At her suggestion, Alfred Blalock (1899-1964) and his technical assistant

Vivien Thomas (1920-1985) with Taussig perfected a palliative surgical procedure called the Blalock-Taussig operation for tetralogy and pulmonary stenosis. It was introduced in 1945 and soon was used worldwide. *Congential Malformations of the Heart* was published in 1947. Taussig received the Lasker Prize in 1954 and the Medal of Freedom from President Lyndon Johnson (1908-1973) in 1964.

Pathologist Edith Louise Potter (1901-1993) wrote definitive descriptions of renal diseases in children and adults. She classified the cystic diseases of the kidney and classified newborn diseases associated with oligohydramnios. After an analysis of five thousand newborn autopsies she deciphered the intrauterine events that lead to what is now known as Potter Syndrome or the Potter Sequence.

Gerty Radnitz Cori (1896-1957) trained in medicine at the German University of Prague where she met and married Carl Cori (1896-1984). They became lifelong collaborators in America on research in physiologic biochemistry. In 1947 they shared the Nobel Prize for their elucidation of glycogen metabolism.

A graduate of the College of Physicians and Surgeons at Columbia University and the first woman to be appointed professor there, anesthesiologist Virginia Apgar (1909-1974), after twelve years of study and observation, in 1953 published her formula that has become the standard method for evaluating newborns – the Apgar Score. Five variables – heart rate, respiratory effort, muscle points and totaled to ascertain the infant's vitality score.

Dorothy Whipple (1901-1995) graduated from Johns Hopkins School of Medicine in 1929, practiced pediatrics in Virginia for forty years and taught pediatrics at Georgetown University. In contrast to the prevailing wisdom of nurture espoused by Luther Emmet Holt (1855-1924) that advocated strict and spartan principles, Whipple championed the converse. In 1944 she published a book that advocated a more flexible approach to child rearing two years before Benjamin Spock's (1903-1998) famous *Baby and Child Care*. "Be natural and easy with your baby," Whipple counseled in her book *Our American Babies*. Whipple published a series of pamphlets for the Federal Government dealing with child care and everyday hygiene. In 1950 she published concepts on normal childhood growth in *Euthenic Pediatrics*.

Barbara Evelyn Clayton (1922-2011) was Professor of chemical pathology at the Great Ormond Street Hospital. Among her many contributions to the field was the investigation of lead poisoning in children and the development of microchemistry techniques that allowed metabolic assessment of prematures employing tiny quantities of blood. She evolved a heel-prick program to diagnose phenylketonuria and worked with nutritionists to develop special diets for these babies. Her analytic methods employing these micromethods revolutionized the field of neonatology.

One of the founders of the American Society of Clinical Oncology was African-American Jane Cooke Wright (1919-2013). She was a pioneer in cancer surgery and chemotherapy, devising protocols in specified manners for the administration of anticancer drugs.

Working on physiologist John Clements' (b. 1923) observation of surfactant, Mary Ellen Avery (1927-2011) discovered that newborn respiratory distress syndrome (RDS) – also called hyaline membrane disease – was due to a lack of pulmonary surfactant. She compared the lungs of RDS babies to healthy lungs and published her data in 1959. Picking up on her work, Tetsuro Fujiwara (b. 1931) experimented for 15 years until he found a method to deliver surfactant to the sick newborn via intratracheal instillation.

Jacqueline Anne Noonan (b. 1921), a graduate of the University of Vermont, in 1963 described the syndrome that carries her name, Noonan syndrome, which is marked by a characteristic physiognomy and pulmonary valve stenosis.

Rita Levi-Montalcini (1909-2012) studied medicine at the University of Turin and, in hiding during the Nazi occupation of Italy, did research in neurology. After the war she accepted a faculty position at Washington University in St. Louis, and in the early 1950s began experiments with chicken embryos and cancer cell cultures to isolate nerve growth factor. She is the co-recipient with Stanley Cohen (b. 1922) of the 1986 Nobel Prize.

Dorothy Mary Hodgkin (1910-1994) developed protein x-ray crystallography, advancing the physical chemistry study of the three-dimensional structure of molecules and *inter alia*, she determined the structures of penicillin, vitamin B-12, and insulin.

Rosalind Elsie Franklin (1920-1958) conducted research on the microstructure of carbon compounds, and in the last five years of her life worked on the structure of plant viruses. Famously, after studying Franklin's x-ray crystallography, James Watson (b.1928) and Francis Crick (1916-2004) elucidated the molecular structure of DNA in 1953 and, in 1962, were awarded the Nobel Prize. Nobel Prizes are not given posthumously and, having died in 1958, Franklin's work was not honored by the committee. Crick, however, is on record as having acknowledged that he and Watson could not have discovered the structure of DNA without Franklin's seminal work.

At first denied acceptance, Barbara McClintock (1902-1992) studied plant genetics at Cornell University (Ph.D. 1927). It took years for the importance of her work in cytogenetics to be recognized as essential to understanding human biology. In 1983 she was awarded the Nobel for her discovery of genetic chromosomal transposition.

Swiss born and educated, with a medical degree from Zurich University (1957), Elisabeth Kübler-Ross (1926-1994) trained in psychiatry in New York, where she focused on the treatment of the terminally ill. Her famous book, *On Death and Dying,* published in 1969, discussed what is now known as the Kübler-Ross model of the six stages of death. The book's success earned her worldwide fame and twenty honorary degrees, and her theories remain the standard for understanding the psychodynamics of dying.

Rosalyn Sussman Yalow (1921-2011) received a doctorate in nuclear physics from the University of Illinois – the sole woman in a class of four hundred. She was the first woman recipient of the Lasker Prize in 1976 and the first American woman to win, in 1977, the Nobel Prize in Medicine and Physiology with Solomon Berson (1918-1972) for their work in developing the radioimmunoassay (RIA) technique.

Since 1983 there have been seven additional Nobels awarded to women (all shared): biochemist and pharmacologist Gertrude Belle Elion (1918-1999) shared the prize in 1988 for the development of innovative methods in producing new drugs, among them azathioprine, allopurinol, trimethoprim and acyclovir. Biologist Christiane Nüsslein-Volhard (b. 1942) won the 1991 prize for work on the genetic control of embryonic development. In 2004 biologist Linda B. Buck (b.1947) shared the prize for novel work on olfaction. Virologist Françoise Barré-Sinoussi (b. 1947) with Luc Montagnier (b. 1932) were recipients of the Nobel in 2008 for their work on the human immunodeficiency virus. The 2009 prize was shared by three winners, two of them women – Elizabeth Helen Blackburn, (b. 1948) and Carolyn Widney Greider (b.1961) – for ground-breaking work on telomeres and telomerase. Mary Britt Moser shared the 2014 prize for elucidating cells that control positioning in the brain.

"The Glass Ceiling" women confronted evolved as a concept only in the later part of the 20th century after women had made inroads in all professions. In the past, women's struggles to pursue goals in every field tended to be lonely and singular sagas of courage and tenacity in the face of almost universal rejection and humiliation. In this 21st century, their great battles can be – should be – relegated to the dusty pages of ancient history, no longer relevant to our modern and presumably ever more enlightened society.

IX: Twentieth Century Medicine

Timeline:

1900 Boxer rebellion
1902 US Public Health Service
1906 San Francisco earthquake
1909 Orthodontia introduced
1912 Titanic sinks
1914 World War I
1918 Spanish influenza pandemic
1927 Lindberg crosses the Atlantic
1929 The Great Depression
1932 Tuskegee Study
1934 Adolf Hitler: Chancellor of Germany
1939 WW II begins
       Paul Müller develops DDT
1941 US enters WW II
1946 Nuremberg trials
1948 World Health Organization
1949 NATO formed
1959 Microchip: modern computer
1961 Yuri Gagarin in space
1969 Man on the moon
1981 AIDS is named
1980 Small pox eliminated
1990 PCR technology comes of age
1993 Maastricht Treaty: the EU
1999 The human genome

I represent a party which does not yet exist: the party
of revolution, civilization. This party will make the twentieth
century. There will issue from it first the United States of
Europe, then the United States of the World.
    Victor Hugo (1802-1885) *Place des Vosges, Paris*

Sparta must be regarded as the first Völkisch State. The
exposure of the sick, weak, deformed children, in short, their
destruction, was more decent and in truth a thousand times
more humane than the wretched insanity of our day which
preserves the most pathological subject, and indeed at any
price, and yet takes the life of a hundred thousand healthy
children in consequence of birth control or through abortions,
in order subsequently to breed a race of degenerates burdened
with illnesses.
    Adolph Hitler (1889-1945): *Zweites Buch* (1928)

The health of the people is a public concern; ill health
is a major cause of suffering, economic loss, and dependency;
good health is essential to the security
and progress of the nation....
    Franklin D Roosevelt (1182-1945)
    National Health Program (1945)

Whereas mankind owes to the child the best it has to give,
Now, therefore, the General Assembly proclaims this
Declaration of the Rights of the Child to the end that he may
have a happy childhood and enjoy for his own good and for
the good of society the rights and freedoms herein set forth,
and calls upon parents, upon men and women as individuals
and upon voluntary organizations, local authorities and
national governments to recognize these rights and strive for
their observance by legislative and other measures....
    United Nations General Assembly:
    The Rights of the Child (1959).

Twentieth Century: A chronology of achievements

The 20th century poses the biggest challenge when writing a concise history of medicine. The accomplishments of an extraordinary one hundred years in which virtually every year was marked by astounding discoveries, original descriptions and innovations, extend well beyond the scope and intent of this book's objective to be comprehensive in a concise format. Therefore the highly complex transformative advances in medicine are here posited succinctly, consistent with the format of this book.

One approach to this end would be to simply list all the winners of the Nobel Prize in Medicine and Physiology. Such a list in fact is presented (Appendix E), and several Nobelists are discussed in the body of the text, but the interconnections and cooperation amongst disciplines and the vital work of vast numbers of researchers and clinicians extended well beyond those few who became instantly world acclaimed as winners of a prestigious prize. Importantly, the comprehension of the enormity of accomplishments made in the century would be incomplete if only Nobel Prize recipients were mentioned and the contributions of legions of extraordinary scientists were to be overlooked.

Another approach, to write about scientific movements, is not pertinent as was the case with the 19th century, in which it was possible to examine spheres of influence that dominated the scientific landscape of the Schools of Paris, Dublin, Vienna, London and Berlin. No such cohesive pedagogical forces marked the 20th century. The endeavors had universally evolved into an Age of the Laboratory, and the century was celebrated by exponential – almost logarithmic – leaps within disciplines such as hematology, infectious diseases, immunology, endocrinology and surgery.

The concession is to aim for an instructive elaboration of the major advances within each discipline in a narrative that attempts to integrate a timeline of discoveries while at the same time illustrating how new insights were at times embraced by another – or several other – disciplines. Inevitably and to possible dismay, some observations, discoveries and even names of importance will be missed, and in a few instances the narrative may be repetitive, but the cohesion should endure and an overall mural of 20th century medical attainments should edifyingly emerge. What lies ahead in this 21st century is anyone's guess, but, with certainty, scientific researchers and clinicians should refer in all of their enquires to their predecessors' work to whom they are indebted.

Two extraordinary late 19th century discoveries in physics that had epochal influence in the 20th century were the x-ray by William Conrad Roentgen (1845-1923) in 1895 and radium in 1898 by Marie Curie and Pierre Curie (1859–1906). Antoine Henri Bequerel's (1852-1908) work on natural radioactivity in uranium influenced Marie and Pierre Curie's studies. Their research isolated two new elements, polonium and radium. The discovery of radium was a monumental achievement that issued in a new era of research. Studies of the physics of radiation and its properties during the course of the century made unparalleled breakthroughs that contributed to imaging and diagnostic scintigraphy, radio-immunoassays and cancer therapies. All of these complex, multifaceted modalities of treatment employed not only traditional surgical excision, but also borrowed from other sciences to produce an arsenal of chemotherapeutics, radiation and immunotherapy. Heralded new medical specialties, oncology and radiation oncology for example, emerged with requisite knowledge and insights that advanced further astoundingly original research and treatments.

The public response to Roentgen's discovery was as a whimsical curiosity, and all were bedazzled by the human transparency that uncovered living skeletal forms behind the fluorescent screens. Scientists such as physiologist Walter B. Cannon (1871-1945) immediately grasped the clinical and experimental importance of the invention, and as early as 1897 used oral radio-opaque bismuth to study under x-ray the anatomy and functional motility of the gastrointestinal tract from mouth to bowels to rectum.

In the 20th century the x-ray was at first used to study the most immediately evident body structure – the osseous system. But with increased use, subtleties of non-osseous tissues became more and more evident, and it was not long until the x-ray was employed to study the lungs, heart and viscera. Imaging techniques gradually advanced in sophistication and subtlety, so that by 1955 research efforts, using another phenomenon of physics – the sound wave – resulted in the development of another exceptional diagnostic procedure: sonography. Ultrasound technology to create images enabled clinicians to avoid overusing x-ray, by now known to have deleterious effects due to excessive radiation exposure. X-ray continued to be a useful tool, but one to be used sparingly.

X-ray pictures of the body remained two-dimensional until Godfrey Newbold Hounsfield (1919-2004) conjoined the computer with x-ray technology to assemble multiple images of x-rays that generated cross-sectional images of the body. With more sophisticated software, three dimensional pictures of bone and soft-tissue of internal organs became possible, and, with intravascular contrast agents, made visible the entire circulatory system, both normal and abnormal. Hounsfield called the process he invented computerized axial tomography, known ubiquitously as the CAT scan (1971). In 1979 Hounsfield shared the Nobel Prize with Allan Cormack (1929-1998), the physicist who explicated the mathematical principles behind the extraordinary medical imaging process.

Significant exposure to radiation using the CAT scan, however, was a known danger. Further research in the physics lab mitigated this problem with the invention and clinical application of nuclear magnetic resonance described by Raymond Vahan Damadian (b. 1936). Its clinical application, better known as magnetic resonance imaging (MRI), was developed in 1973 by Paul Lauterbur (1929-2007) and Peter Mansfield (b. 1933). With no radiation, the MRI enabled computerized interpretation of electro-magnetically manipulated cell nuclei hydrogen to produce clear and distinctive images of all tissues, fluids and contrasting air spaces (Fig. 26).

The fact that, by the end of the 20th century, within one hundred years of the inception of research into its possibility, a non-invasive complete map of the human body that can explore even the intricacies of the brain without violating the chamber of the skull portends advances in the future beyond current imaginings.

Hematology emerged in the 19th century with effectually no remarkable antecedents. Swammerdam and van Leeuwenhoek had both described red blood cells in the 17th century. William Hewson (1739-1774), who worked alongside the Hunter brothers, demonstrated that red cells were discoid rather than spherical and rendered further definition of white blood cells. He also isolated fibrin and showed that coagulation was a function of plasma rather than the red blood cell. Microscopist Alfred Donné (1801-1878) mistook platelets for fat globules, leaving it to Osler in 1874 to recognize them as the "third element of blood." The function of platelets in the coagulation process was described in 1882 by Giulio Bizzozero (1846-1901) who also identified them as a separate cell line in marrow. Having described these elements in the blood, however, none understood their physiological significance. Nor was their information coalesced until Ernst Newmann (1834-1918) described nucleated red blood cells in marrow and concluded that erythropoiesis (red cell production) and leucopoiesis (white cell production) took place in bone marrow and that all these cell lines were essential to life.

It was long known that significant loss of blood resulted in cardiovascular collapse. The patient who experienced catastrophic bleeding, whether because of an accident, trauma, a postpartum or internal hemorrhage, would slip into shock and certain death. As early as the 17th century there were experiments with transfusion. Richard Lower in 1669 performed dog to dog transfusions, and German surgeon Matthäus Gottfried Purmann (1648-1721) in 1694 wrote about animal to human transfusions in his *Chirurgia Curiosa*. Philip Syng Physick performed a human to human exchange in 1795 without success. Obstetrician James Blundell (1791-1878), at St. Thomas' and Guy's Hospitals in London, was inconsolable as, helpless, he watched young mothers slowly exsanguinate from post-partum hemorrhages. Between 1818 and 1829 he used only human blood in his transfusion experiments. He transfused ten patients, with a fifty percent survival rate. A statistical compilation by 1873 of other experimental transfusions demonstrated an overall mortality of fifty-six percent.

The work of three prominent investigators, Karl Landsteiner (1868-1943), Alexander Wiener (1907-1976) and Richard Lewisohn (1875-1961), identified the key properties of blood that made safe transfusion possible, a goal that had eluded clinicians for centuries. About 1900 Austrian Karl Landsteiner, working with human blood, noted that some samples agglutinated (clumped together) when mixed. His experimentation over the next two years resulted in the recognition of different kinds of blood types, and he classified them into groups: the now universally known A, B, and O blood types. Alfred von Decastello (1878-1936) and Adriano Sturli (1873-1964) in 1902 discovered the AB type. Rhesus factor determination would not be understood for another three decades (see ahead). In 1907 Ludvig Hektoen (1863-1951) of the University of Chicago demonstrated that safe transfusion was possible once blood compatibility of patient and donor were matched. His research revealed that type O blood was the universal donor type that could in an emergency be administered. Successful direct donor to patient transfusions were finally possible. It was a revolutionary advance in treatment.

With the introduction of newly innovated cannulas the injection of blood via syringes became standard. A donor no longer had to be an active presence during the procedure. Attempts, however, were often frustrated because of gelatinous lumps of clots that formed. Richard Lewisohn of Mt. Sinai in New York examined the impasse and searched for a method to inject blood on demand that did not clot, an imperative in an acute hospital situation. A known anticoagulant, sodium citrate (a calcium chelator), had been introduced by Oswald Robertson (1886-1966) and it worked well in the laboratory but was toxic when administered. It was used as a one percent solution to keep blood stable. Lewisohn speculated a smaller concentration would be safe and effective. In 1915 he developed a zero point two (0.2) percent solution that was non-toxic. In England, Patrick Mollison (1914-2011) modified the formula by acidification to make acid citrate dextrose which required smaller volumes of anticoagulant and allowed blood storage for up to three weeks. Stored blood for acute blood loss was finally available in the operating room, the obstetric theater and the emergency room.

Alexander Wiener, together with Landsteiner, made an important refinement in blood typing in 1937 with the elucidation of the Rh factor. Wiener received the Lasker Award in 1946 for subsequent achievements in developing the exchange transfusion for newborns with Rh incompatible hemolytic disease.

African American Charles Richard Drew (1904-1950), a noted researcher and surgeon, improved techniques for storing blood plasma and developed blood banks which, in World War II, saved countless lives. Drew successfully demonstrated that plasma in an emergency could be substituted for whole blood transfusion for a patient in shock. The first blood bank was established in Chicago's Cook County Hospital in 1935 and, by 1945, banked blood was being tested for syphilis. In subsequent decades, testing for other blood-borne diseases such as hepatitis B, C and HIV, etc. was developed. Globally today, 81 million units of blood are transfused annually.

Intravenous therapy became almost simple and routine with the introduction in 1950 of the sterile and disposable plastic needle invented by David J. Massa (1923-1990) of the Mayo Clinic, and, in what is perhaps the archetype of transfusion, the bone marrow transplant was introduced in 1956 by E. Donnell Thomas (1920-2012), which offered a revolutionary modality of treatment for intractable anemias and cancers. It also introduced a new disease concept, a threat to all transplantation, that of graft vs. host disease.

The work of bio-chemist Linus Pauling (1901-1994) on sickle cell disease initiated revolutionary work in molecular hematology. Over four hundred different hemoglobin variants are now known. Pauling was awarded two Nobel prizes – in 1954 in Chemistry for protein structure research, and, in 1962, the Peace prize for opposing nuclear testing.

One more dramatic use of blood emerged that employed only a few drops of blood: newborn screening for metabolic syndromes. It was first initiated by Barbara Clayton (1923-2011) and Robert Guthrie (1916-1995) as a screening for phenylketonuria, a cause of retardation discovered by Ivar Følling (1888-1973) in 1934. The testing was introduced in the late 1950s, but by the beginning of this century, newborns were routinely screened for hypothyroidism, galactosemia, fatty acid oxidation disorders, endocrinopathies, organic acidemias, aminoacidopathies, storage diseases – in all, some thirty different ailments – facilitating early treatment protocols for the newborn.

Advancements in the treatment of heart diseases began with electrophysiology and interventional therapy. In 1903 Willem Einthoven (1820-1927) devised the electrocardiogram (EKG), an apt example of how innovations most commonly evolve because of the cumulative genius of many: in 1794 Galvani made a dissected frog leg contract with electrical stimulation → in 1872 Gabriel Lippmann (1845-1921) measured electrical differences in animal hearts → August Desire Waller (1856-1922) in 1887 did the same with the human heart by attaching brine electrodes on the chest and back of a patient → Einthoven, having witnessed this experiment, was inspired to work on and perfect the modern EKG machine. The device was immediately put to clinical use by Thomas Lewis (1881-1945) who in 1903 used it to define different arrhythmias. Åke Senning (1915-2000) conceived of the internal pacemaker in 1958, and it emerged as a reliable device for controlling abnormal rhythms. American engineer Wilson Greatbatch (1919-2011) miniaturized the pacemaker and, in 1956, approached surgeon William Chardack (1914-2006) to make the device clinically applicable. After animal trials in 1960 they implanted the pacemaker successfully in a human. It has become the preferred treatment for patients with life-threatening arrhythmias.

Studies in cardiac physiology during the first half of the 20th century paved the way for avant-garde therapeutic interventions. One of the earliest procedures benefited children born with tetralogy of Fallot. The palliative Taussig-Blalock shunt (1945) ameliorated the cyanosis associated with pulmonic stenosis in blue-babies. In 1948 Russel C. Brock (1903-1980) of Guy's Hospital, London, performed intracardiac surgery and repaired a stenotic pulmonary valve. Ambitious cardiac surgery was made possible by the cardiac bypass technique first introduced at the University of Minnesota in 1954, and the ultimate cardiac intervention measure, the heart transplant, was dramatically achieved in 1967 by Christian Barnard (1922-2000).

In 1929, Werner Forssmann (1904-1979), then a 25 year old intern in Eberswalde, Germany, proposed the idea of cardiac catheterization. Forbidden by his professors to experiment on animals or patients, he successfully performed the procedure on himself, and introduced a new modality for vascular imaging and the diagnosis and treatment of heart disease. Today, the occluded coronary artery is treated either by employing bypass surgery or by catheterization with the use of stents. Catheterization has become the gold standard of diagnostic methods and, for some maladies, the therapeutic intervention. These cardiac modalities became possible because of sophisticated imaging, modern pharmacological agents to control cardiac rhythm and contraction and agents that modify coagulation.

Vascular imaging lent itself to study other organs and earlier, in 1927, Egas Moniz (1874-1955) from the University of Portugal injected the carotid artery with sodium iodide to visualize the cerebral arterial system and thereby study vascular anatomy, identify aneurysms, tumors and anomalies. In 1931, a serendipitous delay in imaging resulted in the first cerebral venous phase study. At first all studies were via carotid injections, but during the 60s, transfemoral approach supervened and with the introduction of the CAT scan in the 70s the use of invasive angiography of the head greatly diminished.

The Mendelian concept of heredity progressed from trait observation to an elucidation of the molecular science of genetics. In 1869, while at the University of Tübingen, Swiss physician Johannes Friedrich Miescher (1844-1895) isolated nucleic acids from white blood cells, which he called "nuclein." He published his results in 1871 and raised the idea of their association with heredity. Then, in 1878, Walther Flemming (1843-1905) found a cellular structure – chromatin – which absorbed basophilic dyes and which he associated with microthreads in the nucleus. These threads would later be named chromosomes by Wilhelm von Waldermeyer-Hartz (1841-1923). They were observed independently by Edouard van Beneden (1846-1910). Flemming ultimately observed the mitotic process, so that by 1890, the chromosome was recognized as the cellular unit of genetic inheritance. In 1905 William Bateson (1861-1926) coined the term "genetics."

The concept of genes as markers or units of heredity was proposed by Dane Wilhelm Johannsen (1857-1927) and it followed that the study of their locations would be next. Thus, in 1911, while working on the fruit fly *Drosophila* Thomas Hunt Morgan (1866-1945) published gene maps of their chromosomes. The gene concept led Archibald Garrod (1857-1936), who was studying alkaptonuria, to propose the notion of inborn errors of metabolism inherited along Mendelian laws. Oswald Avery (1877-1955), Colin MacLeod (1909-1972) and Maclyn McCarty (1911-2005), working with pneumococcus in 1944, demonstrated that DNA was the source of genetic transmission and Erwin Chargoff (1905-2002) in 1950 described the four bases of DNA and the rules of paring for adenine with thymine and guanine with cytosine. The model of DNA followed some three years later (see Watson and Crick). In 1963, Jacques Monod (1910-1976) and François Jacob (1920-2013) linked DNA with messenger RNA, and during the 1970s David Baltimore and Howard Temin discovered reverse transcriptase, converting RNA to DNA and opening a new phase of genetic understanding that led to revolutionary treatments for HIV and HBV infections, as well as enhancing new applications of PCR reactions.

Dialysis is the electrochemical gradient diffusion of molecules in solution through a semipermeable membrane to keep the intra and extracellular milieu in balance. The use of peritoneal and hemodialysis in the treatment of acute and chronic renal failure became the preferred medical modalities in the 20th century. John J. Abel (1857-1938) and colleagues in 1913 published the results of experiments with dialyzed animals whose blood was circulated outside the body through semipermeable collodion membranes and returned to the animal. For anticoagulant he used hirudin from leech saliva, which had been first isolated in 1880 by John Haycraft (1859-1923). Hirudin, however, proved to induce significant allergic reactions and when Georg Haas (1886-1971) began human dialysis in 1924 he therefore employed mammalian heparin which had been isolated from dog livers by Jay McLean (1890-1957) in

1916. Haas' dialyzers used a modified version of the Abel machine for his studies. None of Haas' patient survived, most likely because dialysis was not started until they were in critical condition, but in 1945, Willem Kolff (1911-2009) successfully treated a 67 year old woman with a rotating drum model that employed cellophane membranous tubes wrapped around a wooden slate drum spinning in electrolyte dialysate. After the War the Kolff machine crossed from the Netherlands into America and the Peter Brent Brigham in Boston where it after technical modifications was named the Kolff-Brigham kidney. It met with much success particularly during the extreme conditions of the Korean War when Major Paul Teschan (b. 1923) used it to treat post-traumatic acute renal failure. Further refinement added "ultrafiltration," which facilitated the removal of edematous fluid overload as well as metabolic toxins. Swede Nils Alwall (1904-1986) successfully modified the dialyzer to accomplish this task. In 1960, Norwegian Fredrik Kiil (b. 1921) produced the parallel plate-dialyzer that sent blood and dialysate through alternating layers of membrane – a modification that remained in use throughout the 1990s. These early patients were hemodialyzed for acute renal failure for several days after which the process quickly exhausted arterial and venous access. The treatment of chronic renal failure, therefore, was untenable until the arteriovenous shunt was developed. Belding Scribner (1921-2003) and Wayne Quinton (b. 1921) used Teflon to create a reusable arteriovenous access for these patients. This was an exteriorized access, a process improved in 1966 by employing a subcutaneous forearm fistula designed by James Cimino (1928-2010) and colleagues.

With increasing numbers of chronic renal failure patients now undergoing dialysis, home treatment programs were started employing peritoneal dialysis that used the Henry Tenckhoff (b. 1930) catheter, a soft tunneled catheter left in place under the abdominal skin that communicated with the peritoneum, eliminating the need for repeated peritoneal taps thus lowering the risk of infection. The dialysate was infused into the peritoneum where it remained for a period of time removing toxins and then was drained back into a bag for disposal. This allowed the patient several toxic-free days before the process was repeated, generally 2 to 3 times per week. Currently, about 10% of chronic renal failure patients use the peritoneal method, but the ultimate treatment of renal failure, once immune-rejection was understood, was transplantation (see ahead).

Arguably, the advances in the field of infectious diseases have most benefited mankind globally. While the astounding and gripping drama of open heart surgery or organ transplantation bespeaks remarkable technical advances, it is the appropriate, now routine, use of antibiotics that has had the most efficacious impact on world health.

The direct and astounding evolutionary course of antibiotic development traces to the work of Paul Ehrlich (1854-1915) in the 19th century. Ehrlich is credited with the discovery of the basophile (1877), acid-fast bacillus (1882), vital staining (1886) and the protein complement (1899) (Fig. 22). He originated the concept of the minimal lethal dose in experimental pharmacology and the side-chain theory of neutralization. His work on lead poisoning demonstrated certain tissues possessed selective affinity for specific compounds. Together with Sahachiro Hata (1873-1938), he conducted experiments using anilines on rabbits and monkeys. In 1910 their work with arsphenamine, labeled compound 606, proved efficacious in the treatment of syphilis and was marketed as Salvarsan. The organism responsible for syphilis, *Treponema pallidum*, was described in nerve tissue by Hideyo Noguchi (1876-1928) in 1913. Noguchi also was fascinated with the subject of tropical infectious diseases and went to Africa to conduct research, where he succumbed to yellow fever.

Between 1917 and 1945 malariotherapy was used for tertiary syphilis. Patients were infected with *Plasmodium vivax* in the belief that high fevers averted the effects of the bacteria. Nobel laureate Julius Wagner-Jaureg (1857-1940) was the major proponent of this modality which was followed by a course of quinine. However, by the mid-forties, penicillin became the treatment of choice.

Ehrlich's studies suggested that other organic compounds could possess antibacterial properties and inspired additional research by many others. In 1932 pathologist and bacteriologist Gerhard Domagk (1895-1964) experimented in Germany with the antibacterial effects of red dye prontosil – a sulphanilamide. He used it successfully to treat his daughter's streptococcus infection. At Queen Charlotte Maternity Hospital in London in 1936 Leonard Colebrook (1883-1967) used the same compound to treat puerperal fever and thereby reduced mortality from twenty to five percent. Domagk won the Nobel in 1939, but Nazis authorities prohibited him from accepting the award. He collected his medal after the war.

The antibiotic most recognized by all is penicillin. The remarkable story of its discovery, commemorated in many books, relates how Alexander Fleming (1881-1955) in 1928 discovered the fungus *Penicillium notatum* inhibited the growth of bacteria. Fleming had published important and original work on nasal lysozyme secretions in 1922, but his discovery of penicillin overshadowed any other of his work. At Oxford in 1941 Howard Florey (1898-1968) and Ernst Chain (1906-1979) extracted and purified penicillin for therapeutic use. They injected mice via the peritoneum with *Streptococcus pyogenese* and observed the extraordinary successful response to the penicillin. With Fleming they shared the 1945 Nobel Prize in Physiology and Medicine.

In 1943, Albert Schatz (1922-2005) a graduate student in Selman Waksman's (1888-1973) laboratory at Rutger's University found an agent produced by *Actinomyces griseus* that was active against *E. coli* as well as other gram-negative organisms and the ancient and pernicious affliction, tuberculosis. Both men published two papers on the agent, now named streptomycin, and jointly received a patent. Two years later, Waksman began a public relations campaign against Schatz to diminish his contributions and as a result only Waksman received the Nobel Prize in 1952. In time, the tuberculosis bacillus soon developed resistance against streptomycin, but further studies would demonstrate that, when conjoined with para-aminosalicylic acid or isoniazid, it controlled the infection.

The immeasurable success of antibiotics and other medicines developed during the catastrophic World War II was a catalyst to develop other antibiotics. As streptomycin resistant tuberculosis has illustrated, bacteria are invidious organisms capable of changing their genetic makeup, rendering them resistant to antibiotics. Overuse and misuse of antibiotics have accelerated those processes, necessitating the constant ongoing search for new agents.

Amidst these remarkable advances in infectious diseases two infamous instances of unethical human experimentation smoldered unnoticed – one for decades. In Tuskegee, the United States Public Health Service studied the natural progression of untreated syphilis among rural African-American men from 1932 until 1972. The men all had contracted the disease before, and believed they were receiving treatment. Despite the fact that by 1947 penicillin had become the standard of care, the study continued unchanged. In 1972 a leak in the press exposed the scandal that terminated the study. In 2010, while researching the Tuskegee experiment, Susan Reverby (b. 1946) uncovered that a similar study was conducted in Guatemala from 1946 to 1948 among prisoners, sex-workers and soldiers infected not only with syphilis but also gonorrhea and chancroid. They too, were unaware they were guinea pigs for an unprincipled team.

Antiserums and vaccinations against common diseases became routine in the 20th century. In 1890 Emil von Behring (1854-1917) and Shibasaburo Kitasato (1853-1931) had developed a diphtheria antitoxin, and in 1892 an early tetanus antitoxin. Kitasato is credited as co-discoverer with Alexander Yersin (1863-1943) of the agent of bubonic plague. In 1897 Almoth Wright (1861-1932) had formulated a killed bacilli vaccine against typhoid. Albert Calmette (1863-1933), a pupil of Pasteur, and Camille Guérin (1872-1961) successfully had propagated a nonvirulent strain of tuberculosis which was used in 1921 to produce an antituberculosis vaccine – the BCG.

Although many major infections were controlled and even eliminated, other contagions remained inexplicable: yet unnamed viruses* that had escaped detection in the porcelain Chamberland filter became the next focus and challenge. The existence of infectious particles had been empirically suspected through observation, and the contagious nature of diseases, such as childhood exanthemas, smallpox, rabies, polio, etc. The causes, however, were a mystery subject to vigorous investigation. The new science of bacteriology was not useful in advancing insights, although animal studies supported the existence of non-bacterial infection, and as far back as 1899 Friedrich Loeffler (1852-1915) had proved that foot and mouth disease of ungulates was caused by a non-filterable agent.

It was the electron microscope, the instrument that revealed minute agents of infection, invisible by light-wave microscopy, but made evident and studied through magnetic field focused electrons within a vacuumed chamber that finally made rejectamenta of all that was miasma theory. Only when visualization and successful cultivation of viruses were achieved in the 1930s, could prevention, the next clinical objective, become possible. Safe propagation of viruses in cell cultures allowed investigators to experiment with attenuated and killed viruses to induce immunity. The yellow fever vaccine was developed by Max Theiler (1899-1976) in 1930. The successful experimentation of John Enders (1897-1995), Thomas Weller (1915-2008) and Frederick Robbins (1916-2003) with *in vitro* polio viral cultivation made possible the work of several investigators. Hilary Koprowski (1916-2013) used Max Theiler's vaccine method passing the polio virus through the brain of cotton rats until it was attenuated enough for an oral vaccine (1950). By the end of the 1950s millions in Europe had safely received the vaccine. Jonas Salk (1914-1995) produced an injectable polio vaccine in 1953, and Albert Sabin (1906-1993) received the attenuated virus from Koprowski and in 1960 further attenuated it formulating a new oral polio vaccine that was licensed in the USA and became the preferred vaccine globally.

It made immunization easily and cheaply possible worldwide and all but eradicated polio.** Vaccines against measles, mumps, rubella,

---

*In 1892, Dmitri Ivanosky (1864-1920) while working on the tobacco mosaic disease conceived of such a particle. Six years later, working independently, Dutch microbiologist Martinus Beijernick (1851-1931) first used the word "virus" in 1898 for what he perceived as a new form of infectious agent not visible microscopically.

**In the USA, in 1955, Cutter Laboratories produced a defective batch of polio vaccine that infected over 200 children. Public outcry was great and this accident was the catalyst that ultimately resulted in the passage of the National Childhood Vaccine Injury Act in 1986 which guaranteed compensation to families of children injured by any adverse effect secondary to any mandatory childhood vaccines.

hepatitides and other viral diseases were successfully introduced and added as routine childhood immunizations, along with protection against diphtheria, pertussis and tetanus. In 1980 the World Health Organization (WHO) announced small pox had been eradicated (the last reported case was in Somalia in 1977).

The first effective antiviral agent – Acyclovir – did not appear until 1975 when it was prescribed for herpetic infections. The growing sophistication of immunology (see below) facilitated the identification of numerous additional viral particles responsible for disease. Hepatitis, for example, simply known as "infectious" and "serum," became specifically classified as types A and B, with the suspicions that there existed a third – the nonA-nonB. Stephen M. Feinstone (b. 1944) together with Robert Purcell (b. 1935) and Albert Kapikian (1930-2014) developed an assay for the HAV (infectious hepatitis) and Baruch Blumberg (1925-2011) identified the serum hepatitis HBV. Together with Irving Millman (1923-2012) he developed the HBV vaccine. Feinstone and Harvey Alter (b. 1935) pursued the concept of the third hepatitis agent and proved its existence, and Michael Houghton and colleagues in 1989 delineated the virus now called HCV. HDV, HEV, and HGV were subsequently discovered, with more possibly to be classified.

Tropical hemorrhagic fevers, such as Ebola and Lassa, were identified by scientists and remain untreatable and under investigation. (A major African epidemic outbreak of Ebola in 2014 led to the introduction of several experimental vaccines). In 1984 Luc Montagnier (b.1932) recognized the human immunodeficiency virus (HIV). Robert Gallo (b. 1937) expounded on HIV as the cause of AIDS. Currently third-generation anti-retroviral agents, together with prevention programs, are being used to treat and curtail the spread of the debilitating, and cachectic immune-weakening disease.

In 1990 polymerase chain reaction (PCR) became a practical clinical tool in microbiology and immunology. It was elaborated by biochemist Kary Mullis (b. 1944) who received the Nobel in Chemistry in 1993. The invention makes possible the identification of infectious agents from even the tiniest of samples, and has become an absolute requisite in molecular microbiology.

At the Rockefeller Institute Peyton Rous (1879-1970) in 1910 studied fowl sarcoma by cell-free filtrate and successfully passed the tumor through multiple inoculations – the first demonstration of a virus induced tumor. Rous was the editor of the *Journal of Experimental Medicine* for forty-six years and received the Nobel Prize for his work in 1966. This was the beginnings of what would evolve into the study of oncoviruses, infective organisms that cause animal cell cancer.* Renato Dulbecco (1914-2012), Howard Temin (1934-1994) and David Baltimore (b. 1938) were awarded their Nobel Prizes in 1975 for demonstrating oncoviruses incorporated their genes into host-cell genome leading to tumor transformation as mediated by reverse transcriptases.

Over the next few decades many cancers were believed to be viral induced, but in 1960 Peter Nowell (b. 1928) and David Hungerford (1927-1993) took notice that patients with chronic myeloid leukemia had a very small chromosome, dubbed the Philadelphia chromosome. A decade later, Janet Davison Rowley (1925-2013) identified the chromosome as a translocation from 9 to 22, which was the first to reveal cancer as a genetic disease. Now, translocations are found in lymphomas, sarcomas, prostate, lung and other cancers.

The natural progression from gross or macroanatomy to microanatomy was, as we have come to appreciate, an offshoot of the compound microscope. The intracellular structures early microscopists observed became further defined by electronmicroscopy (EM). Optical microscopy still had great clinical and research usefulness but the new electron instrument became an extraordinary laboratory tool. In 1928 Ernst Ruska (1906-1988) and Max Knoll (1897-1969) produced an instrument capable of 17x magnification. Four years later their instrument had been improved to a magnification of 400x. The instrument James Hillier (1915-2007) and Albert Prebus (1913-1997) designed increased magnification to 7,000x, and in 1937 Manfred von Ardenne (1907-1997) pioneered the scanning instrument. By 1939 Vladimir Zworykin's (1889-1982) device could reach a magnification of up 2,000,000.

Cellular anatomy now is defined by organelles. These structures can be seen and purified by fractionation and the eukaryotic cell (nucleated) is particularly rich in them. In 1833 Brown (1773-1858), of Brownian motion fame, observed and described the cell nucleus. Over the next half-century other intracellular structures were seen under light microscopy. Walther Flemming (1843-1905) observed the chromatin of chromosomes in 1875 and Karl August Möbius (1825-1908) first made mention of little intracellular organs (1884). Further refined observations defined them as membrane-bound structures that included nucleus, mitochondria, endoplasmids, Golgi complex, lysosomes and peroxisomes. Mitochondria were first described by Richard Altmann (1852-1900) in 1890. He called

---

*Exceptions abound in nature. Despite skepticism from colleagues, as late as 1984, Barry Marshall (b.1951) demonstrated the bacterium *Helicobacter pylori* – visible by light microscopy – was a cause of gastritis, gastric ulcers and linked to stomach cancer.

them "bioblasts," but it was Carl Benda (1857-1932) who, observing their heterogeneous shapes, named them mitochondria (*mitos*-thread; *chondrion*-granule). These organelles are the powerhouses generating most ATP and cellular respiration. In 1897, Camillo Golgi described the cellular endomembrane system that now bears his name, little packets that process protein function both for secretion and intracellular use. In 1883 Edouard van Beneden (1846-1910) and in 1888 Theodor Boveri (1862-1915) first observed the centriole which is involved in formation of mitotic spindles and intracellular architecture. A more refined, minute and extraordinarily imaged probing came with EM.

In the 1940s, using cell fractionation and EM, Christian René de Duve (1917-2013) identified packets that stored intracellular enzymes, naming them lysosomes. George Palade (1912-2008) refined fractionation further and was able to isolate mitochondria, Golgi apparatus and the endoplasmic reticulum which he first observed in 1955. Peroxisomes were described by J. Rhodin in his 1954 doctoral thesis and subsequently were confirmed in 1967 by Duve. Peroxisomes were found to catabolize long chain fatty acids, aminoacids and phospholipids. With the exception of the nucleus these organelles were at the limits of light microscopy. Today, cells have lost all intimacy due to the probing eye of the electron microscope.

From early studies of infection, nascent immunology began to understand cellular and humoral reactions. Elie Metchnikoff (1845-1916) and Jules Bordet (1870-1961) made observations that demonstrated the role of white cells in infection and the humoral response that is now called antibodies. Bordet described the phenomenon of red cell hemolysis and discovered that bacteriolysis by specific antibodies is enhanced by complement. The antibodies themselves became the key to diagnosis. In 1896 Fernand Widal (1862-1929) developed an agglutination test for typhoid fever, and in 1906 August von Wasserman (1866-1925) devised one for syphilis. Edmund Weil (1880-1922) and Arthur Felix (1887-1956) created a test for rickettsial diseases in 1915. The 1972 Nobel Prize was awarded to Gerald Edelman (1929-2014) and Rodney Porter (1917-1985) for elucidating the structure of antibodies. Edelman also discovered cell adhesion molecules that allow cells to stick together.

From these initial phases of immunology evolved a science that explored complex cellular responses, not just to infectious agents, but to all foreign particles and proteins including human grafts. Frank Macfarlane Burnet (1899-1985) conducted seminal work on the serological variations of the influenza virus, the cellular cultivation of viruses and the phenomenon of hemagglutination. However, it was his 1949 work on graft rejection, together with British zoologist Peter Medawar (1915-1987), and their discovery of acquired immune tolerance, that became fundamental to the practice of tissue and organ transplantation. For this work they shared the Nobel in 1960. Experiments in transplantation followed. Alexis Carrel (1873-1944), collaborating with Charles Guthrie (1880-1963), had won the 1912 Nobel for achievements in suturing and transplanting vessels, but of equal significance, in 1935 he kept organs viable outside the body, establishing one of the prerequisites for transplantation. In 1950 R.H. Lawley executed the first kidney transplant, but the first successful kidney transplant, from one twin to another (skirting immune-rejection), was performed in 1954 in Boston by surgeon Joseph E. Murray (b. 1919). In 1963 Thomas Starzl (b.1926) performed the first liver transplant and, as already mentioned, Barnard performed the first heart transplant. It should be noted that Norman Shumway (1923-2006) performed the animal experiments that provided the strategy – cooling and leaving the aortic stalk *in situ* – that allowed for a successful cardiac transplant. Barnard had visited Shumway's lab.

These early efforts commonly were met with failure due to graft rejection, but pharmacologic agents were gradually developed that altered the immune cellular response mounted against grafts. Cyclosporin, which inhibits T-cell proliferation, dramatically improved one year survivals to 90%, but side-effects of neurotoxicity and diabetogenesis brought about the development of new agents, among them tacrolimus and other inhibitors of calcineurin. Methods of organ preservation also improved with the knowledge that cells, in the absence of circulation, quickly switch from aerobic to anaerobic metabolism. Cooling – which halves metabolic rates – and preservation solutions were designed for specific organs. Additionally, when it became possible for tissue typing to identify the best possible donor-recipient matches, organ transplants increased, and by the last quarter of the 20th century the success of organ transplants was routine,* enabling focus to shift to another immune phenomenon – autoimmune disease.

Innumerable dedicated investigators have contributed to the fund of knowledge of cellular immunology. Several outstanding individuals in the field should be singled out for their work.

Rudimentally, the autoimmune system has two major components, the B lymphocyte, which produces antibodies – the humoral response – and

---

*These efforts were all and mostly remain allotransplants. Today xenotransplants, particularly from the pig, are common. Currently heart valves, ligaments, intestinal submucosa (bladder repair) are used as structural tissue from which pigs cells have been removed. Some are designed to become populated with host cells.

the T lymphocyte, which musters the cellular response. Perhaps the earliest and most novel observations with respect to B cells came from Ogden Bruton (1908-2003) who in 1952 reported on a patient unable to generate mature B cells, and Max Cooper (b. 1933) who in1974 identified the precursors of the B cell. With respect to the T cell, major kudos belong to Jacques Miller (b. 1931) who elucidated thymic function and the T-cell subset, and to a giant of immunology, Robert Good (1922-2003). Good independently, but along parallel lines with Astrid Fagraeus (1913-1997) established the lymphocyte as the major antibody producer. Good also differentiated lymphocyte subsets and showed that bone marrow transplantation could correct severe immunodeficiency disease. With the breakthrough work by these scientists, it became known that the immune system normally attacks only foreign proteins. In some individuals, however, the process becomes aberrant and attacks the body's own proteins (autoimmune disease). Examples are multiple sclerosis, Hashimoto's thyroiditis, rheumatoid arthritis, lupus and primary biliary cirrhosis. In experimental animals Georges Mathé (1922-2010) demonstrated that bone marrow transplantation would succeed only if the recipient was irradiated to inactivate the immune system. In 1958 a radiation accident in a nuclear reactor overexposed several Yugoslav physicists. Using his prior protocols, Mathé gave them donor marrow transplants with relative success, but in some he noted a secondary generalized wasting which would come to be known as graft-vs-host disease (GVH). The disease was carefully delineated in 1953, and in 1964 sophisticated T and B cell cooperation was demonstrated.

As the 19th century drew to a close, the discipline of endocrinology progressed beyond the "internal milieu" of Bernard into specific molecules. The most important of these molecules was the hormone, a term derived from the Greek *hormonta* – to arouse. As a messenger molecule, the word was coined in 1902 by physiologists William M. Bayliss (1860-1924) and Ernest Starling (1866-1927). Together they discovered secretin and its relationship to gut peristalsis.

Starling also authored the eponymous Law of the heart that states the strength of the heart's systolic contraction is directly proportional to its diastolic expansion with results that under normal physiological conditions the heart pumps out of the right atrium all the blood returned to it without letting any back up in the veins.

In 1891 George R. Murray (1865-1939) successfully treated myxedema with animal thyroid extract, but it was not until 1914 that Edward Kendall (1886-1972) isolated the active substance – thyroxin. In 1894 Edward Sharpey-Schafer (1850-1935) demonstrated that adrenal extracts produced hypertension, and in 1901 Jokichi Takamine (1854-1922) isolated and purified the active component – adrenalin or epinephrine. Kendall capped his triumphs in endocrinology by isolating cortisone in 1935. Philip S. Hench (1896-1965) and his endocrinology team at the Mayo Clinic in Rochester, Minnesota, in 1949 began to use cortisone in the treatment of rheumatoid arthritis.

Doubtlessly the most dramatic story in the evolution of endocrinology relates to insulin. In 1889 Joseph von Mering (1849-1908) and Oskar Minkowski (1858-1931) determined that pancreatectomy in dogs led to fatal diabetes and in 1910 Edward Albert Sharpey-Schafer (1850-1935) hypothesized that diabetes resulted from the deficiency of a single pancreatic chemical. He named the chemical insulin (after the Latin for island – *insula*) in reference to the pancreatic islet cells of Langerhans. Then in 1921 Frederick G. Banting (1891-1941) and Charles Best (1899-1978) worked on diabetes and the role of insulin. These were studies that made possible injectable insulin in the treatment of diabetes. Twenty-nine year old Banting had convinced Toronto physiology professor J.J.R. Macleod (1866-1935) to set up a lab for the extirpation of the dog pancreas. He had been joined in this work by honors medical student Charles Best. Biochemist J.B. Collip (1892-1965) was enlisted in the effort and devised different methods for extracting pancreatic insulin. On January 11, 1922 the team successfully injected insulin into a fourteen year old diabetic boy who was in a terminal state – the first instance in which insulin extract was used to treat a patient. Only Banting and Macleod were awarded the Nobel Prize for Medicine due to a bureaucratic oversight finally acknowledged by the Nobel committee in 1972: "Although it would have been right to include Best among the prize-winners, this was not formally possible, since no one had nominated him…." Both Banting and MacLeod voluntarily shared their prize money with Best and Collip in recognition of their contributions to the development of insulin therapy. From 1929 on Best continued his research at the university as head of the physiology department, experimenting with heparin to dissolve clots. He succeeded Banting as director of the Banting-Best Department of Medical Research (1923) after his mentor's death in 1941.

The beginnings of modern psychiatry are rooted in the work of Pinel in 1792, and the word "psychiatry" was coined in 1808 by Johann Christian Reil (1759-1813). Two schools of thought surfaced at odds with each other: somatology and psychology. German Wilhelm Griesinger (1817-1868) asserted mental illness resulted from organic brain lesions. Emil Kraepelin (1856-1926) of Leipzig also belonged to the somatology school of thought. His publication, *Diagnosis of Dementia Praecox* (1896) was based on the study of thousands of patients. He introduced the terms "manic-depressive psychosis" and "paranoia," and experimented on the effects of various drugs on the central nervous system. Kraepelin developed a profound interest in psychosis and gradually began to favor psychological etiologies, as did Pierre Janet (1849-1947) who focused on neuroses and obsessive disorders. Both men considered these afflictions stemmed from an interruption of normal psychological functions. In Italy, somatology was favored. Enrico Morselli (1852-1929) from Genoa founded a laboratory of experimental psychology and the journal *Rivista di psichologica scientifica* in 1885. Leonard Bianchi (1848-1927) established a course in psychiatry in Naples in 1890 and authored more than twelve books on psychiatry and diseases of the brain. Cesare Lombroso (1836-1909) of Verona initiated what was to evolve as a separate field of study – criminology – with his books *Genio e follia* (1864) and *L'umo deliquente* (1876). Into Lombroso's somatotyping for causes of criminality, insanity and mental retardation fell left-handedness – all defects which he believed were conducted through the primitive limbic system. He claimed "left-handed people are more numerous among criminals and sensitive left-handed people among lunatics," rendering credibility to the adjective *sinister*. He was not alone. John Hughlings Jackson (1835-1911) posited the "dissolution theory" in which neocortical lesions reversed higher evolution into the lower limbic system, and Bénédict Morel (1809-1873) along with Théodule Ribot (1839-1916) expounded on the "degeneration theory" which posited that some disorders like retardation, depravity, depression, alcoholism and criminality all carried destructive vectors to the nervous system which would eventually become hereditary. In France Jules Joseph Déjerine (1849-1917) and his wife Marie Klumpke (1859-1927) wrote an important neurology text, *Anatomie des centres nerveaux* (1895) in which they focused on the study of psychoneurosis.

Paul Charles Dubois (1848-1918) of Bern believed mental disorders were primarily psychological in nature. In *Les Psychoneuroses et leur traitment moral* (1904) he recommended moral psychotherapy that included hypnosis favored by the Charcot school. Moral treatment advocated good habits, quiet surroundings and a strong doctor-patient bond. Belladonna, aconite (monkshood) and opium also were prescribed.

Polymath Englishman Francis Galton (1822-1911) was a geographer, meteorologist, statistician, eugenicist and the designer of differential psychology. He originated dactyloscopy, a method for classifying fingerprints, that has proved invaluable in forensic science, but his interest in fingerprints was rooted in using them to trace hereditary patterns, intelligence and morals and advance psychological understanding, not crime. He was an unabashed bigot who believed all Negros, Hindu and Arabs were inferior.

In America, the Quaker movement was the first to campaign for compassionate treatment of the mentally ill. Benjamin Rush, influenced by Pinel, had supported the somatology theory of mental disease and predictably advocated his favored treatments of blood-letting and purges.

By 1861 the United States had forty-eight asylums. The growing numbers of the mentally afflicted were attributed to genetics, poverty and social degeneration of depressing urban settlements that emerged with the industrial revolution. Since autopsies commonly failed to show organic lesions, psychological dysfunction was more and more favored. Similar ideation evolved in Germany, France and England. The popularity of the Functional School of Psychology led by William James (1842-1910) and the School of Analytic Psychology promulgated by Carl Gustav Jung (1875-1961) both emphasized exploration of the psyche through mythology, religion, philosophy and dreams. Gradually these movements melded into psychoanalysis theory and the therapeutic techniques evolved by Sigmund Freud (1856-1939) that encouraged free association to unlock repressed memory which, thereafter, according to Freud, made the patient more amenable to treatment. Critical to his therapy was the interpretation of dreams – *Die Traumdeutung* (1899) – written by Freud.

By the beginning of the 20th century neurochemistry experimentation that would vastly influence the field of psychiatry increased. In 1914 Henry Hallet Dale (1875-1968) studied ergot alkaloids and identified acetylcholine, and in 1921 Otto Loewi (1873-1961) demonstrated neurotransmission qualities in the frog heart. For this work they both shared the 1936 Nobel.

New agents in psychopharmacology were gradually integrated into analytic psychiatric intervention, and at the same time psychological testing became sophisticated. One area of psychology – psychological nativism – emerged that contends behavior is hard-wired at birth. This belief was an integral component of the Eugenics movement (inspired by the writings of Galton) that began with the work of Charles Davenport (1866-1944), the director of Cold Spring Harbor Laboratory. Davenport studied human heredity based on the model of inheritance constructed by Gregor Mendel, a hypothesis that discrete factors or genes controlled all heredity. Inheritance was grouped into autosomal dominant, autosomal recessive and sex-linked (x-y chromosomes) modes. By 1910 Davenport had developed his theory of human eugenics, the notion that selective breeding could improve the human species. He founded the Eugenics Record Office that tabulated genetic statistics and in 1911 published *Eugenics.* This text became a major work used as a college textbook for many years, and in parts of the United

States,* was cited to justify the sterilization of the "feeble-minded." Nazi Germany justified eugenics for the creation a white master race.**

Beginning in the late 1960s new insights in neurochemistry and synaptic function evolved the discipline of psychopharmacology. In the decades that followed, highly effective psychotropic drugs such as meprobamate, phenothiazines, tricyclic antidepressants and selective serotonin reuptake inhibitors were standard therapeutics used in psychiatric care.

Nineteen fifty-three was a singular year of achievement in medicine and physiology – a 20th century *anno mirabilis*. Biochemist Stanley L. Miller (1930-2007) performed pioneering experiments on the genesis of amino acid synthesis. His experiments in autotrophic carbon assimilation, began as a synthesis study in which he zapped electricity into a solution of "primordial soup" (CH_4, NH_3, H_2O and hydrogen) that resulted in the spontaneous generation of organic molecules. It was a veritable cosmology of the origins of life from chemical elements. After studying the original x-ray crystallography of Rosalind Franklin, James Watson and Francis Crick elucidated the molecular structure of DNA. Jonas Salk produced the polio vaccine. Following twelve years of study and observation, anesthesiologist Virginia Apgar published her newborn health scoring system. Leroy Hoeck (1912-2009) and Arnall Patz (1920-2010) conducted the first randomized controlled study demonstrating the causative role of oxygen in retrolental fibroplasias of prematurity.

---

*In America between 1909 through the 1950s, 33 states adopted laws that led to the sterilization of over 60,000 disabled persons, the deaf, blind, and anomalous. Most procedures were performed under eugenic statutes in state-run hospitals.

**The Nazis employed the policy as part of its goal to produce a "superior race" of people. In 1939 Hitler's government implemented a program based on eugenic *Rassenhygiene* philosophy. The *Reichsauscchuss zur wissen-schaftlichen Erfassung von erb-und anlagebedingter schwerer Leiden* – "Reich committee for the scientific treatment of severe genetically determined illness" was a pseudo-euphemistic label that both protected the bureaucracy and sanctioned its authority to euthanize "defective" children: children with Down syndrome, microcephaly, hydrocephaly, limb deformities, spina bifida, spastic diplegia – congenital anomalies of all kinds (*missgebildetes*). Children were transported and deposited in twenty-two *Kinderfachabteilungen* – special care wards – and "treated" with a lethal dose of oral chloral hydrate. It is estimated that the so called *Behandlung* program of the *Kinderfachabteilungen* killed over five thousand unwanted German children.

"Heliotherapy" for neonatal jaundice was well-known to nannies for centuries, who simply placed their yellow babies in the sunshine. However, the mechanisms of this modality were not explained until 1958. Following an exchange transfusion for severe newborn jaundice, Richard John Cremer (1925-2014) noted that a post-exchange blood sample that had been inadvertently left in a sunny window had a lower bilirubin level. With this chance discovery he pioneered the use of phototherapy – the blue fluorescent tube – for hyperbilirubinema of the newborn.

Advances in many disciplines have enabled surgery to develop procedures inconceivable before this time. Imaging techniques now allow surgeons to peer with stark intimacy, exactness and precision into the diseased part of the body. Modern anesthesia provides the surgeon with a large and safe block of time for precise handiwork. Physiology and pharmacology have perfected compounds to control shock, and transfusion, anticoagulation and antibiotics have helped to avert complications. New and innovative fields of surgery – neurosurgery, intracardiac intervention, burn care and grafting, transplantation, laparoscopic and robotic surgery – have progressed at a galloping pace.

The new powerful incendiary weaponry employed in WWI resulted in brutal and disfiguring injuries. Harold Gillies (1888-1960) began to experiment with skin grafts and established a facial injury ward. In 1917 at the Queen's Hospital Gillies and associates developed plastic surgery techniques performing over 11,000 surgeries. In 1930 Gillies recruited Archibald McIndoe (1900-1960) who quickly mastered the extant common wisdom of plastic surgery. With the start of WWII, new deep burn injuries became more common as highly flammable aviation fuel powered stronger and faster fighter aircrafts. Survivors of the air warfare injuries were brought to the Queen's Hospital where new grafting techniques were developed.

In cancer surgery the antecedent pathological studies of Morgagni, Hunter, Muller and Virchow had confirmed the errant growth of cells that constituted the leukemia and tumor of cancer, but effective therapy necessitated a more fundamental understanding of the nature of the cells involved, their movements and spread, and their sensitivities – a core of knowledge that would not evolve until this century.

In 1896, Scot surgeon George Thomas Beatson (1848-1933) performed ovariectomy for the treatment of breast cancer, perhaps the first use of "chemotherapy" against cancer. This was followed by Charles Huggins (1901-1997) who in 1939 demonstrated the benefits of orchiectomy for prostatic cancer. These, however, were more like endocrine suppression than chemotherapy as we know it today, which did not emerge until 1946 when Alfred Gilman (1908-1984) and colleagues demonstrated that mustard gas caused the regression of lymphoma. This initiated a vigorous interest in chemotherapy which required a reliable animal tumor model and this became available as a result of the work done in the early 1910s by George Clowes (1877-1958) of Roswell Park Memorial Institute who had developed a transportable tumor in rodents. Shortly after Gilman's work, Sidney Farber (1903-1973) noted that folic acid stimulated the proliferation of lymphoblastic cells and he reasoned that folate antagonists would induce a remission of acute lymphocytic leukemia. His report in 1948 was followed in 1951 by Jane Wright's (1916-2013) demonstration that some solid tumors also responded to this modality.

These early successes motivated Congress to create the National Cancer Chemotherapy Service Center in 1955 which drew the attention of pharmaceutical companies and provided financial incentive for more research. In 1965 Barnett Rosenberg (1926-2009) noted that a current passed between platinum electrodes inhibited bacterial growth, which led to the production of *cis*-platinum salt as an antiproliferative agent. What followed thereafter were *adjuvant therapy* which was used after primary surgical resection of the tumor and *combination chemotherapy* with multiple agents. The major limitation to these approaches was micrometastasis.

Over the next twenty years the number of cancer chemotherapeutic agents multiplied to include the taxanes (antimitotic), nitrosoureas (purine analogues), hormonal modulators like tamoxifen and others. But the ultimate refinement of anticancer molecular therapy began to evolve in this century with the concept of *targeted therapy* such as imatinib which inhibits tyrosine kinase and erlotinib which inhibits epidermal growth factor. To this arsenal have been added human monoclonal antibodies that target specific cancer genes.

Oncogenes, carcinogens, radiation, viruses and other agents have been irrefutably linked to cancer causation. Screening and early detection have become an attainable goal. Now oncology surgeons, teamed with oncologists, have in their anticancer armamentarium not only extirpation, but radiation, chemotherapy, immunotherapy, angiogenesis inhibition, apoptotics and a growing field of tumor-specific killing agents, matched to specific marker genes.

The early endoscopic efforts of Desormeaux have been revolutionized by fiberoptics and the new instrumentation has made laparoscopic surgery the paradigm of intervention for many procedures. Made-man compounds have resulted in artificial vessels, joints, valves, lenses. Refinements in cellular manipulation bring to mind the genetic engineering of *Brave New World* (1932) envisaged by Aldous Huxley (1894-1963). In 1978 Patrick Steptoe (1913-1988) and Robert Edwards (1925-2013) introduced *in vitro* fertilization (IVF) that resulted in the birth of baby Louise Brown. In 1996 the lamb famously known as "Dolly" was born as a result of somatic cell nuclear transfer (SCNT), and in 1999 the human genome, the sequence of chemical base pairs that make up DNA, and approximately 20,000-25,000 genes of the human genome were assembled by a team of international researchers whose work is ongoing. The technological triumphs and development of effective drugs in the 20th century resulted in an exponential growth and use of the *Index Medicus,* now digitized.

The tragic and destructive wars of the century also prodded the medical community to achieve major advances in every field from surgery to psychiatry, and enormous progress was made in medical treatment with transfusions, antibiotics – even vitamins and hormones – and in rehabilitation measures and prostheses for the wounded. The new world of genetics, artificial organs, transplants and life supports now extend life expectations beyond ever imagined. Telemedicine has made the consultation immediate and the computer age has facilitated the instantaneous dissemination of medical knowledge.

At the 20th century's *fin de siècle,* a revived neo-Hippocratic clinical approach reestablished the philosophy that the well-being of the whole patient is the prime consideration in medical study and practice. Scottish physician Archibald Cocrane (1909-1988) advocated the modern concept of evidence-based medicine sustained on randomized clinical trials, a passion he elaborated at length in *Effectiveness and Efficiency* (1971). New research and insights into causes of disease at the beginning of this millennium continue as a springboard for current and future investigative endeavors and new treatment forms.

The financial wealth of many nations has initiated a new focus in medicine, from diseases of poverty to diseases of affluence: obesity and syndrome X, with hypertension, diabetes, fatty liver and atherosclerosis; longevity and associated cancers, chronic degenerative diseases and the dementia named after Alois Alzheimer (1864-1915); narcotic addiction and their psychic scars; tobacco and alcohol and the destructive cellular residue they leave behind.

It can be said that the current scientific community outpaces its social environment. Poverty and disease remain major problems in the developed world, and in the Third World are often an overwhelming challenge. The deprivation experienced by a majority of the population world wide – in Central and South America, all of Africa, all of the Middle East and the sub-Asian continent – is daunting. Progress is slow, but crises are like the tsunamis we have witnessed in the recent past. There are political, social, economic and medical problems that seem insurmountable. From the history in the West, as this book demonstrates, people in the past experienced like conditions and in many instances far worse, but nevertheless have survived, as in the play written by Thornton Wilder

(1897-1975), *By the Skin of Our Teeth*. As this is being written, teams of scientists, medical personnel, social workers, people in all fields dedicated to ameliorating demoralizing and life threatening conditions in the world from all causes are at work. The scientific community has the ability to meet the current medical problems that exist, and, with perseverance and persistence, will make significant – major – strides in all parts of the globe and particularly in the Third World, where the top nine causes of mortality have been and remain, in order of frequency, pneumonias, HIV, malaria, childhood diarrhea, tuberculosis, measles, pertussis and meningitis – all preventable and all treatable. The will and the dedication are there to make progress. A shift in societal and in political and economic powerhouses' priorities are the key to ensuring this progress takes place.

In the meantime, the environment has become a critical concern for the general scientific community (as well as the general population) as the planet's ills – pollution, climate change, water shortages, El Niño instability, etc., have emerged as genuine threats to the world's inhabitants.

These and new challenges of world "eco-health" that now confront society, in conjunction with unsolved etiologies and treatments of diseases, will set the course and vector for medicine in the 21st century, as will indeed epigenetics that examines gene expressions which alter DNA phenotype (such as DNA methylation) without changes in the nucleic acid sequences. Translational medicine, or the adaption of basic science discoveries to clinical medicine, will allow epigenetic analysis to design specific and individual boutique protocols for the treatment of disease. Already patients are having individual cancer treatments designed for them based on their epigenetic phenotype and tumor-specific markers. All this brings to mind Shakespeare's insight:

What's past is prologue....
The Tempest II: i

Authors' Note

In writing histories of medicine and pediatrics, we have read hundreds of books on the history of science and medicine. Those listed below are in our opinion the most readable and enjoyable. For a facile exposure to the movements of medicine we suggest Duffin or Nuland; for the most thorough history read Castiglioni or Garrison, and for the social interactive aspects of medicine turn to Porter. Those interested in child health will profit from Colón. Women in the history of medicine is well discussed by Magner and for the sheer wonder about the instincts to heal immerse yourself in Majno's extraordinary opus.

One final admonition for the student of medicine: read poetry, such as that of physician William Carlos Williams (1883-1963). If you have no affinity for poetry, then read William's essays.

> It's the humdrum day-in, day-out, everyday work that is the real satisfaction of the practice of medicine; the million and a half patients a man has seen on his daily visits over a forty-year period of weekdays and Sundays that make up his life. I have never had a money practice; it would have been impossible for me. But the actual calling on people, at all times and under all conditions, the coming to grips with the intimate conditions of their lives, when they were being born, when they were dying, watching them die, watching them get well when they were ill, has always absorbed me.
> Williams, *The Practice* 1951

Castiglioni, A. 1958. *A History of Medicine*. New York: Knopf.

Colón, A.R., Colón P.A. 1999. *Nurturing Children: A History of Pediatrics.* Westport: Greenwood Press.

Duffin, Jacalyn. 1999. *History of Medicine*. Toronto: University of Toronto Press.

Garrison, F. 1929. *An Introduction to the History of Medicine.* Philadelphia: Saunders.

Haggard, H. 1934. *The Doctor in History.* New Haven: Yale U Press.

Lindberg, D. 1992. *The Beginnings of Western Science.* Chicago: U Chicago Press.
Magner, Lois. 1992. *A History of Medicine.* New York: Marcel Dekker.
Majno, G. 1975. *The Healing Hand.* Cambridge: Harvard U Press.
Nuland, Sherwin B. 1988. *Doctors.* New York: Knopf.
Porter, R. 1997. *The Greatest Benefit to Mankind.* New York: Norton.

Finally, in the interest of keeping you humble, remember, most patients get better despite the doctor.

Appendix A: The Hippocratic Oath* (Reference p. 16)

I swear by Apollo Physician and Asclepius and Hygeia and Panacea and all the gods and goddesses, making them my witnesses, that I will fulfill according to my ability and judgment this oath and this covenant:

To hold him who has taught me this art as equal to my parents and to live my life in partnership with him, and if he is in need of money to give him a share of mine, and to regard his offspring as equal to my brothers in male lineage and to teach them this art—if they desire to learn it—without fee and covenant; to give a share of precepts and oral instruction and all the other learning to my sons and to the sons of him who has instructed me and to pupils who have signed the covenant and have taken an oath according to the medical law, but no one else.

I will apply dietetic measures for the benefit of the sick according to my ability and judgment; I will keep them from harm and injustice.

I will neither give a deadly drug to anybody who asked for it, nor will I make a suggestion to this effect. Similarly I will not give to a woman an abortive remedy. In purity and holiness I will guard my life and my art.

I will not use the knife, not even on sufferers from stone, but will withdraw in favor of such men as are engaged in this work.

Whatever houses I may visit, I will come for the benefit of the sick, remaining free of all intentional injustice, of all mischief and in particular of sexual relations with both female and male persons, be they free or slaves.

What I may see or hear in the course of the treatment or even outside of the treatment in regard to the life of men, which on no account one must spread abroad, I will keep to myself, holding such things shameful to be spoken about.

If I fulfill this oath and do not violate it, may it be granted to me to enjoy life and art, being honored with fame among all men for all time to come; if I transgress it and swear falsely, may the opposite of all this be my lot.

*There is no definitive proof of authorship. Some scholars believe the oath may have been composed by the School of Pythagoras which categorically opposed suicide, abortion and contraception. Interestingly, the famous dictum *primum non nocere* is not part of the oath. It may have come from *On Epidemics*.

> The physician must be able to tell the antecedents,
> know the present, and foretell the future – must
> mediate those things and have two special objects
> in view with regard to disease, namely to do good
> or to *do no harm*.

The Oath places emphasis on diet and non-toxic modalities, with surgery as a last resort and only by those skilled in the art, a sentiment expressed his *Aphorisms*.

> Those diseases which medicines do not cure, iron
> cures; those which iron cannot cure, fire cures; and
> those which fire cannot cure, are to be reckoned
> wholly incurable.

Today there are many versions of the Oath. Most commonly they delete abortion, euthanasia and surgery proscriptions, and all have deleted the polytheism.

Appendix B: A medieval code of conduct for the physician written by Archimathasus of Salerno. (Reference p. 51)

"When the physician goes to visit his patients he should place himself under the protection of God and of the angel who accompanied Tobias. On his way he will try and learn from the person who came to fetch him as much as possible of the condition of the patient in order to put himself au courant of the affliction he will have to treat, so that if, after having examined the urine and felt the pulse, he cannot soon learn the nature of the illness, he can by means of the facts previously ascertained at least inspire confidence in the patient by proving to him that he has divined something of the nature of his sufferings. It is well that the sick man before the arrival of the physician should confess himself or undertake to do so, because if his doctor finds it necessary for him he will believe his case desperate, and the inquietude will aggravate his illness, whereas more than one sick man who provides against the reproaches of his conscience recovers because of his reconciliation with the Great Physician....

On his entrance the physician makes his salutations with a grave and modest demeanor, seats himself to take breath, praises, if opportunity affords, the beauty of the location, the elegance of the mansion, the generosity of the family, in this way gaining the good will of those present and giving the sick man time to regain his composure....

On departing the physician promises the patient he shall recover; to those who are about the sickbed, however, he must affirm that the patient is very ill; if the patient recovers the physician's reputation will be enhanced, should he die the physician can state that the outcome was as he predicted. He should not allow his eyes to fix themselves upon the wife or daughter, however beautiful they may be, for that would forfeit his honor and compromise the welfare of the patient by drawing upon the household the anger of God. If he is requested to dine, as is the custom, he must show himself neither indiscreet nor greedy. Unless he is forced he should not take the first place at the table, although that should be reserved for the priest or physician. If in the house of a peasant he should taste everything without finishing it, remarking on the rusticity of the food; if, on the contrary, the table is delicate, he should not yield to the pleasure of the appetite. He should ask for information as to the state of the patient from time to time, who will be charmed to find that he is not forgotten amidst the pleasures of the repast. Upon leaving the table the physician must go to the bedside of the patient, assure him how well he has fared, and above all must not forget to show solicitude as to the regulation of the diet of the sick man."

From *Introduction to L'Ecole de Salerne* by Ch. Meaux Saint-Marc (fl. 14th century) as quoted in *The School of Salernum: Regimen Sanitatis Salernitanum* by Sir John Harington. New York: Paul B Hoeber, 1920. pp. 18-21.

Appendix C: Some of the popular "medical poems." (Reference p. 70)

POEM	DATE	AUTHOR	LANGUAGE
Physica	c.1170	Hildegaard	Latin
Regimen Sanitatis	c.1260	School of Salerno	Latin
Versehung des Liebs	1491	von Louffenburg	German
Syphilis	1530	Fracastoro	Latin
L'Esperon	1532	Anton du Saix	French
Puerile ad Pueros	1536	Nicholas Bourbon	Latin
La Balia	1550	Luigi Tansillo	Italian
Paedotrophia	1559	Giulio Alessandrini	Latin ?
Hebammen Buch	1580	Jacob Rueff	German
Paedotrophia	1584	Scevola St-Marthe	Latin
de Custodienda	1590	Jacob Truncon	Latin
Callipaedia	1655	Claude Quillet	Latin
Infancy	1774	Hugh Downman	English

Appendix D: The vitamins (Reference p. 159)

1912 Vitamin A (retinol): Elmer McCullom (1879-1967) et.al., Thomas Osborne (1859-1929)
1912 Vitamin B1 (thiamin): Christiaan Eijkman (1858-1930), Casimir Funk (1884-1967)
1912 Vitamin C (ascorbic acid): Axel Holst (1860-1931)
1918 Vitamin D (calciferol): Edward Mellanby (1884-1955)
1920 Vitamin B2 (riboflavin): D.T. Smith and E.G. Hendrick
1922 Vitamin E (tocoherol): Herbert Evans (1882-1971)
1926 Vitamin B12 (cyanocobalamin): George Minot (1885-1950), William Perry, George Whipple (1878-1976)
1928 Vitamin C (isolated hexuronic acid: Albert Szent-Gyorgyi (1893-1986)
1929 Vitamin K (phylloquinone): Henrik Dam (1895-1976) and Edward Doisy (1893-1986)
1931 Vitamin B5 (pantothenic acid): Roger Williams (1893-1988)
1931 Vitamin B7 (biotin): Albert Szent-Gyorgyi (1893-1986)
1931 Vitamin B6 (pyroxidine): Paul Gyorgy (1893-1976)
1933 Vitamin B9 (folic acid): Lucy Wills (1884-1964)
1936 Vitamin B3 (niacin): Conrad Elvehjem (1901-1962)

Appendix E: Nobel Prizes in Medicine-Physiology (Reference p. 181)

In 1895 Alfred Nobel (1833-1896) established "prizes to those who, during the preceding year, shall have conferred the greatest benefit on mankind." He designated five areas for awards: physics, chemistry, literature, peace and physiology and medicine. The list of those awarded the Nobel Prize in Physiology and Medicine follows:

1901: Emil Adolf von Behring – serum therapy against diphtheria.
1902: Ronald Ross – malaria and methods of combating it.
1903: Niels Ryberg Finsen – treatment of diseases with light radiation.
1904: Ivan Petrovich Pavlov – physiology of digestion.
1905: Robert Koch – investigations into tuberculosis.
1906: Camillo Golgi and Santiago Ramon y Cajal – structure of the nervous system.
1907: Charles Laveran – the role of protozoa in disease.
1908: Ilya Mechnikov and Paul Ehrlich – immunity studies.
1909: Emil Theodor Kocher – physiology, pathology and surgery of the thyroid.
1910: Albrecht Kossel – cellular chemistry, proteins and nucleic acids.
1911: Allvar Gullstrand – dioptrics of the eye.
1912: Alexis Carrel – vascular suture and transplantation of blood vessels.
1913: Charles Robert Richet – anaphylaxis.
1914: Robert Bárány – physiology and pathology of the vestibular apparatus.
1915-1918: Money was allocated to a special fund.
1919: Jules Bordet – discoveries related to immunity.
1920: Schack August Steenberger Krogh – discovery of capillary motor regulation.
1921: Money allocated to a special fund.
1922: Archibald V. Hill and Otto F. Meyerhof – muscle physiology.
1923: Frederick Banting and John Macleod – discovery of insulin.
1924: William Einthoven – discovery of the mechanisms of the EKG.
1925: Money allocated to a special fund.
1926: Johannes Fibiger – discovery of Spiroptera carcinoma (Gongylonema neoplasticum).

1927: Julius Wagner-Jauregg – therapeutic value of malaria for dementia paralytica.
1928: Charles Jules Henri Nicolle – typhus.
1929: Christian Eijkman and Frederick Hopkins - vitamins
1930: Karl Landsteiner – classification of human blood groups.
1931: Otto Heinrich Warburg – discovery of respiratory enzymes.
1932: Charles Scott Sherrington and Edgar Douglas – functions of neurons.
1933: Thomas Hunt Morgan – role of chromosomes in heredity.
1934: George Whipple, George Minot and William Murphy – liver therapy for anemia.
1935: Han Spemann – the organizer effect in embryonic development.
1936: Henry Dale and Otto Lowei – chemical transmission of nerve impulses.
1937: Albert Szent-Györgyi – discoveries in oxidation, vitamin C and fumaric acid.
1938: Corneille Heymans – role of sinus and aortic mechanisms in respiration.
1939: Gerhard Domagk – discovery of antibiotic effects of prontosil.
1940-1942: Money allocated to special fund.
1943: Henrik Peter Dam and Edad Doisy – vitamin K.
1944: Joseph Erlanger and Herbert Gasser – the nature of single nerve fibers.
1945: Alexander Fleming, Ernst Chain and Howard Florey – penicillin.
1946: Hermann Joseph Muller – discovery of mutations by X-ray radiation.
1947: Carl Cori and Gerty Cori née Radnitz – the catalytic conversion of glycogen.
1948: Paul Müller – DDT activity against arthropods.
1949: Walter Hess and Antonio Caetano de Moniz – brain-viscera interaction and therapeutic value to leucotomy in certain psychoses.
1950: Edward Kendall, Tadeus Reichstein and Philip Hench – adrenal cortex hormones.
1951: Max Theiler – yellow fever and how to combat it.

1952: Selman Waksman – streptomycin and tuberculosis.
1953: Hans Krebs and Fritz Albert Lipmann – citric acid cycle and co-enzyme A.
1954: John Enders, Thomas Weller and Frederick Robbins – growth of polio virus in cell cultures.
1955: Alex Theorell – nature and mode of action of oxidation systems.
1956: Andre Cournand, Werner Forssmann and Dickinson Richards – heart catheterization and pathological changes of circulatory system.
1957: Daniel Bovet – discovery of compounds affecting vascular and muscular systems.
1958: George Beadle, Edward Tatum and Joshua Lederberg – genes and genetics of bacteria.
1959: Severo Ochoa and Arthur Kornberg – the biological synthesis of RNA and DNA.
1960: Frank MacFarlane Burnet and Peter Medawar – discovery of acquired immune tolerance.
1961: George von Békésy – physical mechanisms of stimulation within the cochlea.
1962: Francis Crick, James Watson and Maurice Wilkins – molecular nature of nucleic acids and translation in living material.
1963: John Eccles, Alan Hodgkin and Andrew Huxley – ionic mechanisms of nerve cell membranes.
1964: Konrad Bloch and Feodor Lynen – mechanisms of cholesterol and fatty acid metabolism.
1965: François Jacob, André Lwoff and Jacques Monod – genetic control of enzyme and virus synthesis.
1966: Peyton Rous and Charles Huggins – tumor inducing viruses and hormonal treatment of prostatic cancer.
1967: Ragnar Granit, Haldan Hartline and George Wald – physiology and metabolism of the eye.
1968: Robert Holley, Har Khorana and Marshall Nirenberg – the genetic code and protein synthesis.
1969: Max Delbrück, Alfred Hersey and Salvador Luria – replication mechanisms and genetic structure of viruses.
1970: Bernard Katz, Ulf von Euler and Julius Axelrod – humoral transmitters in nerve synapses.

1971: Earl Sutherland – discoveries concerning the mechanism of action of hormones.
1972: Gerald Edelman and Rodney Porter – on the chemical structure of antibodies.
1973: Karl von Frisch, Konrad Lorenz and Nikolaas Tinbergen – organization and elicitation of individual and social behavioral patterns.
1974: Albert Claude, Christian de Duve, George Palade – structural and functional organization of the cell.
1975: David Baltimore, Renato Dulbecco and Howard Temin – interaction between tumor viruses and cell genetics.
1976: Baruch Blumberg and Carleton Gajdusek – new mechanisms on the origin and dissemination of infectious diseases.
1977: Roger Guillemin, Andrew Schally and Rosalyn Yalow – brain peptide production and radioimmunoassay of peptide hormones.
1978: Werner Arber, Daniel Nathans and Hamilton Smith – restriction enzymes and application to molecular genetics.
1979: Allan Cormack and Godfrey Hounsfield – development of the CAT.
1980: Baruj Benacerraf, Jean Dausset and George Snell – genetic cellular structure regulating immune responses.
1981: Roger Sperry, David Hubel and Torsten Wiesel – specialization of cerebral hemispheres and processing of the visual system.
1982: Sune Bergström, Bengt Samuelson and John Vane – prostaglandins and related biological substances.
1983: Barbara McClintock – discovery of mobile genetic elements.
1984: Niels Jerne, Georges Köhler and César Milstein – theories concerning the immune system and production of monoclonal antibodies.
1985: Michael Brown and Joseph Goldstein – regulation of cholesterol metabolism.
1986: Stanley Cohen and Rita Levi-Montalcini – discovery of growth factors.
1987: Susumu Tonegawa – discovery of the genetic principle on generation of antibodies.

1988: James Black, Gertrude Elion and George Hitchings – principles for drug treatment.
1989: Michael Bishop and Harold Varmus – cellular origins of retroviral oncogenes.
1990: Joseph Murray and Donnall Thomas – organ and cell transplantation.
1991: Erwin Neher and Bert Sakmann – function of single ion channels.
1992: Edmond Fischer and Edwin Krebs – reversible protein phosphorylation.
1993: Richard Roberts and Phillip Sharp – discovery of split genes.
1994: Alfred Gilman and Martin Rodbell – G-proteins and cellular signal transduction.
1995: Edward Lewis, Christiane Nüsslein-Volhard and Eric Wieschaus – genetic control of early embryonic development.
1996: Peter Doherty and Rolf Zinkernagel – specificity of cell mediated immunity.
1997: Stanley Prusiner – discovery of prions.
1998: Robert Furchgott, Louis Ignarro and Ferid Murad – NO signaling in the cardiovascular system.
1999: Günter Blobel – discovery that proteins have signals governing cellular transport.
2000: Arvid Carlsson, Paul Greengard and Eric Kandel – signal transduction in the nervous system.
2001: Leland Hartwell, Timothy Hunt and Paul Nurse – key regulator of cell cycle.
2002: Sydney Brenner, Robert Horvitz and John Sulston – genetic regulation of organ development and programmed cell death.
2003: Paul Lauterbur and Peter Mansfield – discoveries on magnetic resonance imaging.
2004: Richard Axel and Linda Buck – odorant receptors and organization of olfaction.
2005: Barry Marshall and Robin Warren – Helicobacter pylori and role in gastritis and peptic ulcer disease.
2006: Andrew Fire and Craig Mello – discovery of RNA interference and gene silencing by double-stranded RNA.
2007: Mario Capecchi, Martin Evans and Oliver Smithies – specific gene modification by use of embryonic stem cells.

2008: Harald Hausen, Francoise Sinoussi and Luc Montagnier – discovery of human papilloma virus cervical cancer and discovery of HIV.
2009: Elizabeth Blackburn, Carol Greider and Jack Szostak – discovery of how chromosomes are protected by telomeres and enzyme telomerase.
2010: Robert Edwards – invitro fertilization.
2011: Bruce Beutler, James Hoffman and Ralph Steinman – innate and adaptive immunology.
2012: John Gurdon and Shinya Yamanaka – cloning, and cellular pluripotentials.
2013: James Rothman, Randy Schekman, Thomas Südhof - regulation of cellular vesicles.
2014: John O'Keefe, Mary Britt Moser, Edvard I. Moser – cells that control positioning in the brain.

Appendix F: Origins of National Health Insurance (Reference - p. 115)

In Western medical history, the genesis of health insurance – the "3rd party system" of our day – can be traced to 1601 and the Elizabethan Poor Relief Act which mandated Parishes responsible for the welfare and health of the poor. The medieval structure of monastic health care, having vanished after the dissolution of the monasteries (1536-1541) by Henry VIII, left the poor essentially without recourse to health care. Parochial care for the poor filled the void for decades. Always financially onerous, parishes finally began to form medical care collectives that required mandatory premiums for those with some means, with frequent amendments to the Poor Relief Act.

In 1757 parliament decreed the Thames coal-heavers be required to establish funds for medical care by requiring employers to withhold from workers' wages two shillings for each pound earned. The system was widely abused by employers, and, twelve years later, in 1770, the act was abolished. Twenty-three years passed before England's parliament in 1793 enacted the George Rose (1744-1818) Plan that authorized the establishment of societies to collect funds to be used for medical necessities for its members. Societies such as these grew in number, and, by 1872, there were between two to four million people enrolled in approximately 32,000 collectives. To ensure against the financial collapse of any of these societies, the Act of 1875 placed them under government supervision and guaranteed the funds therein. The Act of 1834 provided medical care for the indigent with 'Poor Law doctors' who received fixed salaries and case-load supplements and facilitated the establishment of infirmaries and dispensaries.

On the continent, voluntary insurance plans also began to evolve. In France, the glass industry and the gravediggers guilds collected medical care premiums. In Germany, a *Krankenkassen* evolved that collected dues from workers. By the end of the 19th century Germany, Austria, Hungary and France had compulsory health insurance for workers funded by obligatory premiums. In England, after decades of proposals and patch-work laws, Clement Attlee's (1883-1967) postwar government, in 1946, established the National Health Service. The whole of Europe and Canada embraced the philosophy that health care was a public right that should be supported and managed by the State.

Early efforts to guarantee health care emerged in America by 1799, when the Congress established the Marine Hospital system that required all sailors to buy health insurance. In 1850, the Franklin Health Assurance Company of Massachusetts offered injury insurance for railroad and steamship worker accidents. Several other companies began to offer similar insurances in other industries. But these plans benefited a very small number of the general population.

Universal health care was a vision of President Theodore Roosevelt (1858-1919) when, in the election of 1912 his Progressive Party endorsed health insurance for all in its platform. Roosevelt, of course, lost the election. In 1915, the American Association of Labor lobbied for compulsory health insurance, but, with the advent of World War I, the effort waned. The Sheppard-Towner Act of 1921, with a federal appropriation of seven million dollars, aimed to reduce infant and child mortality by providing state planned and administered health clinics for prenatal and preventative pediatric care, and public health nurses to instruct mothers on nutrition and child-care. Senator James Reed of Missouri (1861-1944) was one of several dissenting voices who, without foundation, regarded "the fundamental doctrines on which the bill is founded were drawn chiefly from the radical, socialistic, and Bolshevistic philosophy of Germany and Russia." In 1922 at its annual association meeting, the pediatric branch of the American Medical Association (AMA) supported the Sheppard-Towner Act, despite much rancor and criticism from the general membership. Before the day was over the AMA House of Delegates vindictively condemned the Act. The conflict and disagreement festered for years until, in 1929, after intense pressure from various groups including the AMA, the law was allowed to expire. A year later, in 1930, no longer able to tolerate fundamental philosophic differences, a schism group of AMA members, strong advocates of children's rights, established the American Academy of Pediatrics.

In the early 1930s Franklin Delano Roosevelt's (1882-1945) administration studied health care policies. There was strong opposition, fiercely voiced by physicians and members of Congress to any national health care proposal. Morris Fishbein (1889-1976) of the American Medical Association echoed the general view that such an entity "would socialize if not communize one phase of American life. We shall become a nation of automatons, moving, breathing, living, suffering and dying at the will of politicians and political masters."

During the 'Great Depression' Roosevelt managed to persuade Congress to pass the landmark Social Security Act in 1935. The legislation restored much of the Sheppard-Towner programs for children. Concerned, however, that a debate about National Health Insurance (NHI) would jeopardize the Social Security Act, the administration and Congress tread lightly and did not endeavor to further expand health care coverage. In anticipation the Social Security Act would be signed into law, physicians organized the first Blue Shield Insurance Plan to assure what they erroneously perceived as threat to their autonomy. Over the next several decades numerous profitable private health insurance companies were established.

Just before the second World War, Senator Robert Wagner (1877-1953) introduced a NHI bill that died in committee. Following World War

II Harry Truman (1884-1972) tried to resurrect the objective of NHI, but a national AMA campaign against any such proposed legislation effectively dismantled the effort. Between 1943 and 1950 several NHI bills were introduced in congress and in 1947 the AMA began its lobbying against what it called "socialized medicine" and "fascist" health care. Ironically, the iconic painting by Luke Fildes (1843-1927) – *The Doctor* – which the British NHS used to commemorate its semi-centennial was used by the AMA to inflame sentiment against a NHI (Fig. 27). With the exception of the AFL-CIO (1957), there was no support for NHI until the passage of the 'Great Society's Medicare-Medicaid legislation signed into law in 1965 by then President Lyndon B. Johnson (1908-1973), with Harry Truman at his side.

In 1993 President William Clinton (b. 1946) proposed a universal coverage plan with individual mandates administered by "managed competition" – a convoluted plan replete with government regulators that splintered congressional support. The bill was soundly rejected. Not until 2006, when Massachusetts passed legislation to provide health care to all state residents through insurance mandates, did a NHI concept began to be seriously imagined nationwide, albeit with ongoing strong opposition. President Barack Obama (b. 1961) cajoled out of the Congress the most far reaching and innovative health care coverage ever experienced in America – the Affordable Care Act in 2010. It extended healthcare coverage to the poor through Medicaid expansion and to the middle class by mandatory insurance exchanges. Insurance health plans no longer could deny coverage for any reason, whether it be a pre-existing condition or a job change and 80% of premiums had to be spent on patients. Fully implemented in 2014, the Act made health insurance available to nearly everyone in the country. The closest the United States of America has ever come to NHI was signed into law on 23 March of 2010 nearly fifty years after the rest of the industrialized nations of the world had enacted NHI for its citizens. The sentiments Virchow expressed in his Silesia report (1848) still reverberate today: "Every individual has the right to existence and health, and the State is responsible for ensuring this."

Appendix G: Ophthalmology (Reference p. 40)

In 1247 Peter Hispanus (c. 1215-1277) was professor of medicine and ophthalmology at the University of Siena, where he wrote *De Oculis*, a compendium of classical and Arabic ocular knowledge. Three hundred years later, little else had evolved in the field until Georg Bartisch (1537-1607) published *Ophthalmodoulein das is Augendienst* in 1583, which described both operative interventions and conservative measures such as ocular movement exercises and eye patching.

An understanding of the mechanisms of vision began with Felix Platter (1536-1614), who described the convex nature of the eye lens. Johann Kepler (1571-1630) and Jesuit, Christoph Scheiner (1573-1650), both surmised that an inverse image was projected on the retina instead of the commonly held opinion that the image was upright, and that papillary constriction occurred with light and convergence, with near sight.

As the 18th century began, Antoine Maitre-Jan (1650-1725) on dissection demonstrated that a cloudy lens was a lenticular cataract. In 1745 Jacques Daviel (1696-1762) performed the first extra capsular cataract extraction, a technique improved by Guillaume Pellier de Quengsy (1751-1835) from Montpellier who also devised a technique for correcting a scarred cornea.

An original text on eye disease and glaucoma – *Traite de la Cataracte et du Glaucome* – was published by Charles Saint Yves (1667-1731) in 1722, but it was Englishmen John Taylor (1703-1772) and John Thomas Woolhouse (1650-1734) who recognized the destructive nature of glaucoma.

Vienna's fame as a center for the treatment of eye diseases began in 1812 with the first department of ophthalmology headed by Georg Joseph Beer (1763-1821). About this time Johann Wolfgang von Goethe (1749-1832) – whose oeuvres include epic poetry, prose, aesthetic criticism and treatises on botany and anatomy – advanced a theory about the perception of color which was experiential rather than physical. It was critically examined by John Dalton (1766-1844) who was himself color-blind and who recognized the hereditary nature of the condition.

An exciting era of ophthalmology began in the mid-19th century as new instruments and a better understanding of eye anatomy evolved. Von Helmholtz described the ophthalmoscope, and Frans Cornelis Donders (1818-1889) analyzed anomalies of refraction and accommodation. Iridectomy for glaucoma pathology was explained by Albrect von Graefe (1828-1870), but pilocarpine for the non-surgical treatment of glaucoma was not isolated until 1874. Three years later, Adolf Weber (1829-1915) recognized its value for decreasing intraocular pressure. Carl Koller published on cocaine for corneal anesthesia (1884) facilitating operative procedures, and the first successful corneal transplant was done by Eduard

Zirm (1863-1944). The slit lamp for segmental examination of eye chambers was invented by Allvar Gullstrand (1862-1930), which made possible more detailed description of pathological mechanisms.

Jules Gonin (1870-1935) of Switzerland studied the vitreous body, and, from 1902 to 1921, revolutionized the treatment of retinal tears through *ignipuncture*. Hans Goldmann (1899-1991) designed the semicircular perimeter for visual field examination as well as a new tonometer. Ragnar Granit (1900-1991) and Gösta Karpe (1908-1990) both introduced retinal electrophysiology examination, and in 1946, Gerhard Meyer-Schwickerath (1920-1992) advanced the treatment of retinal tears with light coagulation. Later this would be accomplished by the laser. In 1950, Harold Ridley (1906-2001) performed the first intraocular lens implantation followed by new and more stable clip-on designs. By the end of the 20th century the routine care and treatment of two of the most common eye ailments – glaucoma and cataracts – were routine.

The focus on treatment of sight loss due to macular degeneration – the juvenile form and age-related forms that generally begin after the age of 60 – began with Karl Stargardt (1875-1927) who described the juvenile form in 1901. Both juvenile and age-related macular degeneration are now considered the most common causes of blindness and visual impairment. The prevalence is about 30% in patients between the ages of 75 to 85 years. The causes, risk factors, genetics and treatments of macular degeneration are in the forefront of ophthalmology research and study.

Appendix H: Spices (Reference p. 45)

The historiography of healing spices begins with all ancient cultures* and their extant records of *re medicamentosa*. The common thread in these ancient texts is that bad odors were associated with illness and sweet odors with health and joy. Rooms therefore were suffused with the wafting smoke of gums, resins and spice, a fumigation of pleasant aromas *per fumus* – perfume. Poultices saturated with the vapors of bdellium (*Commiphora mukul*), mustard and sesame were placed over wounds. Apothecaries mixed sweet honey syrups of violets and roses spiced with ginger, pepper, nutmeg and many other spices. All had specific indication and contraindications. Through the ages, the great plant pharmacopeias of the *Susruta*, Dioscorides, Theophrastus, ibn al-Baitar, Lin Shih Chen, Paracelsus, and ethnobotanicals of New World informed the treatment of disease. Today, twenty-five percent of the medications employed are still of botanical origin, and, there was a time before the pharmaceutical industry when all medications were defined by the Dioscoridian classification (p. 33) and employed by long established indications and guidelines.

Geographer Strabo (c. 63 BCE-24 CE) wrote that Roman fleets annually sailed to India using a piloting guide – the *Periplus* – that described each navigation juncture across what was referred to as the Erythraean Sea (the Red Sea, Persian Gulf and Indian Ocean). These annual journeys were conducted to obtain *pigmenta* – spices from the Moluccas – that were part of the *materia medica* of the apothecary long before they entered culinary chemistry, and thus were described in ancient pharmacopeias. In the physician's cupboard, spices were labeled *armarium pigmentorum*.

Under the humoral theory, some ailments considered to have cold and wet properties were treated with spices deemed to have hot and dry qualities. Therefore, considering the principles of *contraria contrariis curantur*, spices were employed to treat dyscrasias of melancholic humors. Cinnamon, nutmeg, pepper, cloves were considered hot and dry; ginger and galangal were considered hot and wet. Of all the spices, the most prescribed was pepper – *Piper nigrum*. The fifth century *Syriac Book of Medicine* recommended pepper corns placed in the canal for earaches, in the

---

*Egyptian papyri (c. 1500 BCE) list cumin, garlic, thyme and fennel as curative. Tutankhamen's tomb had garlic scattered about. Sumerians (c. 5000 BCE) also employed garlic and thyme. Hippocrates prescribed garlic for uterine cancer and licorice for asthma and mouth ulcers. Chinese Emperor Huang Ti recommended *Ginko biloba* for stamina, galagal for abdominal pain, nutmeg for diarrhea and cinnamon for colds. The *Ayurveda* used turmeric for jaundice, basil for heart ailments, maca for diarrhea and ginger for nausea and vomiting.

mouth for oral abscesses or toothaches, and taken internally for intestinal worms and for dysentery. Both Venerable Bede (672-735) and Alcuin (c. 735-804) prescribed pepper, cassia and cinnamon for the plague and disorders of the bowel. Hildegarde von Bingen treated pleurisy with pepper, heartburn and halitosis with galagal, and used cinnamon for fevers. Spices were graded by potency and, for example, the Salernan *Regimen Sanitatis* advised one nutmeg as salubrious, but two as dangerous and three as fatal.

Spices were particularly used for disorders associated with aging, poisoning and sexual dysfunction. Growing old was considered a process of gradual heat loss, a slow decay from the cooling of the body, terminating in death. The aging patient, it was noted, always complained of "feeling cold" and had cold extremities. Frequently they overdressed – a clear indication of heat loss. Aging therefore, it was thought, could be mitigated by hot spices. Roger Bacon advocated cloves, nutmeg and mace to slow the process. (Mace and nutmeg both come from *Myristica fragans* whose fruit upon ripening splits open to release a brown nutmeg in a membrane of red mace). Arnold of Villanova recommended licorice root, nutmeg and galangal for the same purpose. (Galangal, the root of *Alpina offinarum* is related to ginger). Like aging, poisons were believe to kill by cooling, albeit, in the contrast, rather acutely. Spices, therefore, in the absence of bezoars or unicorn horn,** were considered antidotes to be administered with immediacy. Theophrastus (c. 372-287 BCE) prescribed pepper against hemlock, while Dioscorides preferred ginger for almost all poisons, and Galen favored cinnamon.

For sexual dysfunction, a most unexpected manual comes from the Benedictine Constantine Africanus, whom we first encountered in the great translational movement, during which time he translated thirty-seven books from Arabic into Latin. Constantine wrote *De coitu*, that prescribed electuaries (cane sugar based preparations) of ginger, pepper, galangal and cinnamon as aphrodisiacs, and in the morning, milk flavored with cloves to sustain sexual vigor. For frank impotence, he added arugula and carrots, with their phallic connotation, to the mix. Both al Jazzar and Avicenna believed ginger was aphrodisiacal and also increased fertility. Spices occasionally were prescribed for visual and anal disorders.

**The belief that bezoars mitigated poisoning dates back to Mithridates VI (c. 132-63 BCE), king of Pontus, who experimented with antidotes. He exposed himself to so many poisons that he developed resistance and when fate led him to suicide he had to order his own bodyguard to run him through. He lent his name to Mithridatum, an ingredient of *Theriac magna* (p. 42). As a poison semaphore, medieval kings often kept a unicorn horn (narwhale) in their dining rooms, believing that the horn "sweat" in the presence of poison.

Peter Hispanus recommended a poultice of pepper placed over the eyes for dimming vision, as did the *Herbarium de Apuleius*. Such a recipe must have inevitably resulted in irritation, some degree of conjunctiva injection and pupillary constriction (an artificial squint that temporarily sharpened vision). Albertus Magnus prescribed the insertion of peppercorns for hemorrhoids and Juan Gil de Zamora (1241-1318) inserted peppercorns in the nose of patients with epilepsy.

Spices were considered dried and aged substances, differentiated from herbs, which were generally green and fresh. Botanical in origin, they could be buds like cloves, roots like ginger or galagal, seeds like cumin, poppy or sesame, berries such as peppercorns or stigma like saffron. But other dried and age ingredients entered the armamentarium of the apothecary. Thus tutty, chimney scrapings from Alexandria, was classified as a spice and used as a panacea. Momie or mumia were dried and pitch-like desiccated Egyptian corpse *material* – specifically from the head or spine, and used to stem bleeding from the nose or gums. Medicinal perfumes were concocted from frankincense, balsam, myrrh, ambergris (sperm whale gastric content), castoreum (beaver), musk (Tibetan deer) and civet (wild cat) and all used to avert diseases associated with miasma.

Appendix I: Figures referred to in the text.

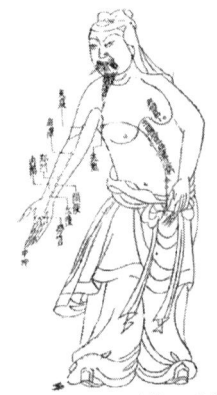

Fig. 1: Acupuncture meridians, Ming period. Courtesy Wikimedia Commons.

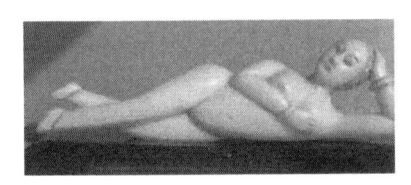

Fig. 2: "Doctor's Lady" (5 x 15 cm) c. 19th century. Collection of the authors.

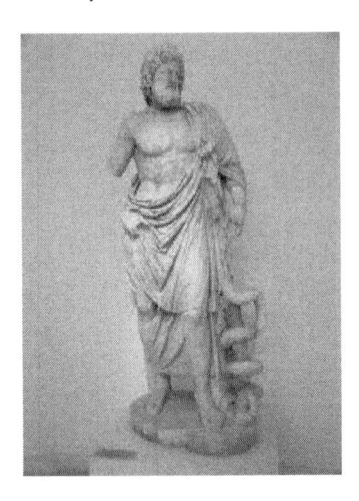

Fig. 3: Asklepios. Note his staff with entwined snake. Courtesy Wikimedia commons.

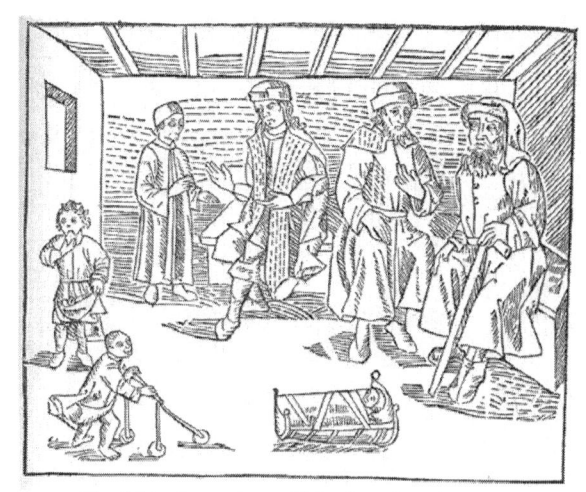

Fig. 4: The Seven Ages of Man from Bartolomeus Anglicus *La proprietaire des choses*, Lyon 1497. Courtesy Wikimedia commons.

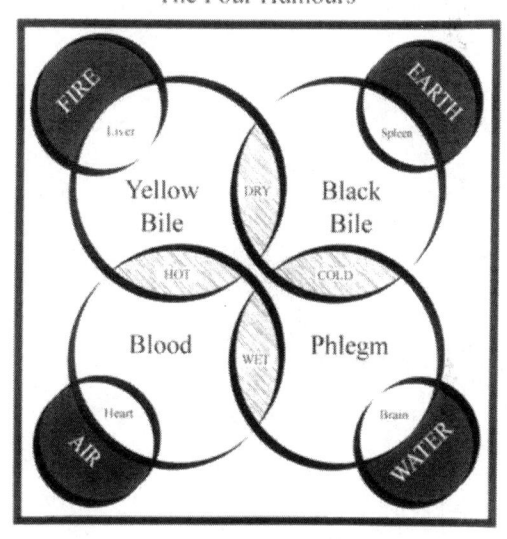

Fig. 5: The Four Humors, elements and attributes. From *Nurturing Children*.

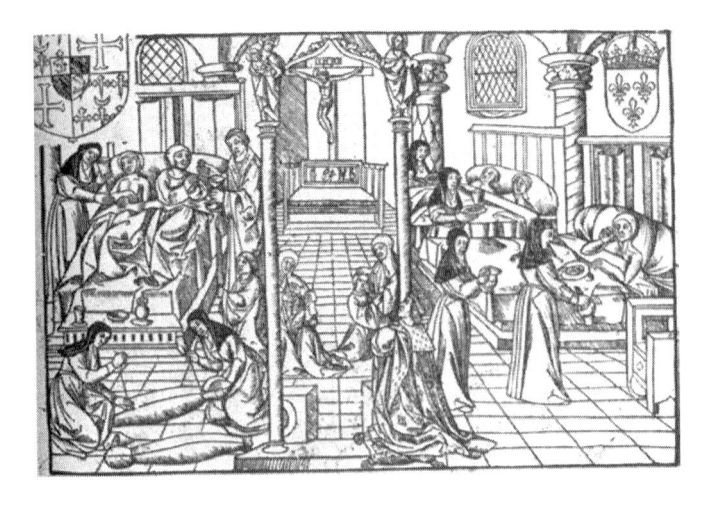

Fig. 6: *Hotel Dieu*. Note the Christian iconography and the dead being enshrouded in linen. The nuns are of the Augustinian order. GNU free documentation license.

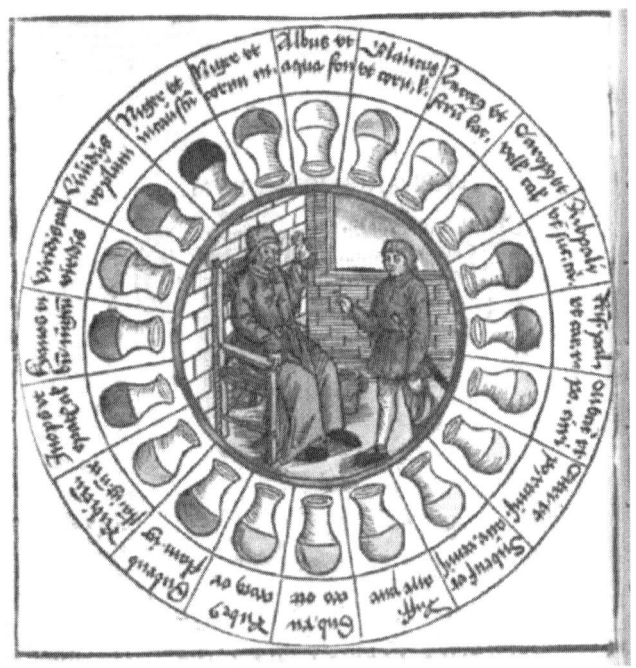

Fig. 7: Urine color wheel. Note the physician examining a matula. *Fasciculus medicinae*, Venice 1496. Courtesy Library of Congress.

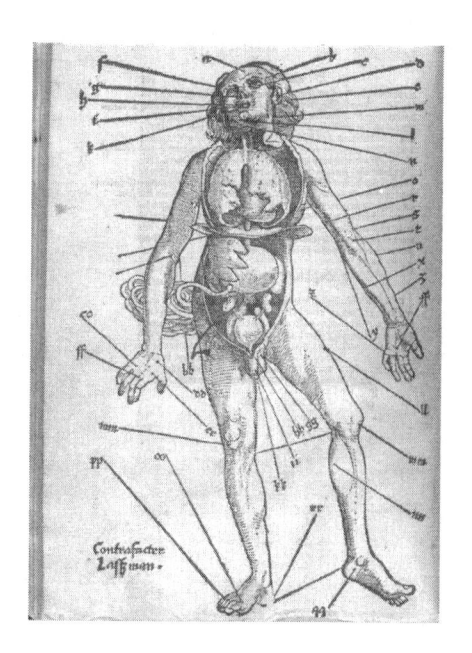

Fig. 8: Phlebotomy man that illustrates the sites for bleeding. Courtesy NLM-IMH

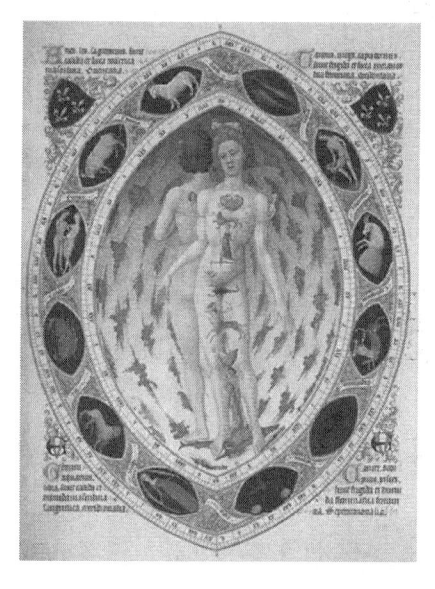

Fig. 9: Astrologic or Zodiac man. Duc de Berry Psalter (14th century). Courtesy Wikimedia commons

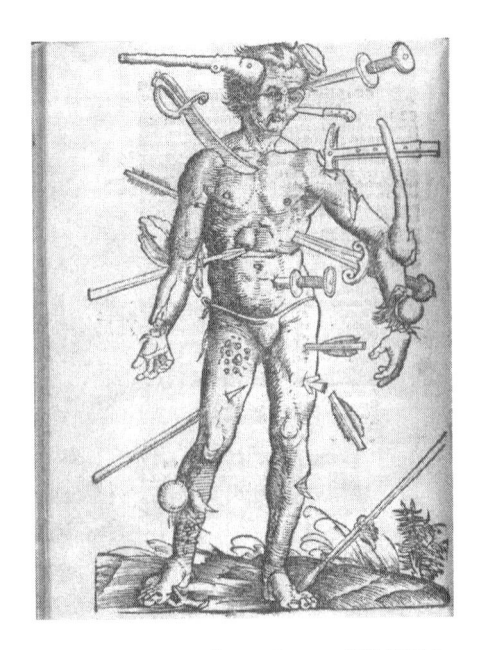

Fig. 10: The Wound man. Courtesy NLM-IHM.

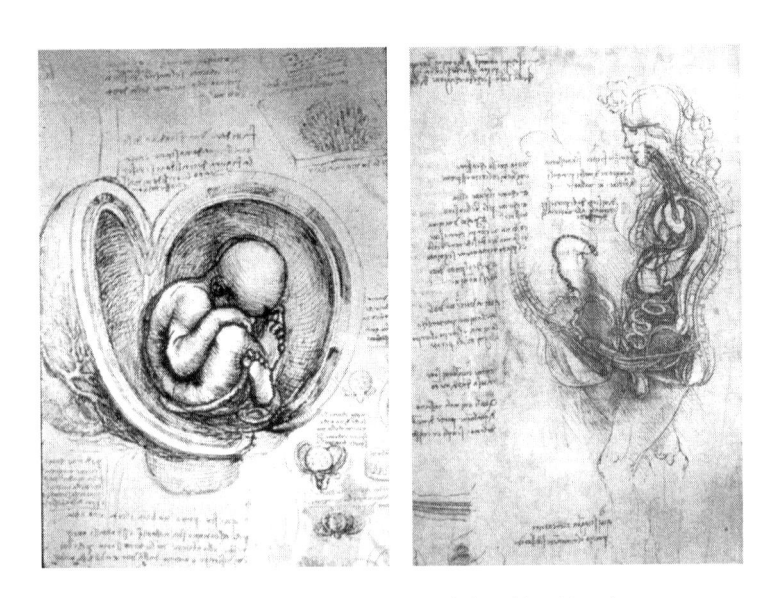

Fig. 11: Da Vinci's fetal depiction and couple in coition. Note the [added] darkened highlighted kiveris vein between the uterus and the woman's breast. Courtesy Wikimedia Commons.

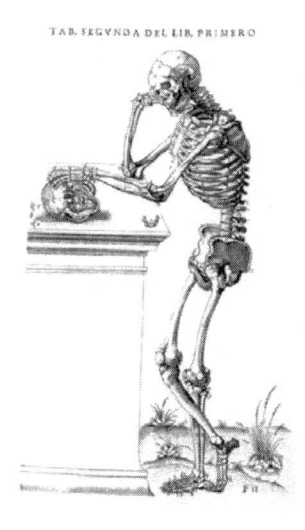

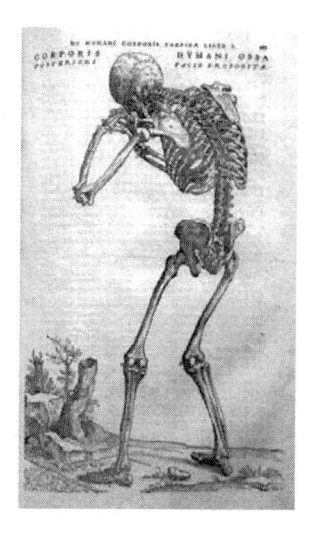

Fig. 12: Illustrations from *De Fabrica Humani Corporis* (1543) by Vesalius. Stephen Kalcar has rendered *contraposto* characteristics and *memento mori* as "death contemplating death" and weeping. Courtesy NLM-IHM.

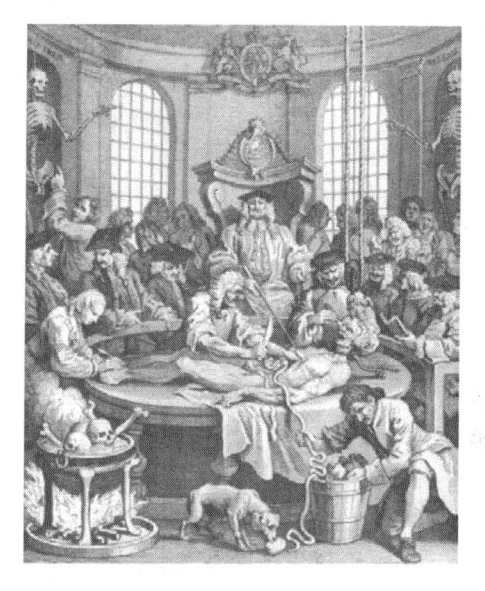

Fig. 13: Hogarth, *The Rewards of Cruelty* (1751). Courtesy NLM-IHM.

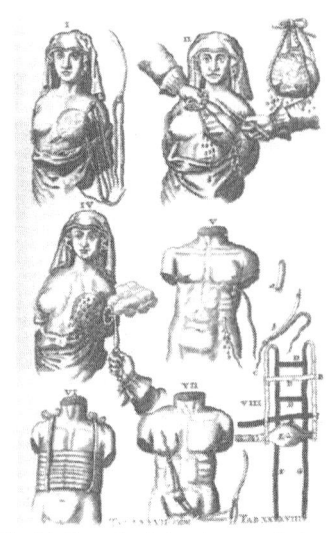

Fig.14: From Scultetus *Armamentarium Chirurgicum* showing mastectomy for cancer and umbilical trusses. Courtesy NLM-IHM.

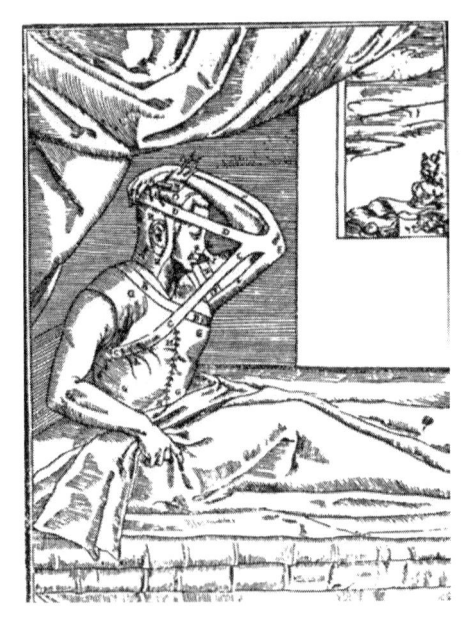

Fig. 15: Rhinoplasty technique of Gaspare Tagliacozzi *Chirurgia curtorum per insitionem* (1597). Courtesy Wikimedia commons.

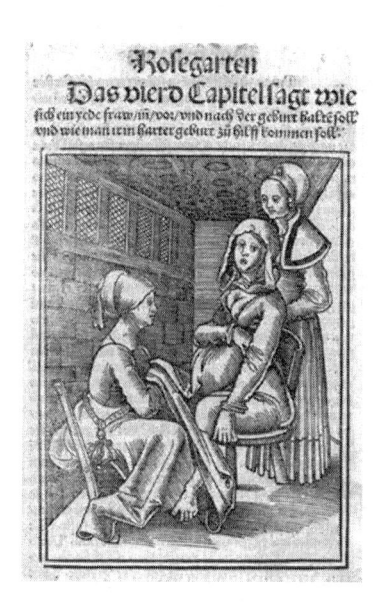

Fig. 16: Birthing woodcut by Conrad Merkel, friend of Dürer, from Roesslin's *Der Swangern frawen und hebammen Rosengarten*. (1512) Courtesy Wikimedia Commons.

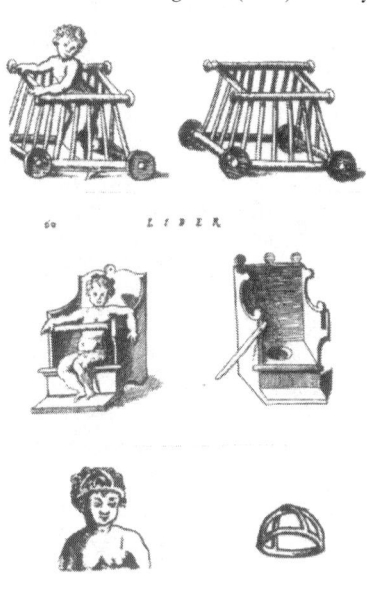

Fig. 17: Omnibus Ferrarius. *De arte medica infantium* (1577). From *Nurturing Children*.

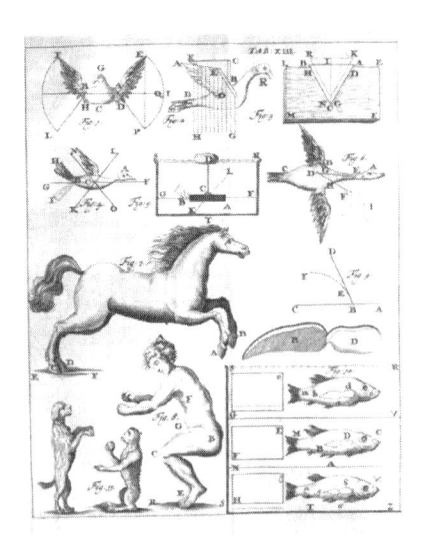

Fig. 18: Iatromechanics of Borelli in *De motu animalium* (1680). Courtesy Wikimedia commons.

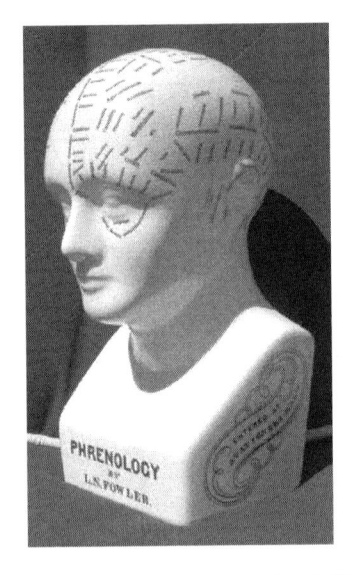

Fig. 19: Phrenology head illustrating Gall's cranial surface analysis. Courtesy Mr. Frank Doyle.

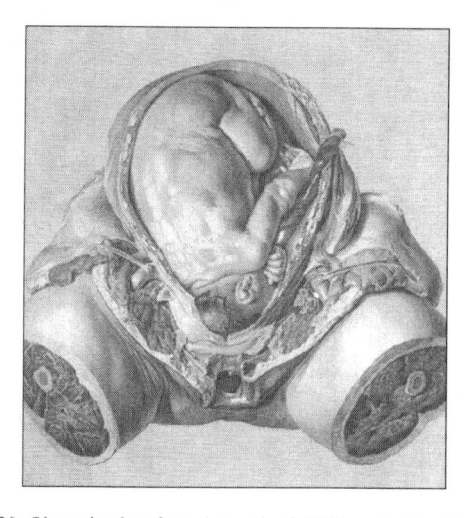

Fig. 20: Obstetric plate from the work of William Hunter. Drawing by Jan van Rymsdyck. Courtesy Wikimedia commons

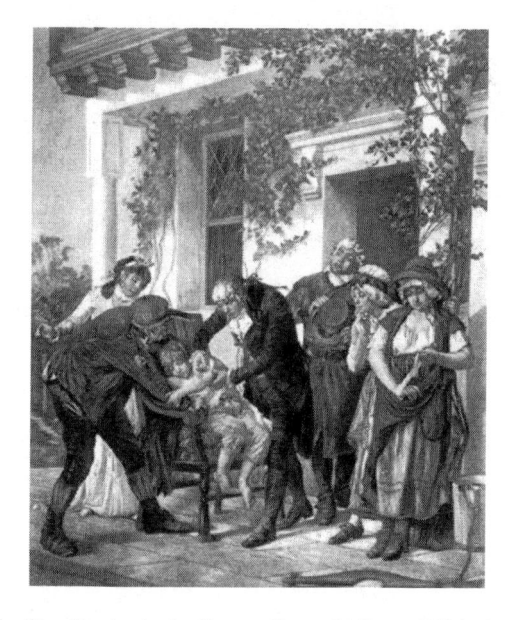

Fig. 21: *The First Vaccination* by Georges Gaston Melingue (1894). Jenner is depicted vaccinating James Phipps with cowpox detritus obtained from milk maid Sarah Nelmes. Collection of the authors.

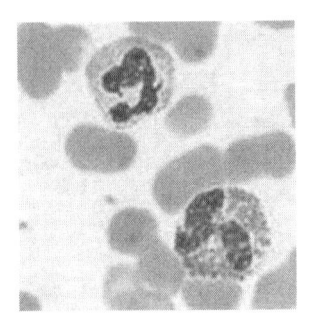

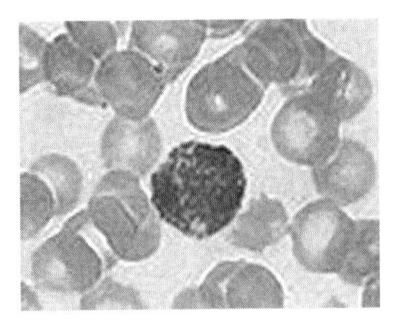

Fig. 22: A neutrophil, eosinophil (red granules) and basophil (blue granules) as stained by Erhlich method. Courtesy Wikimedia commons

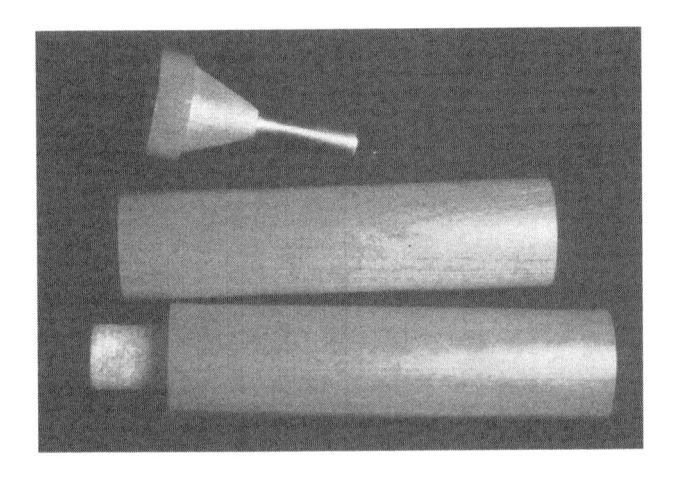

Fig. 23: Model of Laennec's stethoscope. Note how he modeled it after a three part flute for portability. Courtesy Wikimedia commons.

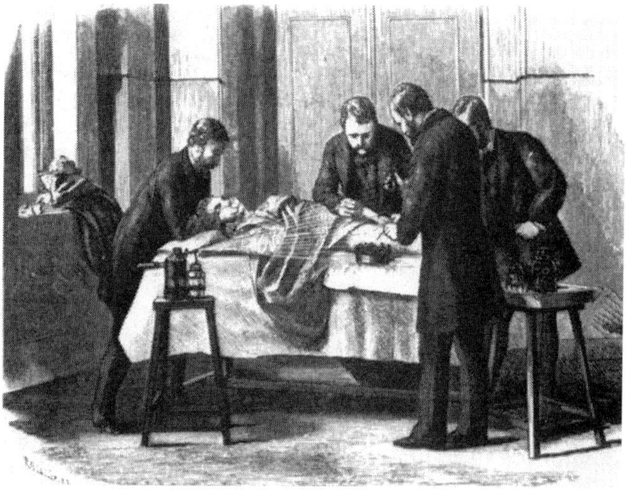

Fig. 24: The use of Lister's carbolic spray over the operative field. The beginnings of asepsis. (Note: no masks, gloves, gowns etc.). Courtesy NLM-IHM

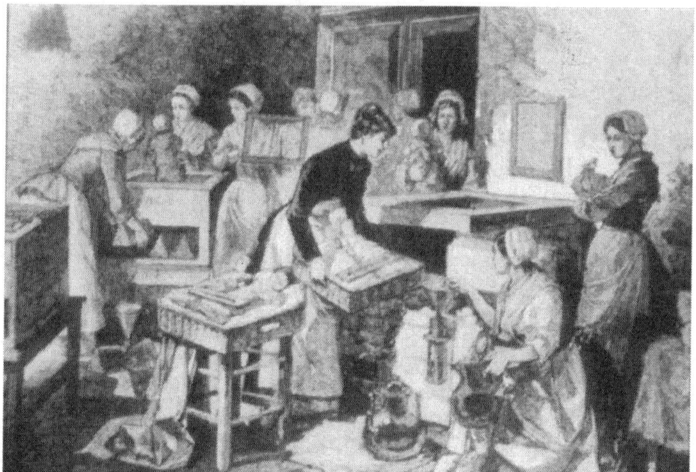

Fig. 25: The incubator designed by Tarnier and Budin, by Eugene Froment (1844-1900). Courtesy NLM-IHM

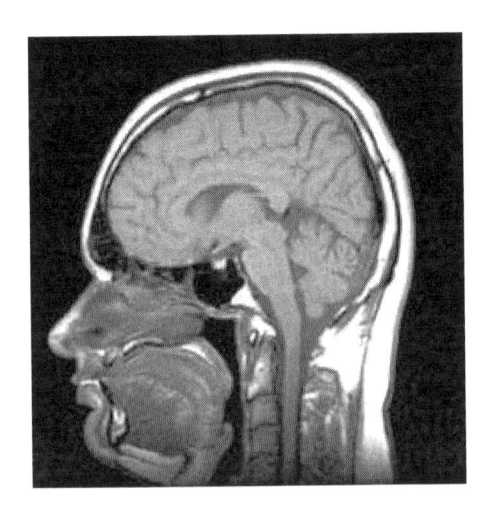

Fig. 26: MRI of a head. Courtesy Wikimedia commons

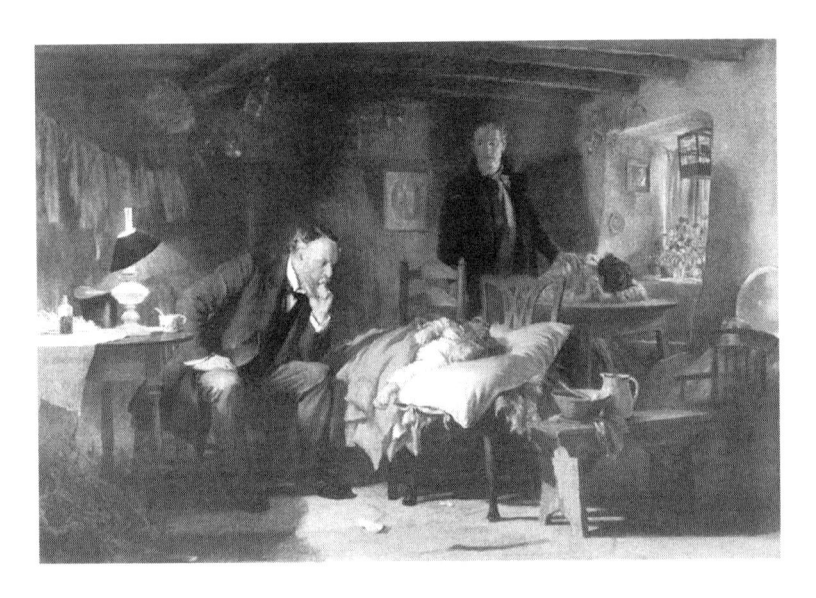

Fig 27: *The Doctor* by Sir Luke Fildes. Courtesy Wikimedia commons.

Bibliography

Ackerknecht, E. 1982. *A Short History of Medicine*. Baltimore: John Hopkins U Press.

Achterberg, Jeanne. 1990. *Woman as Healer*. Boston: Shambhala.

Aragón-Poce, F., et. al. 2002. "History of Opium," *International Congress Series*. 1242. Pp. 19-21.

Baker, J.P. 1991. "The Incubator Controversy." *Pediatr*. 87: 654-662.

Bhagvat Sinh Jee, H.H. 1927. *Aryan Medical Science*. Gondal: Electric Printing Press.

Blake, John E. 1955. "The Development of the American Anatomy Acts," *J of Med Educ*. 30: 431-439.

Brooke, Elisabeth. 1993. *Women Healers Through History*. London: The Woman's Press.

Burch, Druin. 2007. *Digging up the Dead*. London: Vintage Books.

Cairns, T. 1987. *Renaissance and Reformation*. Cambridge: Cambridge U Press.

Castiglioni, A. 1958. *A History of Medicine*. New York: Knopf.

Caulfield, E. 1931. *The Infant Welfare Movement in the Eighteenth Century*. New York: P.B. Hoeber.

Celsus. 1935. *De Medicina*. (Translation: W.G. Spencer). London: Heinemann.

Cockburn, A., Cockburn, E. 1985. *Mummies, Diseases, and Ancient Cultures*. Cambridge: Cambridge U Press.

Colón, A.R., Colón P.A. 1999. *Nurturing Children: A History of Pediatrics*. Westport: Greenwood Press.

------------------------------ 2001. *A History of Children: A Socio-Cultural Survey Across Millennia*. Westport: Greenwood Press.

Duffy, Jacalyn. 1953. *Epidemics in Colonial America*. Baton Rouge: Louisiana State U Press.

Duffin, Jacalyn. 1999. *History of Medicine*. Toronto: University of Toronto Press.

Garrison, F. 1929. *An Introduction to the History of Medicine*. Philadelphia: Saunders.

Gottfried, R. S. 1983. *The Black Death*. London: Free Press.

Granshaw, L., Porter, L. 1989. *The Hospital in History*. London: Routledge.

Gribban, John. 2001. *Science A History 1543-2001*. London: BCA.

Haggard, H. 1934. *The Doctor in History*. New Haven: Yale U Press.

Harington, John. 1920. *The School of Salernum: Regimen Sanitatis Salernitanum*. New York: Paul B Hoeber.

Harper, R.F. 1904. *The Code of Hammurabi King of Babylon*. Chicago: U of Chicago Press.

Hays, J.N. 2005. *Epidemics and Pandemics: Their Impacts on Human History*. Oxford: ABC-Clio.

Herodotus. 1954. *The Histories*. (Translation: A. Selincourt). Middlesex: Penguin Books.

Hippocrates. 1886. *The Corpus*. (Translation: F. Adams). London: Sydenham Society.

Hunter, William. 1829. *Lancet* 12: 769-773.

Jaggi, O.P. 1977. *Medicine in Medieval India*. Delhi: Atma Ram and Sons.

Jones, J.W. 1853. "Observations on the Origin of the Division of Man's Life into Stages," *Archaeologia.* 35: 167-189.

Kramer, S.N. 1981. *History Begins at Sumer*. Philadelphia: U of Pennsylvania Press.

Labat, R. 1951. *Traite Akkadien Diagnostic et Pronostic*. Brussels: Brill.

Lindberg, D. 1992. *The Beginnings of Western Science* Chicago: U Chicago Press.

Lindemann, Mary. 1999. *Medicine and Society in Early Modern Europe*. Cambridge: Cambridge U Press.

MacDonald, Helen. 2005. *Human Remains.* New Haven: Yale U Press.

Magner, Lois. 1992. *A History of Medicine*. New York: Marcel Dekker.

Majno, G. 1975. *The Healing Hand*. Cambridge: Harvard U Press.

Maspero, H. 1978. *China in Antiquity*. Kent: Dawson and Sons.

Masson-Oursel, P., et al. 1934. *Ancient India and Indian Civilization*. London: Kegan Paul.

Mauriceau, F. 1668. *Des Maladies des Femmes Grosses et Accouchees.* Paris: Jean Henault.

Menzies, Gavin. 2002. *1421*. New York: Harper Collins.

Meyerhof, M. 1984. *Studies in Medieval Arabic Medicine*. London: Variorum.

Nuland, Sherwin B. 1988. *Doctors*. New York: Knopf.

---------------------- 2000. *The Mysteries Within.* New York: Simon and Schuster.

----------------------2009. *The Soul of Medicine.* New York: Kaplan.

---------------------- 2005. *Maimonides*. New York: Shocken.

Oribasius. 1876. *Synopsis in Oeuveres d'Oribase*. (Translation: Bussemaker and Daremberg). Paris: Brailliere.
Papyrus Ebers. 1931. (Annotated by Bryan, C.P). New York: Appleton.
Paul of Aegina. 1846. *The Seven Books*. London: Sydenham Society.
Pliny. 1938. *Natural History*. (Translation: W.H.S. Jones). Cambridge: Harvard U Press.
Porter, R. 1997. *The Greatest Benefit to Mankind*. New York: Norton.
---------- 2002. *Blood and Guts.* New York: Norton
---------- 2006. *The Cambridge History of Medicine*. Cambridge: Cambridge U Press.
Precope, J. 1954. *Medicine, Magic, and Mythology*. New York: William Heinmann.
Prioreschi, Plinio. 2002. *A History of Medicine*. Vol.1. London: Horatius Press.
Reynolds, Richard and Stone, John. 1991. *On Doctoring*. New York: Simon and Schluster.
Riddle, J.M. and Estes, J. Worth. 1992. "Oral contraceptives in Ancient and Medieval Times," *American Scientist* 80: 226-233.
Rosenberg, C.E. 1962. *The Cholera Years*. Chicago: U of Chicago Press.
Rosser, Sue V. (Editor). 2008. *Women, Science and Myth.* Oxford: ABC-Clio.
Sena, N. 1901. *The Ayurvedic System of Medicine*. Calcutta: Chatterjee.
Shatzmiller, Joseph. 1994. *Jews, Medicine and Medieval Society.* Berkley: U. California Press.
Sherwood, Joan. 2010. *Infection of the Innocents.* Montreal: McGill Queen's University Press.
Starr, Douglas. 1998. *Blood*. New York: Knopf.
Steuer, R.O., deCusance, J.B. 1959. *Ancient Egyptian and Cnidian Medicine*. Berkeley: U of California Press.
Still, G.F. 1931. *The History of Pediatrics*. London: Oxford U Press.
Tacuinum Sanitatis. 1976. (Compiled by Arano, L.C). New York: George Braziller.
Talmud. 1989. (Translation of Ben Zion Bokser). New York: Paulist Press.
Temple, R. 1986. *The Genius of China*. New York: Touchtone.
Turner, E.S. 1957. *Call the Doctor*. New York: St. Martin's Press.
Turner, Jack. 2005. *Spice*. New York: Knopf.

Viets, H.R. 1977. *Smallpox in Colonial America*. New York: Arno Press.
Watson, C.J., Dark, J.H. 2012. "Organ Transplantation: Historical Perspective and Current Practice," *Brit J Anaesth.* 108: 129-142.
Wise, Sarah. 2004. *The Italian Boy*. London: Pimlico.
Wong, C. 1936. *A History of Chinese Medicine*. Shanghai: National Quarantine Service.
Zimmerman, L.M., Veith, I. 1993. *Great Ideas in the History of Surgery*. New York: Dover.

Proper Name Index

Abbott, Maude (1869-1940) 172
Abel, John J. (1857-1938) 187
Abella (14th cent.) 165
Abulcasis (fl. 936-1013) 43
Addams, Jane (1860-1935) 172
Addison, Thomas (1793-1860).... 148
Adelard of Bath (c.1080-1152)...... 48
Aetius of Amida (fl early 6th C) 34, 52, 163
Agni 9
Agnodice (fl.340) 27, 163
Albertus Magnus - Albert von Bollstaedt (1193-1280). 45, 57, 225
Albinus (Weiss), Berhhard Siegfried (1697-1770) 76
Alcmaeon of Croton (c. 500 B.C.).. 23
Alcuin (c. 735-804) 224
Alderotti, Taddeo (1223-1303) 57
Alessandro di Spina (d. 1313) 55
Alexander Monro I (1697-1767), 104
Alexander of Hales (1185-1245) ... 45
Alexander of Tralles (525?-605?). 34, 52
Alexander the Great (356-323 B.C.) 26
Alhazen (c 965-1039) 43
Alibert, Jean Louis-Marc (1768-1837) 152
Allbutt, Thomas Clifford (1836-1925) 150
al-Ma'mum (786-833) 40
Alpago, Andrea(d. 1522) 80
Alter, Harvey (b. 1935) 192
Altmann, Richard (1852-1900).... 193
Alwall, Nils (1904-1986) 188
Alzheimer, Alois (1864-1915)..... 139, 153, 155, 203
Anaxagoras (500-428 B.C.) 23
Andersen, Dorothy (1901-1963) . 174
Anderson, Elizabeth Garrett (1836-1917) 169
Andry, Nicholas (1658-1742) 113
Apgar, Virginia (1909-1974) 175, 200

Arantius, Giulio Cesare (1530-1589) 80
Archimathasus of Salerno (fl. 15th cent.) 52
Archimedes (287-212 B.C.) 27
Aretaeus of Cappodocia (fl. 55-80 A.D.) 30
Aristotle (384-322), ... 26, 39, 44, 57, 68, 70, 163
Armstrong, George (1719-1789): 113
Arnold of Villanova (1235-1315).. 45, 55, 224
Artemidorus of Ephesus (fl. 2nd cent) 31
Artemisia (d. 355 B.C.) 163
Asclepiades of Bithynia (c 120 B.C.) 29
Aselli, Gaspare (1581-1625).......... 88
Asimov, Isaac (1920-1992) (fn) ... 109
Asklepios (Latinized Aesculapius) c. 429 B.C. 21, 22
Aspasia of Phoenicia (fl 1st cent.) 163
Astruc. Jean (1684-1766) 113
Attlee, Clement (1883-1967) 218
Auenbrugger, Leopold (1722-1809) 110, 115, 121, 160
Auvard, Pierre (1855-1941) 157
Avenzoar (1113-1162) 44
Averroes (1126-1198) 44
Avery, Mary Ellen (1927-2011) ... 176
Avery, Oswald (1877-1955), ... 187
Avicenna (980-1037)...38, 43, 48, 51, 53, 70, 224
Babes, Victor (1854-1926) 138
Babinski, Joseph (1857-1932) 152
Bacon, Roger (1214-1292) 55, 57, 71, 244
Bagellardus, Paulus a Flumine (?-1492) 69
Baglivi, Giorgio (1668-1706) 90
Baillie, Matthew (1761-1823) 108
Baker, Josephine (1873-1945) 172
Balfour, George (1823-1903), ... 149
Baltimore, David (b. 1938).. 187, 193

Bandiano, Juan (1484-c.1552) 14
Banting, Frederick G. (1891-1941) 197
Barlow, John (1924-2008) 149
Barnard, Christian (1922-2000)...186, 195
Barré-Sinoussi, Françoise (b. 1947) 177
Barringer, Emily Dunning (1876–1961) 172
Barry, James (Miranda Stuart) (1795-1865) 170
Bartholin, Thomas (1616-1680) 88
Bartisch, Georg (1537-1607) 221
Barton, Clara (1821-1912) 171
Bassi, Agostino (1773-1857) 133
Bassi, Laura (1711-1778) 166
Bassini, Edoardo (1844-1924) 145
Bateson, William (1861-1926) ... 120, 187
Bayle, Gaspart Laurent (1774-1816). 121
Bayliss, William M. (1860-1924) 196
Beatson, George Thomas (1848-1933) 201
Beaumont, William (1785-1853). 143
Beddoes, Thomas (1760-1808) ... 140
Beer, Georg Joseph (1763-1821). 221
Beijernick, Martinus (1851-1931) (fn) 191
Bell, Charles (1774-1842)... 123, 125, 127
Bell, John (1763-1820 w)... 125, 143
Bellini, Lorenzo (1643-1704) 88
Benda, Carl (1857-1932) 194
Benedict of Nursia (480-547) 47
Benivieni, Antonio (1443-1502)... 57, 107
Bequerel, Antoine Henri (1852-1908) 181
Berengario da Carpi (1470-1530).. 73
Bernard de Gordon (c. 1307) 60
Bernard of Clairvaux (1090-1153), 51
Bernard of Gordon (?- c. 1320) 54
Bernard, Claude (1813-1878) 132, 196

Berson, Solomon (1918-1972) 177
Bert, Paul (1830-1886) 132
Bertapalia, Leonardo (?1380-1460) 53
Berthildis of Chelles (625-702).... 164
Best, Charles (1899-1978) 197
Bianchi, Leonard (1848-1927) 198
Bichat, Marie François (1771-1802) 108, 147
Bier, August (1861-1949) 141
Billard, Charles-Michel (1800-1832) 125
Billings, John Shaw (1838-1913) . 156
Billroth, Theodor (1829-1894) ... 119, 139, 145
Binet, Alfred (1857-1911) 152
Binz, Karl (1832-1912) 132
Bizzozero, Giulio (1846-1901) 183
Black, Joseph (1728-1799) 103
Blackburn, Elizabeth Helen (b. 1948) 177
Blackwell, Elizabeth (1821-1910) 167
Blackwell, Emily (1826-1910) 167
Blalock, Alfred (1899-1964) 175, 186
Blumberg, Baruch (1925-2011)... 192
Blundell, James (1791-1878) 183
Boccaccio, Giovanni (1320?-1375).... .... 60, 68, 165
Boerhaave, Herman (1668-1738) 110
Bohr, Christian (1855-1911) 132
Bond, Thomas (1712-1784), ... 116
Bonet, Théophile (1620-1689) 108
Bordet, Jules (1870-1961)... 136, 194
Borelli, Giovanni (1608-1679) . 88, 90
Borgognoni, Theodoric (1205-1298) 52
Bouillard, Jean Baptiste(1796-1881), ... 124
Bourgeois, Louise (1563-1636) ... 165
Boveri, Theodor (1862-1915) 194
Bowditch, Henry (1808-1892),.... 124
Boyle, Robert (1627-1691) 71, 92, 131
Boylston, Zabdiel (1679-1766).... 111
Bozzini, Philipp (1773-1809) 155
Bravo, Francisco 114

Bretonneau, Pierre (1778-1862). 122
Bright, Richard (1789-1858) 147
Broca, Paul (1824-1880) 124
Brock, Russel C. (1903-1980) 186
Brown, Isaac Baker (1811-1873) (fn) 146
Brown, John (1735-1785) 102
Brown, Robert (1773-1858), ... 193
Brown-Sequard, Charles (1817-1894) 132
Bruce, David (1855-1931) 136
Brunner, Johann Conrad (1653-1727) 88
Brunton, Thomas (1844-1916).... 132
Bruton, Ogden (1908-2003) 196
Buchan, William (1729-1805): ... 113, 115
Buck, Linda B. (b.1947) 177
Budin, Pierre (1846-1907) 157
Burgdorfer, Willy (1925-2014) 138
Burke, William (d. 1829) 127
Burton, Robert (1577-1640) 96
Cabot, Robert (1868-1939) 149
Cadogan, William (1711-1797): .. 113
Caius, John (1510-1573) 75
Calenda, Constancza (c. 1415) 165
Caliph al-Mu'tasim (794-842) 40
Caliph al-Muqtadir (895-932) 46
Caliph Moawia I (602-680) 40
Calmette, Albert (1863-1933) 190
Calvin, John (1509-1564) 81
Cammann, George (1804-1863) . 122
Canano, Giovanni (1515-1579) 75, 86
Cannon, Walter B. (1871-1945) .. 182
Cardano, Geronimo (1501-1576).. 69
Cardinal Wolsey (1471-1530) 69
Carlyle, Thomas (1795- 1881) 66
Carmenta 28
Carna... 28
Carrel, Alexis (1873-1944)... 145, 195
Carroll, James (1854-1907) 138
Carswell, Robert (1793-1857) 123
Carter, Henry Vandyke (1831-1897), ... 125
Cassiodorus (485-575) 47
Castaglioni, Arturo (1874-1952) ... 68

Cavendish, Henry (1731-1810) .. 103, 109
Celsus (c .30 B.C.-45 A.D.) 20, 27, 29, 53, 67, 113, 164
Cesalpino, Andrea (?1519-1603) .. 80
Chain, Ernst (1906-1979) 189
Chamberland, Charles (1851-1908) 136
Chamberlen, Hugh (1630-1720) ... 95
Chamberlen, Peter (1560-1631). 112
Ch'ao Yuan-fang (550-630 A.D.).... 12
Chapin, Henry (1857-1942) 159
Charcot, Jean Martin (1825-1893) 152
Chardack, William (1914-2006) .. 186
Chargoff, Erwin (1905-2002) 187
Charles II (R. 1660-1685) 55
Chaucer, Geoffrey (1343-1400) ... 38, 54, 55, 60, 164
Cheselden, Willilam (1688-1752)105
Cheyne, John (1777-1836) 149
Ch'i Po.. 10
Chien Lung (1711-1799) 13
Cicero (106-43 B.C.) 20, 29
Cimino, James (1928-2010) 188
Clark, Joseph (1758-1834) 114
Clark, William (1819-1898) 140
Clarke, Edward H. (182-1877) 169
Clarke, Robert (1860-1926) 146
Clayton, Barbara Evelyn (1922-2011) 175, 185
Clements, John (b. 1923) 176
Cleveland, Emeline (1829-1878). 168
Clinton, William (b. 1946) 220
Clowes, George (1877-1958) 202
Cobbett, William (1763-1835) 59
Cobo, Bernabé (1582-1657).......... 15
Cochran, John (1730-1807).......... 111
Cocrane, Archibald (1909-1988) . 203
Cohen, Stanley (b. 1922)............. 176
Cohn, Ferdinand (1828-1898) 135
Cohnheim, Julius (1839-1884) 130
Coit, Henry (1854-1917) 159
Colebrook, Leonard (1883-1967) 189
Colinet, Marie (c. 1560-c. 1640) .. 77, 165

Collip, J.B. (1892-1965) 197
Colombo, Mateo Realdo (1516-1559) 73, 80, 86
Columbus, Christopher (c. 1451-1506) 81
Confucius (551-479 B.C.) 12
Constantine (272-337 A.D.) 31, 33
Constantine the African (c. 1020-1087). 43, 48, 224
Coombs, Carey (1879-1932) 149
Cooper, Astley Paston (1768-1841) 105, 127, 142
Cooper, Max (b. 1933) 196
Copernicus, Nicolaus (1473-1543) 67, 86
Cordus, Valerus (1515-1544) 81
Cori, Carl (1896-1984) 175
Cori, Gerty Radnitz (1896-1957) . 175
Cormack, Allan (1929-1998) 182
Corrigan, Dominic (1802-1880) ... 149
Corvisart, Jean Nicolas (1755-1821) 121
Couney, Martin (1860?-1950) 157
Cranach, Lucas (1472-1553) 73
Crassus (115-53 B.C.) 29
Crede, Karl S. (1819-1892) .. 146, 156
Cremer, Richard John (1925-2014) 201
Creutzfeld, Hans (1885-1964) 155
Crick, Francis (1916-2004) . 176, 187, 200
Crumpler, Rebecca Lee (1833-1895) 167
Cruveilhier, Jean (1791-1874) 123
Crytodemus (4th C B.C.), ... 26
Cullen, William (1712-1790) 102
Cunina 28
Curie, Marie (1867-1934).... 173, 181
Curie, Pierre (1859–1906) 181
Cushing, Harvey (1869-1939)..... 146, 149
Cushny, Robert (1866-1926) 133
Cuvier, Georges (1769-1832) 120
d' Medici, Catherine (1519-1589) . 69
d'Agoty, Gautier (1717-1785) 76
da Vinci, Leonardo (1452-1519).... 72

Dale, Henry Hallet (1875-1968) .. 199
Dalton, John (1766-1844) 221
Damadian, Raymond Vahan (b. 1936) 183
Dante Alighieri's (c.1265-1321) ... 58, 60
Darius III (c. 380-330 B.C.) 27
Darwin, Charles (1809-1882) 104, 119, 120
Davaine, Casimir (1812-1882) 135
Davenport, Charles (1866-1944). 199
Daviel, Jacques (1696-1762) 221
Davy. Humphrey (1778-1829) (fn) 109, 140
de Bordeu, Théophile (1722-1776) 102
de Graaf, Regner (1641-1673) 87, 89, 91
de le Boe Franciscus (Latinized Sylvius) (1614-1672) 91
de l'Epée, Charles-Michel (1712-1789) 114
Déjerine, Jules Joseph (1849-1917) 198
della Croce, Andrea (1514-1624) .. 79
Democritus (460-370 B.C.) 29
Desault, Pierre-Joseph (1744-1795) 107
Descartes. Rene (1596-1650). 31, 85, 90, 97
Desormeaux, Antoine (1815-1894) 155, 202
Diane de Poitiers (1499-1566) 69
Diaz, Ruy (c. 1539) 81
Diderot, Denis (1713-1784) 101
Diocletian (284-305) 33
Dioscorides 50, 52, 53
Dix, Dorothea (1802-1887) 171
Dock, William (1898-1990) 149
Domagk, Gerhard (1895-1964) ... 189
Donders, Frans Cornelis (1818-1889) 221
Donné, Alfred (1801-1878) 183
Down, John Langdon (1828-1896) 156
Draco (4th C B.C.) 26

Drew, Charles Richard (1904-1950), ... 185
Dubois, Paul Charles (1848-1918)198
Duchenne, Guillaume (1806-1875) 154
Ducoudray, Angelique-Marie Leboursier (1712-1789) 166
Dulbecco, Renato (1914-2012) ... 193
Dunant, Jean Henri (1828-1910). 160
Duns Scotus 45
Dupuytren, Guillaume (1777-1835) 141
Dürer, Albrecht (1471-1528)......... 73
Dutton, Joseph (1874-1905) 136
Duve, Christian René de (1917-2013) 194
Eakins, Thomas (1844-1916)....... 144
Eberth, Karl (1835-1926)............. 136
Eddy, Mary Baker (1821-1910) ... 152
Edelman, Gerald (1929-2014)..... 194
Edward II (1284-1327) 55
Edward VI (1537-1553) 75
Edwards, Robert (1925-2013)..... 202
Ehrlich, Paul (1854-1915).... 130, 189
Eijkman, Christiaan (1858-1930). 158
Einthoven, Willem (1820-1927).. 185
Eleonora Maria Rosalia, Duchess of Troppau (c. 1697) 166
Elion, Gertrude Belle (1918-1999) 177
Elizabeth, Countess of Kent (1582-1651) 165
Elyot, Thomas (1490-1546)........... 96
Empedocles of Agrigentum (504-443 B.C.) 23
Emperor Charles V (1500-1558)... 59, 75
Emperor Conrad (c. 990-1039) 51
Emperor Frederick I Barbarossa (1122-1190 51
Emperor Lucius Verus (130-169) .. 33
Emperor Marcus Aurelius Antoninus (121-180) 33
Enders, John (1897-1995) 191
Ent, George (1604-1689) 86
Erasistratos (c. 330-255) 27, 32

Erasmus Desiderius of Rotterdam (c. 1466-1536) 68
Etienne, Charles (1503-1564) 74
Euclid (fl. 300 B.C.) 27
Eudocia (396-460 164
Euripides (c. 480-406 B.C.)............ 24
Eustachio, Bartolomeo (1520-1574) 75
Faber, Knud (1862-1956) 136
Fabiola (?-400) 34, 164
Fabrizio ab Acquapendente (Latinized Frabricius) (1533-1619), ... 44, 75, 86
Fagraeus, Astrid (1913-1997)...... 196
Fahrenheit, Gabriel (1686-1736) 150
Falloppio, Gabriele (1523-1562) ... 76
Faraday, Michael (1791-1867).... 140
Farber, Sidney (1903-1973) 202
Fehleisen, Friedrich (1854-1924) 136
Feinstone, Stephen M. (b. 1944) 192
Felix, Arthur (1887-1956)............ 194
Ferdinand II of Aragona (1452-1516) 47
Fernel, Jean (1497-1588) 68
Ferrari, Ognibene (Latinized Omnibonus Ferrarius) (16th cent.) 82
Fibonacc, Leonardo (c. 1170-1240) 41
Ficino, Marsilio (1433-1499) ... 68, 70
Fildes, Luke (1843-1927)............. 220
Finlay, Carlos (1833-1915) 137
Fishbein, Morris (1889-1976) 219
Fix, Georgia Arbuckle (1852-1918) (fn) 169
Fleming, Alexander (1881-1955). 189
Flemming, Walther (1843-1905) 187, 193
Flexner, Abraham (1866-1959) ... 151
Fliedner, Theodor (1800-1864)... 170
Flint, Austin (1812-1886 149
Florey, Howard (1898-1968)....... 189
Flourens, Marie Jean Pierre (1794-1867) 124
Floyer, John (1649-1734) 95, 115
Følling, Ivar (1888-1973)............. 185

249

Forssmann, Werner (1904-1979) 186
Foster, William (1591-1643) 71
Fracastoro, Girolamo (1478-1553)
.... 66, 81, 133
Fraenkel. Albert (1864-1938)...... 136
Franklin, Benjamin (1706-1790) 100, 115, 116
Franklin, Rosalind Elsie (1920-1958)
.... 176, 200
Fraser, Thomas (1841-1920)....... 132
Frederick II, Holy Roman Emperor (1194-1150) 48
Freud, Sigmund (1856-1939) 152, 199
Fry, Elizabeth (1780-1845), ... 170
Fujiwara, Tetsuro (b. 1931)......... 176
Fuller, Samuel (1580-1633),....... 115
Funk, Casimir (1884-1967).......... 158
Funke, Otto (1828-1879) 131
Fuss, Margarita (1555-1626)....... 165
Gaffky, Georg (1850-1910) 136
Gaius Hyginus (c. 64 B.C.-17 A.D.)
.... 163
Galen, Clarissimus or Claudius (129-216)20, 31, 39, 40, 43, 44, 45, 48, 51, 53, 54, 57, 58, 62, 68, 69, 70, 75, 80, 86, 89, 92, 93, 224
Galileo Galilei's (1564-1642) 8, 90 124, 154
Gallo, Robert (b. 1937) 192
Galton, Francis (1822-1911) 198
Galvani, Luigi (1737-1798), . 104, 185
Gariopontus (d. ca. 1050) 49
Garrison, Fielding (1870-1935) ... 150
Garrod, Archibald (1857-1936) ... 187
Gautier, Marthe (b. 1925)........... 156
Gerald of Cremona (1114-1187).. 41, 43, 48
Gerbert of Aurillac (946-1003)...... 41
Gerhard, William Wood (1809-1872), ... 124
Gibson, George (1854-1913)....... 149
Gilbertus Anglicus (d. 1250).......... 54
Giliani, Allesandra (c.1307-1326).. 57
Gillies, Harold (1888-1960) 201
Gilman, Alfred (1908-1984) 201

Giotto di Bondone (1269-1337).... 60
Glisson, Francis (1597-1677)......... 87
Goldmann, Hans (1899-1991)..... 222
Golgi, Camillo (1843-1926) 154
Gonin, Jules (1870-1935) 221
Good, Robert (1922-2003).......... 196
Gorgas, William Crawford (1854-1920)..38
Graham, Sylvester (1794-1851) .. 151
Granit, Ragnar (1900-1991) 222
Grassi, Giovanni (1854-1925)...... 137
Graunt, John (1620-1674), ... 96
Graves, Robert (1796-1853) 148
Gray, Henry (1827-1861) 125
Greatbatch, Wilson (1919-2011.. 186
Green, Cordelia (1831-1905) 167
Greider, Carolyn Widney (b.1961)
.... 177
Griesinger, Wilhelm (1817-1868) 197
Gross, Samuel David (1805-1884)144
Guarna, Rebecca (13th cent.) 165
Guérin, Camille (1872-1961)....... 190
Guillotin Joseph-Ignace (1738-1814) (fn) 109
Gula 4
Gull, William (1816-1890) 148
Gullstrand, Allvar (1862-1930).... 221
Gurney, Russell (1804-1878)....... 170
Gutenberg Johann (?1400-?1468)59, 67
Guthrie, Charles (1880-1963) 195
Guthrie, Robert (1916-1995) 185
Guy de Chauliac (1300-1360),. 44, 56
Haas, Georg (1886-1971)............ 187
Hadrian (117-138)......................... 30
Haeckel, Ernst Heinrich (1834-1919)
.... 130
Hahnemann, Samuel (1755-1843)31, 103
Hales, Stephen (1677-1761) 109, 147
Halsted, William Stewart (1852-1922) 139, 144, 150
Haly Abbas al-Majusi (930-994) ... 43, 48
Hamilton, Alice (1869-1970) 172
Hammurabi (died c. 1750 B.C.)....... 4

Hansen, Gerhard (1841-1912) 136
Hansmann, Carl (1852-1917) 144
Hare, William (d. 1829)................ 127
Haroun of Alexandria (c. 800) 40
Harris, Walter (1647-1732) 94
Harrison, Tinsley (1900-1978)..... 151
Harun al-Rashid (764?-809) 40, 41
Harvey. William (1578-1657) . 44, 80, 85, 86
Hata, Sahachiro (1873-1938) 189
Havy, Valentin (1745-1822) 114
Haycraft, John (1859-1923) 187
Heberden, William (1710-1801) 110, 119
Hektoen, Ludvig (1863-1951) 184
Hench, Philip S. (1896-1965)....... 197
Henle, Jakob (1809-1885) 129
Henri de Mondeville (1260-1320), 54
Henry II of France (1519-1559)69, 77
Henry VII of England (1457-1509). 69
Henry VIII of England (1491-1547). 69, 218
Hernandez, Francisco (1517-1587) 114
Herodotus (c. 484- 425 B.C.) 5, 6, 23,24
Herophilus (c. 330-260 B.C.), .. 27, 32
Hewson, William (1739-1774) 183
Hidalgo de Agüero, Bartolomé (1531-1597 79
Hilda of Whitby (614-680) 164
Hildanes, Fabricius (1560-1639) ... 79
Hildegarde von Bingen (c. 1099-1179) 51, 224
Hillier, James (1915-2007) 193
Hippocrates (?460-?377) . 16, 20, 24, 31, 39, 40, 43, 48, 51, 58, 61, 68, 97
His Jr., Wilhelm(1863-1934)........ 130
His, Wilhelm (1831-1904) ... 130, 154
Hitler, Adolph (1889-1945) 180
Hodgkin, Dorothy Mary (1910-1994) 176
Hodgkin, Thomas (1798-1866)... 148, 150
Hoeck, Leroy (1912-2009)........... 200
Hoffmann, Friedrich (1660-1742), ... 102
Hogarth, William (1697-1764) 74
Holbein, Hans (1497-1543) 73
Holmes, Oliver Wendell (1809-1894) 124, 138, 139
Holt, Luther Emmet (1855-1924) 175
Homer (c. 9th century B.C.) 22
Hooke, Robert (1635-1703), .. 71, 87, 92, 131
Hopkins, Frederick Gowland (1861-1947) 159
Hoppe-Seyler, Felix (1825-1895) 131
Horace (65-8 B.C.) (fn) 92, 101
Horsley, Victor (1857-1916)........ 146
Hounsfield, Godfrey Newbold (1919-2004) 182
Howe, Julia Ward (1819-1910) ... 169
Hroswitha of Gandersheim (935-1000) 164
Hua Tuo (c. 110-207) 12
Huang Fu (214-282 A.D.)............... 12
Huang Ti (c. 2600 B.C.).................. 10
Huggins, Charles (1901-1997)..... 201
Hugh of Lucca (c 1190). 52
Hugo, Victor (1802-1885) 180
Hungerford, David (1927-1993).. 193
Hunt, Harriot (1805-1875) 167
Hunter, John (1728-1793). 100, 105, 106, 127, 142
Hunter, William (1718-1783)95, 102, 106, 112
Huxley, Aldous (1894-1963)........ 202
Huxley, Thomas (1825-1895) 119
ibn al-Baitar (1197-1248).............. 45
Ibn al-Jazzar 49, 224
Ibn al-Nafis (1213-1288) 80
Imhotep (c. 2990) 6
Isaac Judaeus (?880-?932) 42, 48
Ishtar.. 4
Itard, Jean-Marc (1775-1838) 121
Ivanosky, Dmitri (1864-1920)-(fn) 191
Jackson, Charles (1805-1880) 140
Jackson, Chevalier (1865-1958) .. 156

Jackson, John Hughlings (1835-1911) 154, 198
Jacob, François (1920-2013) 187
Jacobaeus, Han Christian (1879-1937) 155
Jacobi, Abraham (1830-1919).... 119, 156
Jacobi, Mary Putnam (1842-1906) 168
Jakob, Alfons (1884-1931). 155
James, William (1842-1910) 199
Janet, Pierre (1849-1947) 198
Janssen, Zacharias (1580–1638) ... 89
Jenner, Edward (1749-1823)107, 112
Jesty, Benjamin (1737-1816) 112
Jex-Blake, Sophia (1840-1912).... 170
Johannes Mesue of Damascus (777-857) 40
Johannitius (809-873) 40
Johannsen, Wilhelm (1857-1927)187
John Komnenos II (1087-1143) 46
John of Arderne (1306-1390?) 56
John of Gaddesden (1230-1361),.. 55
Johnson, Lyndon B. (1908-1973) 175, 220
Juan de Vigo (c.1450-c.1520) 78
Juan Gil de Zamora (1241-1318). 225
Jung, Carl Gustav (1875-1961).... 199
Justinian (527-565 A.D.)... 34, 35, 39, 61
Kalcar, John Stephen (1500-1546) 73
Kant, Emmanuel (1724-1804) 101
Kapikian, Albert (1930-2014) 192
Kaposi, Moritz (1837-1902)... 152
Karpe, Gösta (1908-1990)........... 222
Keats, John (1795-1821) 107
Kelling, George (1866-1945) 155
Kelly, Howard (1858-1943) 150
Kendall, Edward (1886-1972) 196
Kepler, Johann (1571-1630)........ 221
Key, Charles Aston (1793-1849).. 149
Khosru I (531 to 579). 39
Kiil, Fredrik (b. 1921).................. 188
King Charles II of England (1630-1685) 96

King Charles IX of France(1550-1574) 78
King Clotaire (497-561) 164
King Louis XV of France (1710-1774) 166
King Philip II of Spain (1527-1598) 75
Kircher, Athanasius (1602-1680) . 89, 133
Kitasato, Shibasaburo (1856-1931) 136, 190
Klebs, Edwin (1854-1913) 136
Klumpke, Marie (1859-1927)...... 198
Knoll, Max (1897-1969) 193
Knox , Robert (1791-1862)......... 127
Koch, Robert (1843-1910)... 129, 135
Kocher, Theodor (1841-1917)..... 139
Koeberlé, Eugene (1828-1915) ... 144
Kolff, Willem (1911-2009)........... 188
Koller, Carl (1857-1944)...... 141, 221
Koprowski, Hilary (1916-2013) ... 191
Korotkov, Nicolai (1874-1920).... 147
Kraepelin, Emil (1856-1926) 153, 197
Krebs, Hans (1900-1981) 131
Kübler-Ross, Elisabeth (1926-1994) 177
Kühne, Willy (1837-1900), ... 131
Küntsher, Geghard (1900-1972) . 144
Kussmaul, Adolph (1822-1902)... 154
La Mettrie, Julien Offray de (1709-1751) 91
Labartu.. 4
Laennec, René-Théophile-Hyacinthe (1781-1826)................................ ....108, 115, 121, 122, 147, 160
Lamarck, Jean Baptiste (1744-1829), ... 105
Landsteiner, Karl (1868-1943) 184
Lanfranchi of Milan (d. c. 1306) ... 52, 54
Langerhans, Paul (1847-1888) 131
Lao-Tse (b. 640 B.C.), ... 12
Larrey, Dominique Jean (1766-1842) 79
Lauterbur, Paul (1929-2007) 183
Laveran, Charles (1845-1922) 136

Lavoisier, Antoine Laurent (1743-1794) 100, 109, 131, 157
Lawley, R.H. 195
le Dran, Henri François (1685-1770) 77
Leibnitz, Gottfried von (1646-1716) 71
Leiter. Josef (1830-1892) 155
Lejeune, Jérôme (1926-1994) 156
LeJumeau, Jean Alexandre (1787-1877) 122
Leoniceno, Niccolo (1428-1524) ... 68
Levi-Montalcini, Rita (b. 1909) 176
Lewis, Thomas (1881-1945) 186
Lewisohn, Richard (1875-1961) .. 184
Linacre, Thomas (1460-1524) . 69, 96
Lind, James (1716-1794) 158
Lippmann, Gabriel (1845-1921) .. 185
Lister, Joseph (1827-1912). 139, 143, 144
Liston, Robert (1794-1847) 142
Littre, Alexis (1658-1726) 95
Locke, Frank (1871-1949) 149
Loeffler, Friedrich (1852-1915) .. 136, 191
Loesch, Fedor (1840-1903) 136
Loewi, Otto (1873-1961) 199
Lombroso, Cesare (1836-1909) ... 198
Long, Crawford (1815-1878) 140
Longfellow, Fanny (1821-1891) . 141
Longfellow, John W. (1807-1882) 141
Lopez de Hinajoso, Alphonso 114
Louis, Pierre (1787-1872) 59, 122, 124
Lower, Richard (1631-1691) .. 87, 92, 131, 183
Lucina 28
Ludwig, Karl (1816-1895) 147
Lullius, Raymundus (1232-1315). 140
Lysippus (fl. 4th century B.C.) 24
Macewen, William (1848-1924) .. 146
Macfarlane Burnet, Frank (1899-1985) 194
MacLeod, Colin (1909-1972) 187
Macleod, J.J.R. (1866-1935) 197
Madison, James (1751-1836) 112

Magendie, François (1783-1855) 123, 125,132
Magnus, Wilhelm (1871-1929) ... 146
Maimonides (1135-1204) . 38, 44, 45
Maitre-Jan, Antoine (1650-1725) 221
Malcolmson, John Grant (d. 1844) 158
Malpighi, Marcello (1628-1694) .. 28, 86, 90, 94, 107
Mansfield, Peter (b. 1933) 183
Manson, Patrick (1842-1922) 137
Manzolini, Anna Morandi (1714-1774) 166
Manzolini, Giovanni (1700-1755) 166
Marat, Jean-Paul (1743-1793) 109
Marco Antonio della Torre, Marco Antonio (1478-1511) 73
Marcus Aurelius (121-180) 32
Marie d'Medici (1575-1642) 165
Marie, Pierrre (1853-1940) 152
Mark Anthony (83-30 B.C.) 29
Marshall, Barry (b. 1951) (fn) 193
Martin, Richard (1754-1834) (fn) 123
Maser Djwawah ibn Djeldjal of Basra (fl. Late 7th century) 40
Massa, David J. (1923-1990) 185
Mathé, Georges (1922-2010) 196
Mather, Cotton (1663-1728) 111, 133
Mathijsen, Antonius (1805-1878) 144
Mathilda of Quedlinburg (895-968) 164
Mauriceau, François (1637-1709), 95
Maximian (c. 250-310 A.D.), ... 33
Mayer, Julius Robert (1814-1878) 120
Mayow, John (1643-1679), ... 92, 131
McBurney, Charles (1845-1913) . 145
McCarty, Maclyn (1911-2005) 187
McClintock, Barbara (1902-1992) 176
McCollum, Elmer Verner (1879-1967) 158
McDowell, Ephraim (1771-1830) 143
McIndoe, Archibald (1900-1960) 201
McLean, Jay (1890-1957) 187
Meckels, Johann (1781-1833) 105

Meckels, Johann Friedrich (1714-1774), ... 105
Meckels, Philipp (1756-1803) 105
Medawar, Peter (1915-1987) 194
Meigs, Charles (1792-1869), ... 124, 138, 141, 169
Mencius (372 - 289 B.C.) 12
Mendel, Gregor (1822-1884) 120, 199
Ménière, Prosper (1799-1862) ... 121
Merit Ptah (c. 5000 B.C.) 6
Meskhenit 5
Mesmer, Franz Anton (1734-1815) 102
Metchnikoff, Elie (1845-1916) ... 130, 194
Metlinger, Bartolomaeus (?-1491) 69
Meyer, Karl Friedrich (1884-1974) 134
Meyer-Schwickerath, Gerhard (1920-1992) 222
Michelangelo di Lodovico Buonarroti (1475-1564) 73, 76
Miescher, Johannes Friedrich (1844-1895) 187
Miguel de Servede (Latinized Servetus) (1509-1553) 80
Miller, Jacques (b. 1931) 196
Miller, Stanley L. (1930-2007) 200
Millman, Irving (1923-2012) 192
Minkowski, Oskar (1858-1931) ... 197
Mithridates VI (c. 132-63 BCE) 224
Möbius, Karl August (1825-1908) 193
Moliere (Jean Baptiste Poquelin) (1622-1673) 85
Mollison, Patrick (1914-2011) 184
Mondino de Luzzi (Latinized Mundinus) (1270?-1326) 57
Moniz, Egas (1874-1955) 186
Monod, Jacques (1910-1976) 187
Monro primus, Alexander (1697-1767) 104
Monro secundus (1733-1817) 104
Monro tertius (1773-1859) . 104, 127
Montagnier, Luc (b. 1932) .. 177, 192

Montagu, Lady Mary Worthy (1689-1762) 111
Montaigne, Michel de (1533-1592) 66
Montesquieu (1689-1755) 101
Montessori, Maria (1870-1952) .. 173
More, Thomas (1478-1535) 68
Morel, Bénédict (1809-1873) 198
Morgagni, Giovanni (1682-1775) 107
Morgan, Thomas Hunt (1866-1945) 187
Morselli, Enrico (1852-1929) 198
Morton, Richard (1637-1689) 94
Morton, William Thomas (1819-1868) 140
Mosso, Angelo (1846-1910) 153
Muller, Johannes (1801-1858) ... 129, 130
Mullis, Kary (b. 1944) 192
Murray, George R (1865-1939) ... 196
Murray, Joseph E. (b. 1919) 195
Napoleon Bonaparte (1769-1821) 51, 79, 121, 134, 141
Neisser, Albert (1855-1916) 136
Neith 5
Nemesius, bishop of Emesa (Syria) (c. 390) 33
Nergal 4
Nestorius (c.386-c.451) 39
Newmann, Ernst (1834-1918) 183
Newton Isaac (1643-1727) ... 71, 101, 166
Nicolaus Salernitanus (Praepositus) (fl. 1140) 49
Nightingale, Florence (1823-1910 171
Ninib 4
Nitze, Max (1848-1906) 155
Nobel, Alfred (1833-1896) 212
Noguchi, Hideyo (1876-1928) 189
Noonan, Jacqueline Anne 176
Nordentoft, Severin (1866-1922) 156
Nowell, Peter (b. 1928) 193
Nuland, Sherwin (1930-2014) 108
Nüsslein-Volhard, Christiane (b. 1942) 177

O'Dwyer, Joseph (1821-1898) 124
Obama, Barack (b. 1961) 220
Oribasius of Constantinople (325-405) 33
Osler, William (1849-1919).. 16, 147, 150, 173, 183
Ötzi the Iceman..................... 11, 138
Paget, James (1814-1899)... 129, 142
Palade, George (1912-2008) 194
Palmer, Daniel David (1845-1913) 151
Papanicolaou, George Nicholas (1883-1962)............................ 146
Paracelsus (1493-1541) ... 31, 53, 66, 70, 91, 95, 97, 140
Pare.. 29
Paré, Ambroise (1510-1590).. 29, 56, 66, 70, 77, 165
Parkinson, James (1755-1824)... 153, 155
Pasteur, Louis (1822-1895) 135, 139, 190
Patin, Guy (1601-1672)................ 59
Patz, Arnall (b. 1920) 200
Pauku 10
Paul of Aegina (625-690) .. 34, 44, 52
Pauling, Linus (1901-1994) 185
Pavlov, Ivan Petrovich (1849-1910) 131
Péan, Jules (1830-1898).............. 144
Pechey, Edith (1845-1908).......... 170
Pecquet. Jean (1622-1674) 88
Pedanius Dioscorides (fl 1st c A.D.) 30
Pelletier, Pierre-Joseph (1788-1842) 132
Pellier de Quengsy, Guillaume (1751-1835 221
Pericles (c. 495-429 B.C.) 24, 163
Pesehet (c. 2500 B.C.) 6
Peter Hispanus (c. 1215-1277)..... 50, 221, 224
Peter III of Aragona (1239-1285) .. 55
Peter of Abano (1250-1315) 57
Petit, John-Louis (1674-1750). 77, 95
Petrarch, Francesco (1304-1374).. 68

Petri, Julius Richard (1852-1921) 135
Peyer, Johan Conrad (1653-1712) 88
Phaer, Thomas (1510-1560) 82
Phidias (c. 480-430 B.C.) 24
Philip IV (1268-1314) 56
Phillista (318-272 B.C.)............... 163
Physick, Philip Syng (1768-1837) 143, 183
Piero della Francesca (c.1412-1492) 73
Pincus, Gregory (1903-1967) 173
Pinel, Philippe (1745-1826), 121, 198
Piso, Willem (1611-1678).............. 93
Plato (428- 348 B.C.)....23, 26, 44, 68
Platter, Felix (1536-1614) 221
Pliny Elder (23-79) 20, 21, 28, 30, 68, 101, 163
Pope Benedict XIV (1675-1758).. 166
Pope Clement VII (1478-1534)...... 59
Pope Clement VIII (1536-1605)..... 80
Pope Honorius III (1148-1227)...... 48
Pope Sixtus IV (1414-1484)........... 72
Porter, Rodney (1917-1985) 194
Potain, P.C. (1825-1901)............. 149
Pott, Percivall (1714-1789) . 100, 106
Potter, Edith Louise (1901-1993) 175
Praxagoras of Cos (fl. 340) 27
Praxiteles (c. 400-330 B.C.) 24
Prebus, Albert (1913-1997) 193
Preston, Ann (1813-1872)........... 168
Priestley, Joseph (1733-1804)......(fn) 109, 131, 140
Prout, William (1785-1850) 143
Prusiner, Stanley B. (b. 1942)..... 155
Ptolemy (c. 367-283 B.C.) 27
Purcell, Robert (b. 1935)............. 192
Purkinje, Johannes (1787-1869) . 128
Purmann, Matthäus Gottfried (1648-1721) 183
Pythagoras (?580-?500 B.C.),........ 23
Pythias (c. 365-335 B.C 163
Queen Elizabeth I (1533-1603) 75
Queen Isabella of Castile (1451-1504) 79
Queen Mary (1516-1558) 75
Queen Victoria (1819-1901) 141, 149

Quincke, Heinrich (1842-1922) ... 155
Quinton, Wayne (b. 1921) 188
Quintus Tertullian (163-220), ... 27
Ra 5
Rabelais, François (1483-1553) 68
Radcliff, John (1652-1714) 59
Radegonde (525-587) 34, 164
Ramazzini, Bernadino (1632-1717)95
Ramon y Cajal, Santiago (1852-1934)
 154
Rannut 5
Rayer, Pierre-François-Olive (1793-
 1867) 135, 148
Recorde, Robert (1510-1558) 90
Redi, Francesco (1626-1668) .. 88, 89
Reed, James (1861-1944) 219
Reed, Walter (1851-1902) 137
Reil, Johann Christian (1759-1813).
 197
Remak, Robert (1815-1865) 129
Rembrandt van Rijn (1606-1669).. 74
Reverby, Susan (b. 1946) 190
Rhazes (865-925) ...40, 41, 48, 52, 60
Rhodin, J. 194
Ribot, Théodule (1839-1916) 198
Richard I the Lion Hearted (1157-
 1199) 45
Ricketts, Howard Taylor (1871-1910)
 134
Ricord, Philip (1799-1889) 152
Ridley, Harold (1906-2001) 222
Ringer, Sydney (1835-1910) 130
Riva-Rocci 109
Riva-Rocci, Scipione (1863-1937) 147
Robbins, Frederick (1916-2003).. 191
Robert Curthose (1053-1134) 49
Robertson, Oswald (1886-1966) . 184
Rock, John (1890-1984) 173
Rodrigues Pereira, Jacob (1715-
 1780) 114
Roelans, Cornelius (1450-1525).... 69
Roentgen, William Conrad (1845-
 1923) 181
Roesslin, Eucharius (?-1526). 82, 233
Roger of Palermo (fl 12th cent.) 49
Roger, Henri-Louis (1809-1891).. 150

Rokitansky, Karl (1804-1878) 129,
 139
Roland of Parma (fl 12th cent.) 49
Roosevelt, Franklin Delano (1882-
 1945) 180, 219
Roosevelt, Theodore (1858-1919)
 219
Rose, George (1744-1818) 218
Rosenberg, Barnett (1926-2009) 202
Ross, Ronald (1857-1932) 137
Rotch, Thomas Morgan (1849-1914)
 157
Rous, Peyton (1879-1970) 192
Rousseau, Jean Jacques (1712-1778)
 101
Roux Wilhelm (1850-1924) 130
Roux, Emile (1853-1933) 136
Roux, P.J. (1780-1854) 142
Rowley, Janet Davison (1925-2013)
 193
Rubens, Peter Paul (1577-1640) ... 73
Rueff, Jakob (1500-1558) 70
Ruge, Carl (1846-1926) 144
Runge, Friedrich (1795-1867) 132
Rush, Benjamin (1745-1813) 59, 198
Ruska, Ernst (1906-1988) 193
Rutherford, Daniel (1749-1819).. 103
Sabin, Albert (1906-1993) 191
Sabin, Florence Rena (1871-1953)
 174
Sahagún, Bernardo (1499-1590) ... 14
Saint Yves, Charles (1667-1731) . 221
Saladin (1138-1193) 45
Salicetti, Guglielmo (dotto Saliceto)
 (c 1210-1277) 52, 54
Salk, Jonas (1914-1995) 191, 200
Salvino de Armato (d.1317) 55
Sandstrom, Ivar (1852-1889) 130,
 150
Sanger, Margaret (1879-1966) ... 173
Sanguozhi (2nd C, A.D.) 12
Santorius, Santorio (1561-1636) ... 90
Scarpa, Antonio (1752-1832) 107
Schatz, Albert (1922-2005) 189
Schaudinn, Fritz (1871-1906) 136

Scheele, Carl Wilhelm (1742-1786) (fn) 109
Scheiner, Christoph (1573-1650) 221
Schleiden, Matthias (1804-1881) 129
Schmiedeberg, Oswald (1839-1921) 132
Schwann, Theodor (1810-1882) . 129
Schweitzer, Albert (1875-1965) .. 174
Scribner, Belding (1921-2003) 188
Scultetus. Johannes (1595-1645).. 77
Seacole, Mary Jane (1805-1881). 171
Sechmet 5
Semmelweis, Ignaz (1818-1865). 138
Senning, Åke (1915-2000) 186
Serapion (fl. 9th century) 40
Sertürner, Friedrich (1783-1841). 53, 132
Servetus 80, 86
Seshat 5
Seth 5
Severino, Marco (1580-1656) 94
Shakespeare, William (1564-1616) (fn) 53, 71, 204
Shamash 4
Sharpey-Schafer, Edward Albert (1850-1935 .... 196, 197
Sherrington, Charles (1857-1952)154
Shiga, Kiyoshi (1871-1957) 136
Shippen, William (1736-1808) 105
Shumway, Norman (1923-2006). 195
Sigmund Freud (1856-1939) 31
Simon, Gustav (1824-1876) 144
Simpson, James (1811-1870) 141
Sims, J. Marion (1813-1883) 145
Sin 4
Skoda, Josef (1805-1881).... 122, 139
Smellie, William (1697-1763) 112
Snow, John (1813-1858) 134, 141
Socrates (c. 469 -399 B.C.): 23
Sophocles (c. 496-406 B.C.) 24
Soranus of Ephesus (fl 98-138) 30, 50, 52
Southey, Reginald (1835-1899)... 155
Spallanzani, Lazzaro (1729-1799) 108
Spock, Benjamin (1903-1998) 175
Spoerry, Anne (1918-1970) 174

St Agatha (d. 251) 63
St. Anthony (d. 1231) 63
St. Apollonia (d. 249) 63
St. Blaise (d. 316) 63
St. Dymphna (c. 7th cent.) 63
St. Fiacre (d. 670) 63
St. Jerome (347-420) 164
St. Lucy (283-304) 63
St. Roch (c.1295-1327) 63
St. Sebastian (d. 288) 63
Stahl, George Ernst (1660-1734). 101
Stargardt, Karl (1875-1927) 222
Starling, Ernest (1866-1927). 196
Starzl, Thomas (b.1926) 195
Steell, Graham (1851-1942) 149
Stensen, Neils (1638-1686), ... 87, 91
Steptoe, Patrick (1913-1988) 202
Still, Andrew Taylor (1828-1917) 151
Still, George Frederick (1868-1941) 150
Stokes, William (1804-1878) 148
Stopes, Marie (1880-1958) 174
Strabo (c. 63 BCE-24 CE) 223
Straus, Nathan (1848-1931) 159
Sts.Cosmas and Damian (d. c. 287)63
Sturli, Adriano (1873-1964) 184
Sun Ssumiao (581~682 A.D.) 12
Swammerdam, Jan (1637-1680) .. 89, 91, 183
Sydenham, Thomas (1624-1689). 85, 93, 97, 147
Syme, James (1799-1870) 142
Szent-Gyorgyi, Albert (1893-1986) 158
Taboulay, Mathieu (1860-1913) . 145
Tacitus (56-117) 21
Tagliacozzi, Gaspare (1545-1599) . 80
Tait, Robert (1845-1899) 146
Takamine, Jokichi (1854-1922) ... 197
Tamba, Yasuyori (c. 10th cent.) 13
Tarnier, Stephan (1828-1897) 157
Taussig, Helen Brooke (1898-1986) 174, 186
Taylor, John (1703-1772) 221
Temin, Howard (1934-1994)187, 193
Tenckhoff, Henry (b. 1930) 188

257

Tennent. John (c.1700-1760), ... 115
Teschan, Paul (b. 1923) 188
Thales (624-547 B.C.) 22
Theano (b. c. 546 B.C.) 163
Theiler, Max (1899-1972) ... 138, 191
Themison of Laodicea (fl. 1st century B.C.) 29
Theodosius II (401-450) 164
Theophrastus (c. 372-287 BCE) ... 224
Thessalus (c. 4th C B.C.) 26
Thomas Aquinas (c.1225-1274) ... 45, 57
Thomas, E. Donnell (1920-2012). 185
Thomas, Vivien (1920-1985) 175
Thompson, Mary Harris (1829-1895) 168
Thoth 5
Thycydides (c. 460 - 395 B.C.) 24
Timonius, Emmanuel (1669–1720) 111
Titian - Tiziano Vecellio (1485-1576), ... 73
Tourette, George Gilles de la (1857-1904) 152
Trajan (53-117) 21,30
Trotula (?-1097) 31, 49
Trousseau, Armand (1801-1887) 123
Underwood, Michael (1737-1820): 113
Urso of Salerno (fl. 1160-1200) 51
Valsalva, Antonio (1666-1723) 88, 107
Valverde, Juan de Amusco (c. 1560) 76
van Beneden, Edouard (1846-1910) 187, 194
van Ermengem Emile (1851-1932) 136
van Helmont. Jan Baptist (1577-1644) 91
van Leeuwenhoek, Anton (1632-1723) 88, 135, 183
van Roonhuysen, Roger (c. 1660) 112
van Rymsdyck, Jan (1750-1784) .. 106
Veit, Johann (1852–1917) 144
Venel, Jean Andre (1740-1791) .. 113

Venerable Bede (672-735) 224
Vesalius, Andreas (1514-1564) 70, 75, 78
Virchow, Rudolf (1821-1902) 123, 130, 220
Volta, Alessandro (1745-1827) .. 104, 166
Voltaire - (François-Marie Arouet) (1694-1778) 100
von Ardenne, Manfred (1907-1997) 193
von Baer, Karl Ernst (1792-1876) 130
von Basch, Samuel Siegfried (1837-1905) 147
von Baumgartner, Paul (1848-1928) 136
von Beethoven, Ludwig (1770-1827) 129
von Behring, Emil (1854-1917) .. 136, 190
von Bergman, Ernst (1836-1907) 139
von Bollinger, Otto (1843-1909) . 159
von Decastello, Alfred (1878-1936) 184
von Goethe, Johann Wolfgang (1749-1832) 221
von Graefe, Albrect (1828-1870),221
von Haller, Albrecht (1708-1777) 108
von Hebra, Ferdinand (1816-1880) 139, 152
von Helmholtz, Herman (1821-1894) 129, 131, 221
von Helmont 97
von Hilden, Wilhelm Fabry (1560-1624) 76
von Kölliker, Albert (1817-1907) . 128
von Langenbeck Bernhad (1810-1887) 144
von Leibig, Justus (1803-1873) .. 131, 158
von Leydig, Franz (1821-1908) 131
von Linné, Karl – Linnaeus (1707-1778) 101, 104
von Louffenburg, Heinrich (1391-1460), ... 69
von Mering, Joseph (1849-1908) 197

258

von Nussbaum, Ritter (1829-1890) 139
von Pettenkofer, Max (1818-1901) 131
von Rechlinghausen, Daniel (1833-1910) 130
von Rosenstein, Neils (1706-1773): 113
von Soxhlet, Franz (1848-1926) . 135, 159
von Voit, Carl (1831-1908) 131
von Volkmann, Richard (1830-1889) 144
von Waldermeyer-Hartz, Wilhelm (1841-1923) 187
von Waldeyer, Wilhelm (1836-1921) 131
von Wasserman 194
Wagner, Robert (1877-1953) 219
Wagner-Jaureg, Julius (1857-1940) 189
Wakley, Thomas (1795-1862) 142
Waksman, Selman (1888-1973) .. 189
Wald. Lillian (1867-1940) 172
Walker, Mary Edward (1832-1919) 168
Wallace, Alfred Russell (1823-1913) 120
Waller, August Desire (1856-1922) 185
Wandelaar, Jan (1690-1759) 76
Warburg, Otto (1883-1970) 131
Warren , John Collins (1778-1856) 140, 143
Warren, James (1753-1815) 143
Warren, John (1753-1815) 124
Washington, George (1732-1799) 111
Wassermann. August (1866-1925) 137
Waterhouse, Benjamin (1754-1846) 112
Watson, James (b.1928) 176, 187, 200
Weber, Adolf (1829-1915) 221
Weber, Eduard (1806-1871) 131

Weber, Ernst (1795-1878) 131
Webster, Noah (1758-1843) 137
Weichselbaum, Anton (1845-1920) 136
Weil, Edmund (1880-1922) 194
Welch, William Henry (1850-1934) 150
Welcker, W.H. (c. 1850) 8
Weller, Thomas (1915-2008) 191
Wells, Horace (1815-1847) 140
Wells, Thomas (1818-1897) 145
Wepfer, Johan (1620-1695) 88, 95
Wesley, John (1703-1791). 115
Wharton, Thomas (1614-1673) 87
Whipple, Dorothy (1901-1995)... 175
Whytt, Robert (1714-1766) 114
Widal. Fernand (1862-1929)137, 194
Wiener, Alexander (1907-1976) . 184
Wilder, Thornton (1897-1975).... 204
Willan, Robert (1757-1812) 152
William Harvey 76
William of Occam (c. 1285-c. 1349) 38
William the Conqueror (1027-1087) 49
Williams, Cicely (1893-1992) 174
Williams, William Carlos (1883-1963) 205
Willis, Thomas (1621-1675) 87, 91
Wirsung, Johan (1600-1643) 87
Wiseman, Richard (1625-1686) 94
Withering, William (1741-1799) . 110
Wolff, Kaspar (1733-1794) 130
Wölker, Anton (1850-1917) 139
Wood, H.C. (1841-1920) 133
Woolhouse, John Thomas (1650-1734) 221
Wren Christopher (1632-1723) 91
Wright, Almoth (1861-1932) 190
Wright, Jane Cooke (1919-2013). 176, 202
Wright, Joseph of Derby (1734-1797) 92
Wunderlich, Carl Reinhold (1815-1877) 150, 160

Wynter, Walter Essex (1860-1945) 155
Yalow, Rosalyn Sussman (1921-2011) 177
Yersin, Alexandre (1863-1943) .. 136, 190

Yperman, Jean (1295-1351).......... 56
Zakrzewski, Maria (1829-1902)... 167
Zheng He (1371-1433) 14, 67
Zirm, Eduard (1863-1944)........... 221
Zoser (2980-2900 B.C.) 6
Zworykin, Vladimir (1889-1982) . 193

Subject Index

a capite ad calcem 43, 49
abdominal surgery 145
abortifacient 50
absorbable sutures 44, 143
accoucheur 95, 112
acetylcholine 199
acquired immune tolerance 194
acupuncture 11
acyclovir 192
adhesion molecules 194
adrenal glands 132
adrenalin 197
Affordable Care Act 220
African burial grounds 127
African-American .167, 168, 176, 190
Age of Revolution 101
Ages of Man 25
agglutination test 137, 194
AIDS 192
al-Andalus 44
alchemy 71
alcohol 7, 21
alcoholism 198
Alexandria library 24, 27, 34
alternative medicine 103, 151
Alzheimer disease 153, 155
AMA 168, 220
ambulance 79
American Civil War 168, 171
American College of Physicians .. 105
American Medical Association.... 219
American Red Cross 171
American Revolution 101, 111
amino acid synthesis 200
amniotic fliud 95
amoebic dysentery 136
ampulla of Vater 107
amputation 32, 44, 76, 78, 79, 94, 142, 143
amyl nitrite 132
amyotrophic lateral sclerosis 155
analgesic 15
anatomical models 166

anatomical theater 76
anatomy 56, 87, 95, 104, 125, 166
Anatomy Act of 1831 126
Anatomy Act of 1832 128
anatomy dynasties 104
Ancient Period Summary 15
anemia 93, 165, 185
anesthesia 12, 140
aneurysms 142
anima ....See Soul
animal models 158
Animism 101
anopheles 137
anthrax 60, 135
antibiotic resistence 190
antibiotics 189
antibodies 194
anticoagulant 184, 187
anti-retroviral agents 192
antitoxin 137
antivivisectionist 112
Antonine plague 33
aortic regurgitation 149
Apgar Score 175, 200
aphorisms 41, 55, 110
aphorisms of Hippocrates 25
aphrodisiacs 224
apothecary 66, 105
Appendices 207
appendicitis 69, 148
Arabia's ascendancy 35
Arabic materia medica 45
Arabic medicine 39
Arabic numerical system 41
Arabic surgery 43
Aristotelian naturalism 44, 57
Aristotelian medicine 26
Arnold of Villanova 224
arrhythmia 186
Ars Parva 40
Art and the Great Anatomists 72
art of medicine 20
art of surgery 53, 56

Artemisia	50
arteriovenous shunt	188
artery clamp	144
Articella	40
asepsis	138
ashipu	4
asthma	15, 95, 124
asu	4
atherosclerosis	108
Atomism	29
auscultation	122, 149
auscultatory sounds	122
Austin Flint murmur	149
autopsy	57, 121, 125, 129
autopsy method	107, 129
aviation medicine	132
Aztec	13
Babinski sign	153
baby farming	114
Babylonian culture	5
bacteria	135
balneology	62, 71
barbers	44, 94, 105, 141
Barlow's murmur	149
barometric pressure	132
basophile	189
BCG vaccine	190
Bell's palsy	123
belladonna	198
benign prostatic hyperplasia	49
beriberi	158
bezoar	42, 78
biliary cirrhosis	148
bilirubin	201
Billroth II	145
Bills of Mortality	96
bimaristan	45
biological reductionism	129
biological weapon	111
birthing chair	95
Black Death	61
bladder stone	49
Blalock-Taussig shunt	175
bleeding	58, 106
blindness	69, 114, 222
blood banks	185
blood group	184
blood pressure	109, 147
blood-letting	58, 69, 75, 198
blue-babies	186
body-snatching	127
Bohr Effect	132
bone marrow	183
bone marrow transplant	185
Borrelia	138
botulism	134, 136
Boyle's law	92
brain anatomy	87, 91, 95, 123
brain tumors	146, 147
breast anatomy	142
breast milk	3
Bright's disease	147
Broca's area	124
Brownian motion	193
brucellosis	134, 136
Brunonism	102
Bruton, Ogden (1908-2003)	196
bubonic plague	190
Buddhism	37
bundle of His	130
burn injuries	201
Byzantine Empire	33
Cabot-Locke murmur	149
cacao	14
caduceus	22
caffeine	132
caisson disease	132
calor, dolor, rubor, tumor	29
calorimetry	157
Canada	115
cancer	77, 95, 106, 185, 201
cancer causes	202
cancer chemotherapeutic agents	202
cancri venenum	77
cannabis	9
Canterbury Tales	38
capillary	86, 109
capsicum	14
carbolic acid spray	139
carbon dioxide	103
cardiac arrhythmias	149
cardiac bypass	186

cardiac catheterization 186
cardiac gallop............................. 149
cardiocentricity........................... 26
carotid artery 186
Casa di Bambini 173
CAT..................................... 73, 186
cataract....................................... 221
cataract couching........................ 29
catgut.. 139
cauterization...............43, 49, 52, 78
cell division 129
cell nucleus 193
cells of Langerhans 197
cellular growth............................ 129
cellular organelles...................... 193
cellular pathology 129
centriole...................................... 194
cerebellar ataxia 153
cerebral angiography................. 186
cerebral apoplexy .... *See* Stroke
cerebral pressure........................ 155
certified milk............................... 159
cervical cancer 146
cesarean 77
Chamberland filter.............. 136, 191
chancroid 190
Charaka... 9
Charcot's disease 152
Charcot's joint............................. 152
chemotherapy 176, 201
chest percussion 110
Cheyne-Stokes breathing............ 149
child development 82, 173
child nurturing 175
childbirth in medieval period........ 60
childhood immunizations 192
children....................33, 42, 106, 125
children's plague.......................... 62
chimney sweep 100, 106
Chinese College of Medicine......... 12
Chinese medicine.................. 10, 23
Chinese specialists 12
chiropractic medicine 151
chloroform .... 141, *See* Anesthesia
cholera 134
Christian Science........................ 152

chromatin 187
chromosomes 187
chronic adrenal insufficiency ....*See*
   Addison's disease
chyliferous vessels 88
cinchona 93, 103
circulation 80, 86
circumcision.................................. 8
circumnavigation 67
cirrhosis 108
cis-platinum 202
Cistercians................................... 48
citric acid cycle............................ 131
classical Period............................. 21
cleft palate 142
cleric/physicians 68
climate change............................ 204
clitoridectomy............................. 146
club feet 145
clubbing 153
clysters 59
coagulation 8, 183
coca.. 15
cocaine................................. 15, 221
cocaine anesthesia.... *See* Anesthesia
cocaine skin infiltration............... 140
coccidiomycosis 135
coction 52
code of Hammurabi........................ 4
code of conduct 42, 51
code of conduct for surgeons 53
code of ethics........................ 66, 106
code of ethics for surgeons........... 66
Codex Barberini 14
Colonial medical schools..............*See*
   American medical schools
Colonial Medicine 114
Company of Physicians 69
compilation............................ 33, 40
complement 194
compound fractures 25
compound microscope 89
computerized axial tomography -
   CAT scan 182
congenital anomalies................ 8, 70
congenital cardiac anomalies 173

congenital syphilis (fn) 166
conjunctivitis 2, 3
consultationes 94
contagion .... *See* Germ theory
Continental Army 143
contraceptives 30, 50, 163
contraria contrariis curantur 72, 103
Coombs murmur 149
cornea 221
cortisone 197
cosmology 200
Council in Clemont 48
Council of Albi (1254) 45
Council of Beziers (1246) 45
Council of Lateran 44, 48
Council of Nicaea 34
Council of Rheims 37, 48
Council of Tours 37
Council of Treves (1227) 45
Council of Vienna (1267) 45
cow milk 159
cowpox 112
cranial nerves 123
cretins 72
Creutsfeldt-Jakob disease 155
Crimean War 171
criminology 198
Crohn's disease 59
crusaders 46
C-sections 29
cult of Asklepios 21
cupping 11
cyanosis 186
cystic fibrosis 174
cytodiagnotic vaginal smear 146
dactyloscopy 198
Danse Macabre 61
Datura stramonicum 15
DDT 134
De Humani Corporis Fabrica 75
De motu cordis 86
deafness 69, 114, 121
Decknamen 71
degeneration theory 198
degenerative neuropathy 155
dementia 153

dengue 138
dentistry 106, 127, 140
depression 198
depth of anesthesia 141
Derivationism 59
dermatology 148, 152
development biology 130
diabetes 9, 197
diabetic ketoacidosis. 154
dialectical medicine 57
dialysis 187
diapedesis 130
digitalis 110, 132
diphtheria 2, 3, 60, 94, 122, 136
diphtheria and appellations 122
diphtheria antitoxin 190
dissection 8, 27, 32, 40, 55, 57,
    62, 72, 77, 87, 89, 166
dissolution theory 154, 198
DNA 176, 187, 200
Dock murmur 149
Doctrine of Irritability 108
Doctrine of Signatures 72
Dogmatism 28
Dominicans 48
Down syndrome 156
dracunculus 7
dreams 31
dreckapoteke 6, 71
dropsy 15
dry wound 79
dura 15, 52, 146, 155
dyscrasia 23
dyslexia 154
Ebola fever 26, 192
ectopic pregnancy 146
eczema 15, 152
Egypt 53
Egyptian papyri 5
Egyptian specialists 6
Eighteenth Century Summary 116
EKG 185
electron microscope 191, 194
elephantiasis 137
embryology 130
Empiricism 28

encyclopedists 33
endocrinology 197
endoplasmids 193
endoscopy 155, 202
English Company of Surgeons 105
English Act of 1511 105
English Hippocrates 93
English suffrage movement 169
Enlightenment 97, 101
epidemic of Athens 26
epidemics 7, 133
epidemics and pandemics 60
epidemiology 96, 124, 134
epigenetics 204
epilepsy 8, 24, 54, 60, 146
epinephrine 197
ergotism 60, 199
erysipelas 136
erythropoiesis 183
ether anesthesia 143
Etruscans 28
eucrasis 23
eugenics 180, 199
European Union 180
eustachian tube 76
euthanasia 119
evidence-based medicine 203
exchange transfusion 201
exophthalmic goiter 148
eye lens 221
Father of American Neurosurgery
 146
Father of American Pediatrics 156
Father of Cellular Pathology 128
Father of English Pediatrics 82
Father of Helminthology 89
Father of Modern Chemistry 109
Father of Modern Neuro-surgery.
 125
Federal Vaccine Agency 112
Female Medical College of
 Pennsylvania 167
female testis 87
fennel juice 53
fermentation 135
fetal positions 95

fever 55, 150
fibrin 183
filariasis 137
fingerprints 198
fistula in ano 56
fistulas (fn) 59
Florentine Codex 14
FMCP 168
fontanelles 59
forceps 112, 113
formulary of prescriptions 49
fossils 81
Founder of Modern Neurology ... 152
Founder of Pediatric Cardiology . 174
Four Apostolic Successions of
 Medicine 16
four elements 23
four humors 24
foxglove 110
fracture screws and plates 144
fractures 5, 25, 32, 56, 76, 144
fractures and dislocations 44
Franciscans 48
French medicine 120
French Revolution 101, 107, 109
frozen section 144
Functional School of Psychology . 199
Galen's anatomy 32
gaol fever 134
gastrectomy 145
gastric lavage 154
gastric secretions 143
gastrocutaneous fistula 143
gastroduodenostomy 145
gastroscopy 154
gelders 44
genes 187, 203
genetics 176, 187
germ theory 129, 133
German influence 132
germ-layer theory 130
Gibson murmur 149
gladiators and anatomy 31
glaucoma 221
Glisson's capsule 87

265

glomerulonephritis .... *See* Bright's disease
glycogen metabolism 175
goiter 48, 72
Golgi complex 193
gonorrhea 136, 190
Goths 32
gout.. 15, 93
graft-vs-host disease (GVH) 185, 194, 196
Graham Steell murmur 149
grandmal seizure 3
grave robbers...................... 106, 127
Graves' disease 148
graveyard shift............................ 127
Gray's *Anatomy* 74, 125
Great Fire of London..................... 62
Great Pestilence............................ 61
Greek healing temples *See* Sanitarias
Greek medicine............................. 21
Greek pantheon............................ 21
Greek women in medicine 163
grief.. 96
guillotin (fn) 109
gunpowder 67, 78
gunshot wounds 94
gut motility 182, 196
Guy's Hospital............................ 147
gynecology............................ 30, 145
hallucinogenics 14
harelip.........................9, 12, 56, 145
Harveians 87
HAV.. 192
HBV.. 192
HCV.. 192
health insurance 115
heart failure 110
heart murmurs............................ 149
heart transplant.......................... 186
Hebdomadism 25
Hebraic medicine 6
helio-centricity...................... 67, 86
hemagglutination 194
hematemesis 8
hematology................................ 183
hemipelvectomy 145

hemlock 52
hemodialysis 187
hemoglobin........................ 131, 185
hemoglobinuria 138
hemolysis................................... 194
Henry Street Settlement............. 172
heparin 187, 197
hepatic glycogen metabolism 132
hepatitis..................................... 192
hepatoscopy 3, 28
heredity 199
Hindu/Arabic numerical system ... 41
Hippocratic corpus........................ 24
Hippocratic medicine................. 110
Hippocratic Oath.26, *See* Appendix A
hirudin 187
hirudotherapy.............................. 58
histamine 132
histology 128
HIV 192, 204
Hodgkin's lymphoma, ... 148
holistic medicine 115
Holy Roman Empire 33, 165
home medical encyclopedias...... 115
homeopathy 103
Homeric medicine......................... 22
honorific paintings 74
hormesis 103
hormones 196
hospital 45, 58, 100
hospital archetypes 34
Hospital *Hôtel Dieu* 58
Hospital Santa Maria Novella 58
Hospital Santo Spiritu 58
hospitals as centers of learning .. 120
Huang Ti Nei Ching....................... 10
Hull House 172
human experimentation 190
human genome........................... 203
human immunodeficiency virus . 177
human milk 2
human monoclonal antibodies ... 202
humoral theory,................ 23, 28, 77
humoralism.................................. 29
humors qualities 29
Hundred Years War 37

266

hydrochloric acid	143
hydrogen	109
hyoscyamus	9
hyperbilirubinema	201
hypercholesterolemia	148
hyperthyroidism	148
hypnosis	198
hysterectomy	34, 146
hysteria	30
iatrochemical	91
iatrochemical theory	90
iatromathematical theory	90
iatromechanical theory	90
iatrophysicist theory	90
iatros	24
ignipuncture	222
Iliad	22
immunodeficiency disease	196
immunology	194
in vitro fertilization (IVF)	202
inborn errors of metabolism	187
Inca	15
incantation	14, 51
incubators	156
incubators sideshow (fn)	157
Index Medicus	156, 203
Industrial Revolution	101
infant colic	53
infant tetany	123
infectious diseases	188
Inflammation, classical signs	29
influenza	26, 60, 69
inguinal hernia	145
inheritance	See Genetics
inoculation	111
Insane asylum	121
insect vector	137
insensible perspiration	91
instrument sterilization	139
insulin	131, 176, 197
internal milieu	132
intracardiac surgery	186
intramedullary nail	144
intraocular pressure	221
ipecachuanha,	15, 93
IQ scores	153
Iridectomy	221
Irish famine	149
Ishimpo	10, 17, See Table 2
Islam	46
Islamic hospital	46
isolation of bacteria	See Infectious diseases
isoniazid	190
Ixodes dammini	138
Japanese medicine	13
Jesuits	93
Jewish physicians	45
Johns Hopkins University	150
Justinian	39
Justinian plague	35, 61
Key-Hodgkin murmur	150
kidney	88
kidney transplant	195
King's touch	55, 56
kiveris vein	95
Knight of Malta	47
Knights of St John	47
Knights of the Holy Sepulcher	47
Koch's postulates	135
Koran	37, 43
Korotkov sounds	147
krankenkassen	218
Kübler-Ross model	177
Kussmaul breathing	154
Kussmaul sign	154
kwashiorkor	174
kymograph	147
lachrymal ducts	87
lacteal veins	88
Lady of the Lamp	171
laparoscopic surgery	202
Las Siete Partidas	45
laser coagulation	152, 222
Lassa	192
laudable pus	54, 79, 130
laudanum	93
Law of Bell-Magendie	123
Law of Conservation of Energy	120, 131
Law of Conservation of Mass	109
Law of Natural Selection	120

Law of Specific Nerve Energy 129
lazarettos 46, 60
lead poisoning 172, 175, 189
leeching 58, 164
left-handedness 198
leishmaniasis 15
lens implantation 222
leprosy 34, 60, 136
leptospirosis 135
leucopoiesis 183
leukemia 130, 202
lingual papillae 87
lithotomy 29
Little Mothers' League 172
London cholera epidemic 134
loop of Henle 129
lues (syphilis) 152
lungs 87
lupus 152
Lyme disease 138
lymphoma 202
lysosomes 193
lysozymes 189
macula 131
macular degeneration 222
Magna Carta 37
magnetic poles.............................. 81
magnetic resonance imaging (MRI)
.... 183
maize 15
malaria .9, 32, 93, 136, 137, 138, 204
malariotherapy 189
maleficium 50
mandragora 52
mantula... 58
mastectomy 34, 140
mater puerorum 42
materia medica .... See China
Maya 13
Mayflower 115
measles 42, 60, 93
mechanisms of disease. 107, 130
Meckel's diverticulum 105
meconium 27
medical apprentice system 116
medical chest 115

medical dolls 12
medical journals 116
medical missionary 174
medical poems ....*See* Appendix C
medical systems 101
Medicare-Medicaid 220
medicine 19th century 147
medieval code of conduct .... *See*
Appendix B
medieval theurgics .. Saints as healers
melancholia 96
Ménière's disease 121
meningitis 114
menses 30
mental disease .... *See* Insanitiy
mental retardation 198
Mercator *World Map* 65
meridians 11
mesmerism 102
Mesoamerica 15
messenger RNA 187
metabolic pathways 131
metabolism 27, 90, 131, 157
metastasis 77, 95, 143
Methodism 28, 29
Mexico 114
miasma 133
microchemistry 175
micrometastasis 202
microtome 128, 130
midwife 27, 60, 77, 166
military "medics" 32
milk 135, 159
milk pasteurization 159
milk vein 95
minerals 70
mithridatum 42, 110
mitochondria 193
mitosis 187, 194
modifying elements .... *See* Table 1
monastic medicine 47
Montpellier 68
morphine 53, 132
mortsafes 127
mosquito 137
moxibuxion 11

MRI 73
mulieres Salernitanae 164
multiple sclerosis 123
muscle contraction ..89, 90, 104, 108
myrrh 50
myxedema 196
National Cancer Chemotherapy
   Service Center 202
National Health Insurance 218
natural selection 119
Naturalism 22
Nazi Germany 200
neonatal jaundice 201
neonatology................................ 176
nephrectomy 144
nerve block 141
nerve growth factor................... 176
nervous system........................... 123
neuroanatomy .... See Brain anatomy
neurology.................................... 152
neurophysiology 33
neuroses 198
neurosurgery 146
New World.................................... 13
New York doctor's riot................ 126
New York Hospital 126
newborn 7, 26, 30, 50, 82
newborn metabolic screening ... 175, 185
newborn phototherapy 201
newborn syphilis......................... 166
Nineteenth century medicine 120
Nineteenth century summary..... 160
nitrogen 103
nitrous oxide .... See Anesthesia
Nobel Prizes in Medicine and
   Physiology............See Appendix E
nosokomium 34, 45, 164
nosology 104
nucleic acids................................ 187
nursing 168, 170
nursing bottles............................ 159
nutrition..................... 109, 131, 157
obsessive compuisve disorders .. 198
obsidian 14
obstetric anesthesia.................... 141

obstetric teaching models 112
obstetrics ...30, 70, 95, 106, 112, 145
Occam's razor 38
occupational medicine.... 71, 95, 172
oligohydraminos 175
omphalomesenteric duct............ 105
On Epidemics 208
oncology 182, 202
oncoviruses................................. 192
One Hundred Year War 56
operative instruments 9
ophthalmia neonatorum 146
ophthalmoscope................ 131, 221
ophthamology 40, 221
opium.......................... 52, 56, 198
oplomoclion................................. 76
opposition to education for women
   169
organotherapy 132
orthopedics................................. 113
ovarian follicles............................ 89
ovariotomy 143, 145
ovary 87
oxygen 103, 109, 132
pacemaker 186
Paget's disease 142
pain 57
palmar fascia contractures ....*See*
   Dupuytren contracture
Panama Canal 137
pancreas 87, 132, 197
Pantocrator................................... 46
paper making 41
para-aminosalicylic acid.............. 190
Paracelsian surgery....................... 71
parasite 7, 89
Parkinson disease 153, 155
parotid gland 87
pasteurization............................. 135
pathology.......57,107, 121, 125, 175
pathophysiology 108
Patristic Period medicine............. 30
Pavlovian conditioning................ 131
Pax Romana 32
PCR technology................... 135, 187
pedagogy 148

269

pediatrics 13, 30, 94, 113. 156
pediatric cardiology 172, 174
pediatric *Incunabula* 69
Pediatric textbooks 113
pediatrist 156
penicillin 176, 189, 190
pennyroyal 50
pepper tree 15
perception of color 221
percussion 121, 122
peripheral neuropathy 158
peritoneal cavity 145
peritoneal dialysis 187, 188
peritoneum 108
peritonitis 108
pernicious anemia 148
peroneal muscular dystrophy 152
peroxisomes 193
Peruvian bark 93
PET neuroimaging 154
petri dish 135
Peyer's patches 88
phagocytosis 130
pharmacology 132
pharmacopeia 6, 10, 55, 81
Pharmacy Wares Drug and Stuffs Act of 1540 105
phenylketonuria 185
Philadelphia chromosome 193
phlebotomy .... Bloodletting
phlogiston 103
phosphorus poisoning 172
phrenology 103, 124, 154
physiognomy 154
physiological chemistry .... *See* Biochemistry
physiological threshold 131
physiology 90, 108, 129
physostigmine 132
pilocarpine 221
placenta praevia 95, 165
placental expression .... *See* Crede manuver
plague 9, 43, 56, 60, 61, 68, 135, 136
plasma 185
plaster cast 44, 144

plastic needle 185
plastic surgery 9, 201
platelets 150, 183
pneuma 29
Pneumatism 29
pneumonia 204
polio vaccine 191, 200
polyarteritis nodosa 154
polymerase chain reaction (PCR) 192
polypharmacy 96
polyps 76
Popes of Avignon 56
post-partum hemorrhage 183
potato famine 134
Pott's disease 106
Pott's fracture 106
Potter Syndrome 175
pregnancy 7
premature infants 156, 175
presenile dementia 139
preventive medicine 148
primum non nocere 208
printing press 59, 66, 67
prion 155
protein-calorie malnutrition 174
protoplasm 128
psittacosis 135
psychiatry 30, 69, 154, 177, 197
psychoanalysis 31, 199
psychological nativism 199
psychology 12, 197
psychosis 198
psychosomatic: 71
psychotropic drugs 200
public health 174
puerperal fever 60, 124, 138, 167, 189
pulmonary circulation 80
pulmonic stenosis 186
pulse 10, 48
pulse clock 90, 95, 115
purgatives 59
Pythagorean School 23
qi 10
quadrivium 43, 48, 164
quarantine 61

Queen Anne's lace 50
quinine 15, 93, 132, 138, 189
quinoa 15
rabies 135
radiation therapy 182
radioimmunoassay 177
radium 173, 181
Rational Surgery Movement 56
Rationalism 28
rectal prolapse (fn) 30
red blood cells 89, 183
Red Cross. 160
reformation 74, 86
refraction 221
Regimen Sanitatis Salernitanum
 (c.1260) 49
remuneration 4
renaissance 67, 74, 82
renal failure 187
renal tubules 129
resistence of education of women
 169
respiration 92, 103
respiratory center 124
respiratory distress syndrome 176
resurrection men 127
retina 221
retinal tears 222
retrolental fibroplasia 200
reverse transcriptase 187
Revulsionism 59
revulsives 59
Rh factor 184
Rh incompatible hemolytic disease
 184
rheumatoid arthritis 197
rhinoplasty 9, 80
rickets 158
rickettsial disease 194
river civilizations 3
Rocky Mountain spotted fever ... 134
Roger's murmur 150
Roman Empire decline 35
Roman medicine 28
Roman military medicine 32
Roman pharmacopoeia 30

Roman public health 32
Roman surgery 29
Roman women in medicine 164
Rosa Anglica 55
Royal College of Physicians 69
Royal College of Surgeons 107
Royal Society 92
Royal Society of London 114
rubber gloves 140
ruta 50
sacred serpents 21
Salerno 48
Salerno surgery 49
salivary gland 87
salvarsan 189
sanitaria 21
scabies 60
scamnum 25
Scarpa's nerve 107
Scarpa's triangle 107
School of Bologna 52
School of Dublin 148
School of Edinburgh 104, 148
School of Hippocrates 23
School of Salerno 43
scleroderma 148
scriptorium 47
scrofula 55, 94
scurvy 8, 158
seasonal diarrhea 94
secretin 196
semina cancri 77
senile dementia 153
Separation of medicine and surgery
 44
seton 59
Seventeenth Century Summary 97
Sheppard-Towner Act 219
shock 183, 185
sickle cell disease 185
side-chain theory 189
sign language 114
silk sutures 140
silphion 30
silver nitrate 146

271

similia similubus curantur 14, 72, 77, 103
Sims position................................ 145
situs inversus 108
skin grafts 201
skull fractures 80
slit lamp 221
smallpox 32, 42, 60,93, 110, 115, 192
social activists 172
social Darwinism......................... 157
social reformer 172
socialized medicine..................... 220
societal attitudes on dissection 73
sodium citrate............................. 184
Solidism 29
somatic cell nuclear transfer (SCNT) 203
somatology 197
sonography 182
soporify.................................... 9, 56
soul... 91
South America 13
Southey tube 155
Spanish-American war 137
spectacles 54
sphygmomanometer 147, 149
spinal roots 123
spinal tap 155
spongia somnifera 9, 49, 52
spongiform encephalopathy....... 155
squirting cucumber....................... 50
St. Anthony's Fire (fn) 60
St. Bartholomew Hospital............. 46
St. Thomas hospital 46
St. Thomas Hospital, ... 171
St. Vitus dance.............................. 93
Starling's law 196
statistics..................................... 124
stent... 186
stereotactic guidance 146
sterilization 200
stethoscope 122, 149
Still's murmur 150
streptococcus 139
streptomycin.............................. 190
strychnine 132

subclavian vein 88
sulphanilamide 189
Sumer 53
Sumerian pantheon 4
surfactant 176
surgery 34, 94, 105, 141
surgical amphitheaters 55
surgical guilds 56
surgical instruments 77, 79
surgical residency program......... 144
Susruta..................................... 9, 80
sweating sickness.......................... 61
swill milk 159
swnw.. 3, 6
Sydenham's chorea....................... 93
Sydenham's system of medicine... 94
symbol of medicine...................... 22
syphilis 66, 68, 81, 136, 137, 189, 190, 194
systole.. 109
talisman 54
Talmud....................................... 1, 8
taste... 87
taste organs 88
tauopathies................................ 155
Taussig-Blalock shunt.................. 186
taxonomy................................... 104
teeth 14, 106
ielemedicine 203
telomeres................................... 177
Templars 47
Tenckhoff catheter 188
teosinte cobs 13
testis 87
tetanus............................... 114, 136
tetanus antitoxin 190
tetralogy of Fallot 186
Tetrarch 33
Theriac magna 42, 44, 110
thermometer 90, 150
thiamine..................................... 158
Thirty Year War............................. 79
thoracentesis 123
thoracic duct................................ 88
thyroid 196
thyroxin...................................... 196

272

tick disease	138
Tlaloc	14
tobacco	15
tongue	88
tonics	102
tonsillectomy	34
tonsils.	88
Tonus theory	102
total blood volume	8
Totentanz	61
Tourette syndrome	153
tourniquet	95
tracheotomy	34, 43, 94, 122, 124
trachoma	60
transfusion	92, 185
Translation Movement	39, 41
Translational medicine	204
translocation	193
transplantation	63, 194
trephination	15, 52, 146
trichinosis	142
trisomy 21	156
trivium	43, 48, 164
tropical medicine	137
Trousseau's sign	123
trypanosomiasis	137
trypsin	131
tryptophan	159
tubal pregnancy	95
tubercular meningitis	124
tuberculosis	60, 155, 159, 190, *See* Phthisis, *See* scrofula
tuberculosis vaccine	190
Tuskegee experiment	190
twentieth century medicine	181
typhoid fever	88, 122, 124, 137, 190, 194
typhus	26, 69, 124, 128, 134
ukhedu	6
ultrafiltration	188
ultrasound	182
umbilical cord	76
Unani medicine	43
universal donor	184
University of Montpellier,	51, 54
University of Paris	59
University of Peru	114
urea cycle	131
urinoscopy	4, 48, 58
uterine wandering	30
vaccination	112, 138
Vaccine Injury Act	191
vademecum	40, 58, 93
Vagbhata	9
vaginal speculum	145
vagus nerve	131
vaidya	3
Valley fever	135
Valsalva maneuver	88
vascular anastomosis	145
vasectomy	142
vein valves	75
venous valves	76
virus	191
virus induced tumors	192
Visiting Public Health Nursing Association	172
visual fields	222
Vitalism	102
vitamin A	158
vitamin C	158
vitamin D	158
vitamin K	8
vitamins	158, *See* Appendix D
vitreous body	221
vivisection	85, 123, 42
vivisection (fn)	123
waqf	46
Warburton Anatomy Act of 1836	128
weapon salve	70
wet wound	79
wet-nurse	2, 114, 166
Wharton's duct	87
Wharton's jelly	87
whdw	6, 102
whooping cough	*See* Pertussis
Wirsung's duct	87
woman's suffrage movement	167
women healers	6
Women in the history of medicine	163
World War II	185, 190

wounds 22, 32, 54, 67, 70, 76, 78
WWI 201
WWII 201
x-ray 181
x-ray crystallography 176

yellow fever 134, 137, 189, 191
Yersina pestis 61
Ying-Yang 10
zoonosis 135

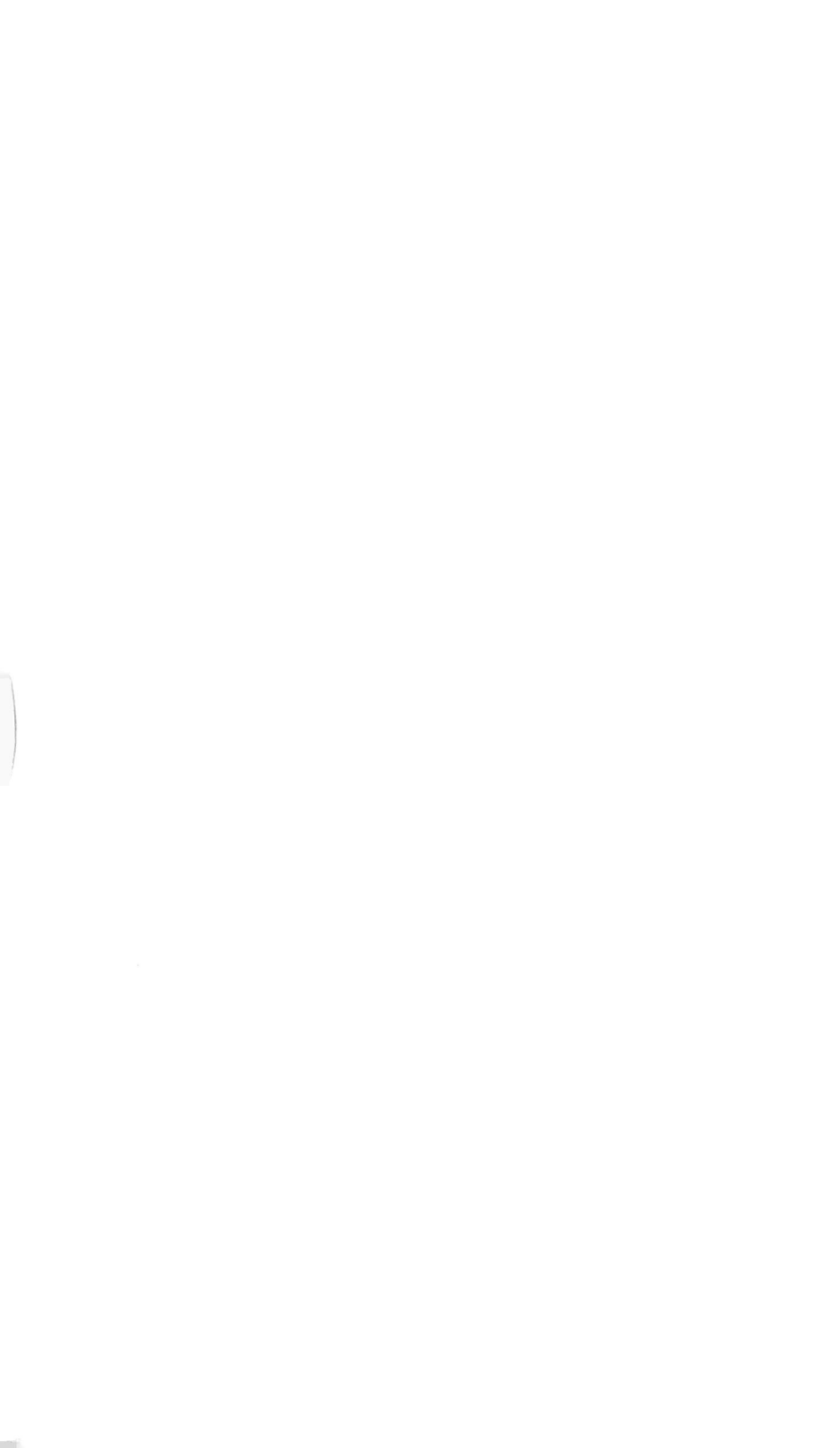

Made in the USA
Middletown, DE
18 March 2016